Natural Healing *for* Women

Susan Curtis has worked with natural remedies since 1979. Originally trained as a homoeopath, she has since studied and used other forms of natural healing including herbs, essential oils and flower remedies. She is the author of several books including *Essential Oils* and co-author with Romy Fraser of *Neal's Yard Natural Remedies*. Susan has two children and lives in Kent.

Romy Fraser founded the innovative and highly successful company Neal's Yard Remedies in 1981. She is now chairwoman of the company, which specializes in natural remedies and cosmetics. Romy also runs courses in natural medicine. Romy has two grown-up children and lives in London.

Natural Healing *for* Women

Caring for yourself with herbs,
homoeopathy & essential oils

Susan Curtis & Romy Fraser

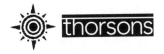 thorsons

Thorsons
An Imprint of HarperCollins*Publishers*
77–85 Fulham Palace Road,
Hammersmith, London W6 8JB

The website address is: www.thorsonselement.com

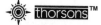

and *Thorsons* are trademarks of
HarperCollins*Publishers* Limited

First published by Pandora in 1991
This edition published by Thorsons 2003

10 9 8 7 6 5 4 3

© Susan Curtis and Romy Fraser 1991, 2003

Susan Curtis and Romy Fraser assert the moral right to
be identified as the authors of this work

A catalogue record of this book
is available from the British Library

ISBN-10   0-00-714591-8
ISBN-13   978-0-00-714591-1

Printed and bound in Great Britain by
Martins The Printers, Berwick upon Tweed

Contents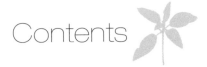

Acknowledgements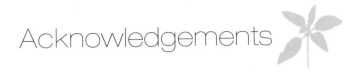

Grateful thanks for their valuable contributions to this book are extended to David Loxley, Rachel Packer, Dragana Vilinac and Rene Burroughs.

Introduction

The most interesting thing about natural medicines is what lies behind them, the way of life that incorporates them. The reawakening of interest in natural medicine in the western world is part of the process of re-evaluation of technology and materialism that has been occurring in the past few decades. As our respect for the earth as an infinitely complex living organism grows, so we can begin to trust her more to provide what we need. To trust and respect nature is to trust and respect your body, and your body's own healing potential.

The same attitude that has allowed us to exploit resources and pollute the earth has led us to fill our bodies with chemicals from drugs and our food. The ecosystems of the earth are suffering from pollution, destruction of natural habitats and depletion of resources. Our health is suffering from diets which are nutrient deficient and affected by chemical toxicity and the stress of living in inhospitable environments. These problems are of a chronic nature; they did not arrive overnight, and they will not disappear without a lot of effort and re-education.

The rapid advancement of genetic engineering is yet another step away from living closer to nature. It works against biodiversity and choice, the choice of farmers and poorer countries especially. Developing alongside genetically modified organisms are gene therapies. As medical treatments become ever more sophisticated, so do diseases. This is a trend that can only be reversed by building healthy bodies based on the basic principles of nature.

Using natural remedies is one of the ways in which we can make a positive step towards improving the quality of our life and health. What is exciting about natural remedies is that they can be used by everyone, on themselves. This is very empowering. Once we have access to our own healing we can take fuller responsibility for our lives as a whole.

The first step towards natural healing may well be visiting a practitioner. A good practitioner will encourage you to become involved in your own healing whilst using their knowledge and skill to help you overcome your present symptoms. Later, by learning yourself about natural remedies, through courses, reading books like this one and, above all, by trying out the remedies, you can begin to make your own decisions about what you need.

If at any time you feel stuck in an uncomfortable frame of mind, or with a particular set of symptoms, despite attempts to treat yourself, then it is probably time to accept that you may need to consult a practitioner. Being healthy is not about cutting yourself off from other people, avoiding difficulties, or even setting yourself up in an ideal environment on an organic farm in the middle of the countryside. It is about being prepared to change and grow as a person and developing a greater contact with your purpose for living – your spirit, if you like.

Ultimately, it may well be that we no longer need even natural remedies because we become so in tune with our needs that we are able to stay in balance without recourse to anything external. But natural remedies are there to help us, they are safe when used sensibly and they are an exciting part of the learning process, so use them.

part I:

The Body's Systems
and their Diseases

Introduction to the Body's Systems

Our body, with all its idiosyncracies and symptoms, is a perfect reflection of who we are. We are each a unity made up of myriad components. You cannot look at your stomach in isolation from the rest of your body, your eating habits and lifestyle, any more than you can look at your physical body without considering the feeling and thinking person that inhabits it.

Modern science has taught us to become accustomed to isolating parts of our body, and its symptoms and illnesses, without considering the interconnected nature of all life. This has led us to develop drugs and surgical techniques that are effective in a particular way, but do not support the organism as a whole. Looking for causes of disease within an individual's life has become neglected, as has a genuine consideration for the overall well-being of the patient.

Natural healing methods should always consider the person as a whole being. The remedies are generally gentler in action than drugs, surgery and genetic techniques, and support the energy of the body, not override it. We can often treat ourselves with natural medicine, thus taking a greater responsibility for our own lives as opposed to placing them in the hands of doctors and experts.

We can look at the different systems of the body just as we contemplate the rivers, mountains and clouds of the earth. This is not to forget that each is part of a whole. The different systems of the body display particular types of symptoms and we can use these to help us trace the cause and the cure of illness. Certain natural remedies have an affinity for particular parts of the body. This was understood in medieval times and used by herbalists to develop the 'doctrine of signatures'. They recognized that certain plants which looked like parts of the body could be used to cure disease in that area. For example, the pansy flower has petals shaped like a heart, and was used to treat diseases of that organ, hence its other name, heartsease.

The remedies that are mentioned here under a particular disease heading are merely suggestions. They should not be used without first looking them up in the *Materia Medica* section and considering their appropriateness in your own case. They are suggested because they do have an affinity for a particular disease, but each disease and each symptom is unique to you as an individual. When we have a disease we have the opportunity to learn something about ourselves. Taking a remedy should be part of that learning process.

1

Accidents and Injuries

Taking full responsibility for our lives as a whole means taking on board all the experiences that come to us, even the unexpected or painful ones. Many of us find it particularly difficult to accept that we create a need for the experience of an accident, and that we cannot simply blame the outside world. However, Freud and many psychologists since have developed the concept that accidents, like slips of the tongue and forgetting things, are actually products of our unconscious intentions. It is actually very empowering to see that we create our own experiences in life, and that we are never simply the victims of it.

To gain an understanding of the role of an accident in your life requires investigating the circumstances and its effects in detail, and applying what you discovered to your current situation. The underlying causes of an accident can be immensely varied, although amongst the most common is the idea that we are resisting or avoiding a change that needs to be made.

By discussing and questioning what might be behind the experience of an accident with trusted friends, or a therapist, it is nearly always possible to come to understand it; and it is remarkable how a person always seems to be able to recognize one explanation that seems particularly appropriate when the various possibilities are explored. A book that throws more light on the role of accidents in our lives is *The Healing Power of Illness* by T. Dethlefsen and R. Dahlke (Element Books, 1990).

See also the First Aid Kit on pages 417–19.

Bites and Stings

Some people are more sensitive to insect stings and bites than others. If symptoms of collapse or breathing difficulties develop, then seek emergency medical advice. The remedies mentioned here will help you to deal with any pain or minor reaction, but it is also important to use methods that prevent infection from developing.

Herbs that will help to relieve pain and inflammation resulting from a bite or sting include CHAMOMILE, MARSHMALLOW and WITCH HAZEL. These should be infused and applied locally. Those that prevent infection and promote healing include MARIGOLD and ST JOHN'S WORT. These should also be infused or used as tinctures to apply locally. ECHINACEA and GARLIC may be taken internally to prevent infection. Herbs may also be used to repel insects – try an infusion or the tinctures of LAVENDER and WORMWOOD. Apply these to the skin, or spray them in a room.

The essential oils of EUCALYPTUS, LAVENDER or MELISSA may be dabbed onto the site of a sting or insect bite to relieve inflammation. BERGAMOT or TEA TREE essential oils may be used to prevent infection. The essential oils that repel insects include CITRONELLA, LAVENDER, LEMONGRASS and PEPPERMINT. These may be diluted in vegetable oil and applied to exposed skin or burnt in a room.

Homoeopathic remedies can be very effective at treating the symptoms of insect bites and stings, and animal bites. Consider the following remedies by looking them up in the *Materia Medica* section: APIS, ARNICA, CALADIUM, HYPERICUM, LACHESIS, LEDUM and STAPHYSAGRIA.

Bruises

A bruise is the result of a blow or fall that causes damage to the soft tissue beneath the skin and breaks the skin capillaries. The skin becomes discoloured where the blood clots in the bruised area.

The two most effective remedies to treat bruising are ARNICA and WITCH HAZEL. These may be applied locally in the form of a lotion or ointment. Other anti-inflammatory herbs that may be used as a compress to relieve bruising include COMFREY, MARIGOLD and YARROW.

Essential oils may also bring relief to the discomfort of bruising. The most effective are LAVENDER and MARJORAM, best applied as a compress.

For more severe cases of bruising, homoeopathic remedies can treat shock, relieve pain and reduce inflammation. The first remedy to consider is ARNICA, although HYPERICUM, LEDUM or RUTA may also be appropriate.

Burns

The correct treatment for a burn depends on how severe it is. Minor burns and scalds can be dealt with safely at home, but the emergency services should be called for more serious burns. In a serious case, do not attempt to remove clothing before getting to Casualty, as this may damage the skin further. Burns resulting from exposure to chemicals should be treated first by bathing the affected area with cold running water for at least five minutes.

When you treat minor or severe burns one of the most important things is to prevent an infection developing. Use only clean gauze and sterile utensils; if these are not available, then leave the burns exposed to the air and take great pains to keep them clean. If blisters form, do not puncture or interfere with them, as they form a protective cushion for the damaged skin.

Internal treatment for shock, for example homoeopathic ARNICA or Bach FIVE FLOWER REMEDY, may safely be given in any case where a burn is involved. Other homoeopathic remedies that may be used in the treatment of burns include CANTHARIS, CAUSTICUM, KALI BICH and URTICA URENS.

The most effective emergency treatment for burns that we know is to pour the essential oil of LAVENDER over the area; this is soothing, prevents infection and promotes new tissue growth. Herbal or homoeopathic tinctures that you may use in the same way are HYPERICUM and URTICA URENS. The juice of the ALOE VERA plant is also effective; grow the plant in your kitchen so that you can break a piece of the leaf off and squeeze the gel onto a burn whenever necessary.

An antiseptic and healing wash can be made by infusing the herbs COMFREY, MARIGOLD and ST JOHN'S WORT and bathing the affected part. COMFREY ointment may be used once the burn has healed over, to reduce scarring.

Eye Injuries

Because the eyes are so delicate, any eye injury should be examined by a physician to assess the damage.

Loose foreign bodies or splashes of chemical substances in the eye should be flushed out with plenty of cool, clean water.

Anti-inflammatory herbs may be used to bathe the eye by cooling down an infusion or diluting the tinctures; consider especially CHAMOMILE, EYEBRIGHT and WITCH HAZEL. Homoeopathic remedies to consider, depending upon the nature of the injury, include ARNICA, LEDUM, SILICEA and SYMPHYTUM. Consult the *Materia Medica* section to find the most appropriate remedy.

Fractures

It can be difficult to tell if a bone is broken – an X-ray may be needed. Then the bone has to be set in plaster to keep it rigid and allow it to heal. Take the homoeopathic remedy ARNICA immediately to treat any shock, reduce bruising and promote healing from the beginning.

The most common sites of fractures are the wrist, ankle and collar bone. Elderly people are more prone to fractures as their bones tend to be more brittle.

The most effective way to promote the healing of broken bones externally is to apply a compress. Make a decoction of the herbs COMFREY ROOT and HORSETAIL to apply locally (obviously this will not be possible until any plaster cast has been removed). COMFREY LEAF may also be taken internally to encourage the healing of the bone. Essential oils may be applied as a compress or diluted in vegetable oil to massage into the area. LAVENDER, MARJORAM, ROSEMARY and THYME will soothe any aching and promote healing.

Homoeopathic remedies to consider to promote healing and ease any symptoms of discomfort include ARNICA, BRYONIA, EUPATORIUM PERF, HYPERICUM, RUTA and SYMPHYTUM. Consult the *Materia Medica* section to see which is most appropriate.

Head Injuries

For any injury to the head that involves a loss of consciousness, however brief, professional medical advice should be sought immediately. Following a head injury the person should be treated as for shock *(see page 9)*.

If the person is unconscious, check that his or her air passages are clear and place him in the 'recovery position': lying on his front or side, with his head turned to the side so that any vomit or secretions drain out of the mouth instead of down into the lungs. The FIVE FLOWER REMEDY may be placed on exposed pulse points while awaiting the emergency services.

If the person is conscious, give her some homoeopathic ARNICA while awaiting medical advice. ARNICA should also be given when concussion follows a blow to the head. The homoeopathic remedy NATRUM SULPH should also be considered after a head injury.

✻ Shock

Physical shock is a reaction that occurs when the blood flow is reduced to below its normal levels. Some degree of shock can occur after any injury, burn or illness that involves the loss of blood or other body fluids. Shock can also occur following coronary thrombosis, allergic reaction, severe infection or malfunction of the nervous system. The characteristics of shock are general weakness; cold, clammy, pale skin; a rapid, weak pulse; reduced alertness; and shallow breathing. Nausea may also be present. Hot sweetened tea will help for minor shock.

You should suspect shock following any accident or injury, and apply first aid measures, then call the emergency services if the injury is severe. The first aid treatment of shock is to reassure the patient; keep him lying down, with his legs higher than his head if he feels faint (except in the case of a head or chest injury where the head should be higher than the feet); and keep him warm.

A herbal infusion that will help with minor cases of shock, or may be administered while you are awaiting emergency medical treatment, can be made from BALM, CHAMOMILE, PEPPERMINT and SKULLCAP. This infusion can be sweetened with honey. Do not give the patient anything to drink before medical investigations in the case of an abdominal injury.

The first homoeopathic remedy to administer for shock is ARNICA. If available, the following homoeopathic remedies can also be useful: ACONITE, CHAMOMILLA, CHINA and IGNATIA.

The essential oils of LAVENDER, MELISSA, NEROLI or PEPPERMINT will alleviate the symptoms of shock. Place a few drops on a tissue so the patient can inhale the vapour, or massage a couple of drops into her temples.

✻ Sprains and Strains

Sprains and strains are caused by an injury that tears or stretches the supporting tissue of a joint. The most common sites of such damage are the ankles, wrists and knees.

Cold water compresses will offer some relief as a first aid measure. If symptoms appear at all severe, seek medical advice to rule out the possibility of a fracture. A supporting bandage may be helpful to take the strain off the affected joint while it heals.

An anti-inflammatory and healing compress can be made by using an infusion, or the diluted tinctures, of the herbs ARNICA, COMFREY or WITCH HAZEL. ARNICA, COMFREY and RHUS TOX are all available as ointments to massage into the site of a sprain, strain or pulled muscle. A compress may be made using the essential oils of EUCALYPTUS, LAVENDER, MARJORAM or ROSEMARY, or add a few drops of one to a warm bath.

Immediately after the injury treat the patient with the homoeopathic remedy ARNICA. Then consult the *Materia Medica* section to see which of the following homoeopathic remedies is best indicated for the particular symptoms: BELLIS PERENNIS, BRYONIA, RHUS TOX and RUTA.

⚘ Sunburn

Prolonged exposure to the sun causes dehydration of the skin, premature ageing, and has been associated with certain types of skin cancer. To prevent painful burning or blistering occurring, keep the skin protected with a sunscreen lotion and only expose yourself to the sun for short periods of time until you become accustomed to it. Wear loose clothing, a hat and keep in the shade as much as possible, especially during the middle of the day.

If you do become sunburned, treat it in the same way as a burn *(see page 7)*. Bathe the area with a cooled herbal infusion or diluted tinctures of CHAMOMILE, ST JOHN'S WORT or WITCH HAZEL. Apply the infused herbal oils of MARIGOLD or ST JOHN'S WORT, or add some CALENDULA tincture to OLIVE OIL and apply that to the burned skin. ALOE VERA gel will have a cooling and healing effect. The essential oils of BERGAMOT or LAVENDER may be diluted in vegetable oil and applied locally.

If a person becomes severely overheated and the cooling mechanism of the skin fails, then sunstroke will occur. The skin becomes hot and dry with sunstroke, and the body temperature rises; this can be dangerous and you should get medical advice. Other symptoms of sunstroke are feelings of dizziness, nausea or feverishness, and a severe headache. The first aid treatment for sunstroke is to cool the person off by bathing her in cool water, and giving her a glass of cool water with half a teaspoon of salt in it to promote perspiration.

The most important homoeopathic remedies that may be indicated after too much sun or sunstroke are BELLADONNA and GLONOINE. The Australian Bush Flower Essence SOLARIS should also be considered.

Wounds

Wounds may be classified as contused, incised, lacerated, perforated or punctured, and each one needs to be dealt with individually:

CONTUSED
Severe contusions or bruises, for example following a car accident, may indicate serious underlying injury, and the emergency services must be called. Treat for shock *(page 9)* as a first aid measure. For minor contusions, *see* Bruises *(page 6)*.

INCISED
Wounds made by cutting, for example with a knife, tend to bleed a good deal and the edges gape. If blood loss is severe, hold a clean cloth tightly against the wound and call the emergency services. After it has been cleaned the edges may need to be stitched together. The wound should heal within a week or two providing there is no infection.

To clean an incised wound, bathe the area with the diluted tincture of HYPERICUM. To promote rapid healing, apply the diluted tincture of CALENDULA. The antiseptic essential oils of BERGAMOT, LAVENDER or TEA TREE may be applied on clean gauze to prevent infection. If the wound becomes weepy, then apply the essential oil of MYRRH in the same way. Immediately after sustaining the wound give the homoeopathic remedy ARNICA; to promote rapid healing, give the homoeopathic remedy CALENDULA.

LACERATED
Torn wounds are the most likely wounds to become infected. These are the most likely to be sustained in a car accident. A severe lacerated wound should be treated by a surgeon, who will clean it thoroughly. Minor lacerated wounds may be treated at home in the same way as incised wounds *(see above)*.

PERFORATING
Wounds that pass through part of the body, for example caused by bullets or fragments of metal, are called perforating. These wounds will need to be treated by a surgeon. As a first aid measure treat for shock *(see page 9)*.

PUNCTURED
Punctured wounds are caused by a sharp object, for example a nail or needle, perforating the skin. Punctures can be dangerous because it may be impossible to tell how far the puncturing object has penetrated; if there is any question of deep penetration call the emergency services. The homoeopathic remedy ARNICA may be given to relieve shock. If the wound is very painful, administer the homoeopathic remedy HYPERICUM. The homoeopathic remedy LEDUM may be used as a prophylactic for tetanus.

2

Breasts and Breastfeeding

Breasts have developed in certain female mammals, including humans, as a method of producing milk to feed their young. Their growth and development are regulated by hormones, first during puberty and then for milk production during pregnancy and childbirth.

Each breast is divided into about 20 compartments containing systems of branching tubes lined by cells that secrete milk. In each compartment, the tubes join together to form a single duct that opens out on the surface of the nipple, making about 20 openings in total. The tissue between the tubes is filled with muscle fibres, fibrous strands and fat.

Traditionally breasts are a symbol of fertility, fecundity and motherhood; they connect humanity with the abundance of nature. However, in western society breasts have become estranged from this symbolism so that they have more to do with sexuality, stimulation and titillation; women have become objects of fantasy and breasts fashion accessories.

Breast Disease

Many women find that their breasts swell and become tender before a period. This process is regulated by our hormones. In the second half of the menstrual cycle, the breast builds up fluid and glandular tissue to prepare for pregnancy. If conception does not occur, the body reabsorbs all this extra substance via the lymph system, which acts as a drain for the breasts.

If the process of fluid and tissue build-up followed by drainage becomes inefficient, congestion will develop, and this may become permanent. Fluids can get trapped in the ducts of the breast to form sacs called cysts or solid lumps called fibroadenomas. When a generally lumpy and swollen condition

Cross-section of the Breast

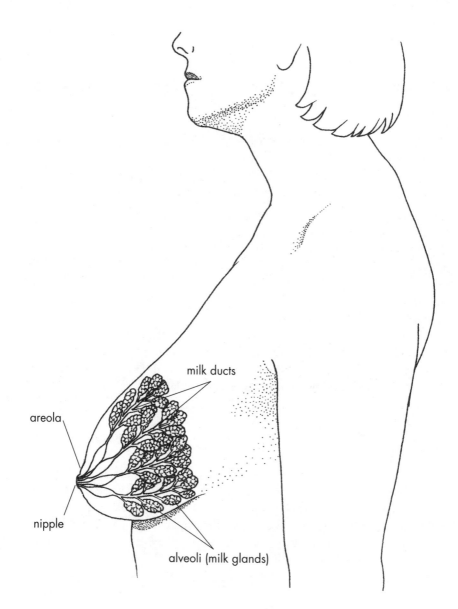

milk ducts

areola

nipple

alveoli (milk glands)

results then it is either fibroadenosis (multiple tiny nodules) or cystic mastitis (fibrocystic disease).

Over 80 per cent of reported cases of breast lumps are caused by one of these 'benign' conditions. Cancer of the breast can also exist as a lump, which is usually hard and may be tender or painless. Symptoms may also include a discharge of bloody or clear fluid from the nipple, flaking or puckering of the skin over the lump or enlarged lymph glands in the armpit.

Around 95 per cent of breast cancers are discovered by the women themselves, and all family planning and health clinics now have leaflets explaining how to do a breast self-examination. This involves examining the breasts visually and by touch for any unusual lumps or skin changes that remain for more than one menstrual cycle. The examination is best carried out at the same time each month, just after your period has finished and when the breasts are no longer swollen.

Orthodox treatment of breast cancer includes surgery, radiation and chemotherapy. Some women prefer to consider alternative systems of medicine such as herbalism, homoeopathy, acupuncture and nutritional or psychological approaches. Many will try a combination of orthodox and alternative treatment. Whichever approach you chose, dealing with the cancer in its early stages is likely to be more successful than when it is well advanced.

Since initial stages of breast disease lie in the lymphatic system's inability to drain and reabsorb waste matter which accumulates during the menstrual cycle, and by an imbalance of the hormones oestrogen and progesterone, it is very important that this system is healthy in order to avoid or treat breast disease. *See* Lymphatic System, beginning on page 72, for suggestions on improving its function.

Caffeine presents a problem for the lymphatic system because it is difficult to eliminate; it is also known to aggravate any tendency you may have to develop fibroids and cysts. Both of these are good reasons to avoid caffeine, whether it is in coffee, cola drinks or chocolate. Try dandelion coffee or herb teas instead. Fresh fruit and fresh green vegetables, preferably organically grown, are good things to eat.

The herbs that are most useful in the treatment of breast disease are those that assist the lymphatic system in its task of drainage. Consider especially CLEAVERS, MARIGOLD, NETTLES, RED CLOVER and YELLOW DOCK. The herb AGNUS CASTUS should also be considered when there is a hormonal imbalance contributing to breast disease.

There is a specialist form of massage known as 'lymphatic drainage'; this is particularly good when it is combined with the right essential oils. Essential oils that encourage lymph drainage, help to regulate any hormone imbalance and relieve symptoms of breast disease include GERANIUM, JUNIPER, LAVENDER and ROSEMARY. These oils can be added to the bath too.

IMPORTANT: None of the lymphatic drainage methods should be used if you have cancer, as it tends to spread via the lymphatic system and speeding up the flow of lymph fluid may encourage secondary sites of the cancer to develop.

EVENING PRIMROSE OIL has been found to be effective for treating symptoms of breast disease, such as swelling and tenderness, that are markedly worse before a period. You can take it in capsule form throughout the cycle or for ten days before each period.

Homoeopathic treatment can be very successful in treating breast disease, but you will probably need constitutional treatment by a qualified practitioner to find the right remedy or remedies that take all the contributory factors into account. Among those homoeopathic remedies to be considered are: BRYONIA, LACHESIS, PHYTOLACCA, PULSATILLA and SILICEA. *See* the *Materia Medica* section of this book. *See also* the information on pre-menstrual tension on page 150.

Breastfeeding

The evidence for the benefits of breastfeeding compared to bottle feeding is so overwhelming that it is a good example of the need to return to a way of life that has more respect for what is natural. Bottle feeding became increasingly popular in the decades immediately following the Second World War. It represented the success of technology over the primitive and natural. Food and drug companies soon invested huge amounts of money in promoting their baby feeds as the best. In more recent years, increased interest in natural health, combined with the realization that breastfed babies are healthier, has led to the recognition that 'breast is best'.

Bottle-fed babies are more prone to allergies, gastrointestinal, ear, respiratory, viral and yeast infections, and from being overweight, than their breastfed counterparts. Breast milk is full of antibodies and antiallergens that protect the baby from disease and infection. It is also easily digestible, as well as warm, fresh, sterile and conveniently available.

Breastfeeding also has benefits for the mother. Suckling after childbirth stimulates the pituitary gland to release oxytocin, the hormone that makes the uterus contract and helps it return to its normal size and shape. Any extra weight gained during pregnancy will be more easily lost at a slow and steady pace while breastfeeding, without the need for dieting. Breastfeeding usually delays the resumption of ovulation and menstruation for some months, although birth control methods should still be used to avoid pregnancy, as you can never be sure when ovulation resumes until after the event (i.e. with menstruation or another pregnancy!)

Breastfeeding should not have any effect on the size or shape of the breasts, as long as a well-made maternity bra is worn to support the extra weight. There is some suggestion that women who have breastfed are at less risk of developing breast cancer, although there are other factors that are more important here (such as family tendency and previous breast disease).

It is possible for nearly all women to breastfeed their babies. The only contra-indications are if the mother has some serious infectious illness, e.g. tuberculosis, or needs to take drugs that will pass through the breast milk to the baby. Inverted nipples will often become more prominent during pregnancy, and this process can be assisted by regularly pulling the nipple out with the fingers and gently squeezing and rolling it around. If the nipple remains inverted you can use a special plastic shield to assist breastfeeding.

It is best to start breastfeeding immediately after the birth, even before the umbilical cord is cut, when the baby's sucking reflex is strongest. Often babies are put to the breast far too late in hospitals, so try to make it clear to the staff that you would like the baby to suckle on the delivery table beforehand. Breastfeeding this early is an important part of the bonding process, it makes use of the baby's early sucking reflex, it stimulates the process of expelling the placenta and uterine readjustment for the mother, and it prevents the breasts from becoming too full and hard, which would make feeding more difficult later on.

If the baby has to be put in an incubator, or has a feeding difficulty (such as a cleft palate), then it is still possible to give breast milk by expressing the milk and giving it to him in a bottle. A breast pump should be supplied by the hospital or midwife to help you do this. You can sterilize an ice-cube tray and fill it with breast milk, then freeze it and store in a plastic bag (e.g. bottle liner).

For the first few weeks of breastfeeding a new baby, feeding on demand is virtually essential. This means feeding the baby when he wants to be fed, instead of trying to impose a regime on feeding times. Most babies thrive on being fed little and often during the first few weeks. Feeding regimes (such as four-hourly feeds) were designed for bottle-fed babies who need to have their feeds carefully measured and timed. Most hospitals these days will allow feeding on demand, but if you come up against a member of staff who does not approve of it, you may need to be quite insistent and determined if this is what you want.

During the last few months of pregnancy your breasts will be making colostrum, and this is what you feed your baby for the first couple of days after the birth. Colostrum is rich in protein, minerals, vitamin A and nitrogen. It also contains antibodies that will help to protect the newborn against infections and diseases such as polio, colds, gastro-enteritis, bronchitis, pneumonia, asthma, eczema, colic and measles. It is impossible to manufacture a complex substance such as colostrum synthetically, and this is one reason why it is so important to breastfeed your baby, even if only for one or two weeks. After two or three days of suckling your baby, the milk proper will come in.

Breasts quite naturally produce milk according to the baby's demands; more frequent suckling at the breast stimulates an increase in the milk produced. If you are advised that your baby is not gaining enough weight, simply let her suckle more often. Breastfed babies usually either stay the same weight in the first week after birth, or lose weight. This is quite normal. If your baby loses weight after the first week, you should seek medical advice.

After the first few weeks you can try to establish a more regular breastfeeding pattern if you find it helpful, such as feeding every three to four hours. After the first month or two, you could try letting someone else give your baby an occasional bottle, but try not to miss two consecutive feeds. If this is successful, when the baby is two or three months old it should be possible to miss one feed during the day regularly and replace it with a bottle. Missing the same feed every day is the key to successful part-time breastfeeding, if this is what you need to establish. The substitute bottles can contain either formula milk or, preferably, pumped breast milk.

Breastfeeding can supply the total nutritional needs of your baby for up to six months, and can supply three-quarters of their needs for up to a year. However, formula milk, correctly prepared, is perfectly adequate to give occasionally after the first couple of months, and solids or cereals can be introduced slowly after about four months. All these suggestions are very general, and one baby will vary very much from another as to his or her feeding wants and needs. Great flexibility is required to establish feeding patterns that are acceptable for the parents and appropriate for the baby.

If you cannot breastfeed, it can be difficult not to feel guilty about it, but instead put your energy into finding out about the best feeds available and creating a pleasant and relaxed feeding environment. Cow's milk is best avoided by babies because it is a common cause of allergies, mucus congestion and colic. Goat's milk is much more similar than cow's milk to human breast milk and is much less likely to cause digestive upsets. There are now goat's milk bottle formulae available to feed infants. Soya milk is not rich enough in iron and calcium to be given on its own, but the unsweetened variety can be mixed with goat's or sheep's milk and bottle formulae are also available.

Nursing mothers require plenty of protein, vitamins and iron in their diet. You do not need to eat any one thing in particular, but ensure that your diet contains plenty of fresh fruit and vegetables, whole grains and protein-rich foods (such as soya beans, cheese, lentils, lean meat, fish, eggs and nuts). If you suspect at any time that you may be anaemic, have a blood test and then follow the advice in this book under Anaemia *(see pages 38–9)*. Dieting can quickly result in a reduction in the milk supply, so do not try any crash diets, but avoid refined sugar and refined carbohydrates (e.g. white flour), and remember that breastfeeding will slowly use up the stores of fat that were laid down during pregnancy for that purpose.

It is important to drink plenty of liquids whilst breastfeeding. Try to drink at least 2 litres (4 pints) of liquid a day.

BREAST ENGORGEMENT

On the third day after giving birth a reflex occurs that stimulates the breasts to produce milk in place of the colostrum that the breasts have been producing during pregnancy. If the milk comes in suddenly, the breasts can feel full, heavy, lumpy and tender. The milk needs to be cleared from the breasts regularly, either by the baby suckling or manually, until things have settled down. If the baby has been encouraged to suckle immediately after labour, and on demand following that, painful engorgement is much less likely to occur.

If the breasts do become engorged and painful, try placing flannels that have been immersed in very cold water onto them. Consider taking the homoeopathic remedy BRYONIA if the breasts are very hard and painful. A compress made using a few drops of the anti-inflammatory essential oils of CHAMOMILE, GERANIUM, LAVENDER or ROSE in warm water can be applied to the breasts at regular intervals to relieve engorgement. Remember to wash any residue of the oils off before feeding the baby again. A compress of herbs made up of MARSHMALLOW and SLIPPERY ELM can be very helpful, or take CLEAVERS and MARIGOLD internally.

Engorgement will also occur if you have to stop breastfeeding the baby suddenly for any reason. If you are only stopping temporarily, you can keep the breasts clear and still produce milk by using a pump to express. If you want to stop producing milk altogether then taking the homoeopathic remedy LAC CANINUM will help you. Try taking just one dose of 200C and only repeat after a couple of days if necessary. You can also drink an infusion of the herb SAGE. Drink a cupful three times a day for several days.

CRACKED NIPPLES

Sore and cracked nipples can be quite agonizing and need to be dealt with promptly if the mother is to be able to continue breastfeeding. Cracks in the nipples can be an entrance point for bacteria, so the nipples should be carefully washed and dried after every feed to prevent any infection developing. Special nipple shields can be worn inside the bra to allow air to circulate around the nipple so that it can dry out between feeds.

If you have delicate skin, or your nipples are sore, try massaging an oil made by adding a few drops of essential oil of ROSE to a vegetable-oil base onto the nipple and surrounding area after each feed. If you get cracked nipples, look up the homoeopathic remedies of CAUSTICUM, GRAPHITES and SILICEA in the *Materia Medica* section of this book to see which one is the most suitable. Also, dilute the tinctures of MARIGOLD and ST JOHN'S WORT in a little boiled water and dap onto the cracked nipples after each feed. COMFREY ointment can also be applied to cracked nipples for a soothing and healing effect. Any substance applied to the nipple should be rinsed off thoroughly using clean water before attempting to feed the baby again. Breast milk is good and healing.

MASTITIS

Mastitis means 'inflammation of the mammaries' (the breasts). Inflammation may occur due to engorgement, a blocked milk duct or if an infection develops (usually by bacteria entering through a cracked nipple). The symptoms of mastitis are a feeling of heaviness and fullness in the breast, combined with tenderness, pain, heat and possibly redness.

To avoid mastitis developing it is important to empty each breast of milk regularly, and also to wash and dry the nipples carefully after each feed. Mastitis can lead to 'milk fever', which was a common cause of death amongst women in the past. Thus it is important to act quickly to reduce the local symptoms of inflammation, and if the symptoms are persistent, particularly if the general temperature of the mother continues to rise after a few hours, seek immediate professional advice.

As soon as any symptoms of mastitis develop, immerse flannels in very cold water and then apply them to the breast. Take the most appropriate homoeopathic remedy after looking the following up in the *Materia Medica* section of this book to see which is most suitable: BELLADONNA, BRYONIA and PHYTOLACCA. A paste can be made by mixing MARIGOLD and SLIPPERY ELM powder with water; this can be spread over the breast and left on for a couple of hours to reduce the inflammation. Alternatively, add a few drops of the essential oils of CHAMOMILE, LAVENDER or ROSE to some warm water, immerse a clean cloth in the water and apply it to the breast as a compress. Anything applied externally near the nipple should be rinsed off before attempting to feed the baby again. BORAGE or FENNEL will encourage the milk to flow. Also, take ECHINACEA for infection.

POOR MILK SUPPLY

Breast milk should smell good, be pure white (almost bluish-white) in colour, flow easily and taste sweet. It is unusual not to produce enough milk for the baby's demands because generally a hungry baby will stimulate the breasts to produce more milk when allowed to suckle more. However, if the quality or supply of milk does need to be improved, a combination of the herbs and seeds of ANISEED, BORAGE, FENNEL and HOLY THISTLE can be made into an infusion. Drink a cupful two or three times a day for a few weeks. If the breast milk seems to cause your baby to have colic then try drinking an infusion made from the seeds of DILL before each feed.

WEANING

The least traumatic way of weaning your baby is to do it gradually. You can try replacing one feed at the same time each day with a bottle feed once the baby is a few months old. Solids can be introduced slowly and made a regular part of the diet once your baby seems able to digest them easily (this time will vary from baby to baby but you can try after four months or so).

Eventually you will probably get breastfeeding down to an evening feed, and probably the odd 'comfort' feed during the night or on a difficult day. Some babies seem quite willing to make the step to not being breastfed from this part-time feeding, whilst for other babies it will seem impossible without causing great trauma to both mother and baby. Some mothers have found that taking the Bach flower remedy WALNUT, and giving it to the baby, helps them both to make the transition go more smoothly.

When you have determined that it is the right time to wean your baby, you can dry up your breast milk by drinking an infusion of the herb SAGE three times a day. Alternatively, take one dose of the homoeopathic remedy LAC CANINUM 200C, and only repeat this after a few days if necessary.

3

Cancer

Cancer is the name given to a group of diseases all characterized by abnormal cell division. Normal cells reproduce in an orderly fashion to carry on their work of tissue growth and repair; cancer cells begin to divide in an uncontrolled way, creating a mass of extra cells or tissue. When the mass of cancerous cells takes on a solid form it is called a tumour.

Cancer may be invasive, that is when it infiltrates and destroys surrounding healthy tissue. It may also metastasize, when it spreads to other parts of the body and forms new growths called metastases. Untreated cancer is often fatal because it displaces healthy tissue and causes organs to cease functioning until the patient dies. However, the disease may go into spontaneous remission, and the symptoms then decrease or disappear altogether.

Cancer can attack nearly all of the body's organs and the disease is often named after the organ where it originated – breast cancer, stomach cancer and so on. In women, nearly half of all cases of cancer affect the reproductive system; of these, breast cancer accounts for about one quarter of cases and cancers of the pelvic area account for the rest.

The causes of cancer appear to be very complex. Some substances are known to be carcinogens and can trigger the disease, for example radiation or cigarette smoke. However, even when we are exposed to carcinogens there is an element of individual susceptibility, because not every heavy smoker will develop lung cancer. There are some indications that certain viruses have a role to play in developing cancer, and there are also indications that there may be a hereditary component. Diet is considered to be another significant factor. A diet high in refined and processed foods and low in fresh vegetables and fibre is considered to be more likely to lead to certain types of cancer.

Psychological factors also have a role to play, probably by increasing an individual's susceptibility to the disease. It is known, for example, that the incidence of cancer rises considerably for an individual in the two years follow-ing the death of a close member of the family. Studies indicate that unassertive people who have difficulty expressing their emotions and forming close personal relationships are more lilkely to develop cancer and are also less likely to respond well to treatment.

With cancer what is happening is that a group of cells is dividing itself off from the rest of the organism and developing without regard for the whole. The cancer cells exploit and eventually threaten the life of the rest of the organism, and thereby of course destroy their own source of existence. The exploita-tion of the well-being of the whole and the alienation from the essential purpose of the organism that occurs with cancer is a revealing metaphor for the problems that are occurring in our society. The increasing incidence of cancer may well be a reflection of the central issues that we need to sort out in order to become a healthier society. For example, many pollutants are known to be carcinogens. Our western diet of refined low-fibre foods is known to contribute to cancer. We live in a society that does not always encourage the expression of emotion and the development of a sense of purpose. A cure for cancer is not going to come about by finding a wonder-drug or more sophisticated surgical procedure. Cancer can only be cured by readdressing the factors that contribute to it on every level – physical, emotional and spiritual.

On an individual basis, the fight against cancer is also more likely to be successful if we reassess all the contributive factors and the patient's whole lifestyle. Whatever approach you take to deal with the physical symptoms of cancer, whether orthodox chemotherapy or radiotherapy or natural remedies such as herbs, homoeopathy or dietary supplements, your chances of recovery will be improved if you also cultivate a positive, transformative attitude to your disease and a sense of purpose for your life.

There are many therapies that can help fight the disease and enhance the quality of your life while doing so. A professional herbalist or homoeopath will be able to select the remedies that are most appropriate to your individual case from those that are known to be effective in the treatment of cancer. Specialized forms of diet have been developed specifically to help eliminate chronic diseases such as cancer, so you might consider consulting a naturopath or dietary therapist for advice. Psychotherapists and counsellors have evolved techniques that are particularly appropriate for cancer sufferers. One of the most widely used is known as 'creative visualization', whereby people are taught to use their imagination, to see themselves fighting off the disease and building a positive image of health.

It is unfortunate that there is so much fear surrounding everything to do with cancer because this tends to undermine our ability to overcome the disease successfully. It is partly a reflection of our society's attitude towards death as something to be afraid of, to hide away from, ignore and avoid, whatever the cost to our quality of life. Any therapist who has treated people with cancer will recognize the profound personal growth and self-learning that they experience. Indeed, like any other disease, cancer can be an exceptional opportunity to reassess what is valuable in life, to develop a less obsessive attitude towards end results, and concentrate on the quality and purpose of our existence.

For an alternative view of degenerative diseases including cancer and case histories of people who have transformed their lives and overcome the disease, the book *The Creation of Health* by Caroline Myss (Bantam, 1997) is an excellent read.

See also Stress *(page 92)*, Shock *(page 9)*, Addiction *(pages 83–5)* and Depression *(pages 86–7)*.

4

Children's Illnesses

The vitality of a normally healthy child is exceptionally strong and children have remarkable powers of recovery. A child can have a high temperature and look very poorly one minute and be running around full of energy, looking completely well again, within the hour. At least, this was the picture until fairly recently. Nowadays, more and more children have begun to suffer from chronic complaints, most notably from allergies.

All practitioners of alternative medicine have numerous cases on their books of children brought by parents who feel that they are not as healthy as they should be. They may have specific complaints, most commonly asthma, eczema or digestive problems, or their parents may have noticed that they do not throw off colds and viruses as quickly as they should.

The main reason for this decline in our children's health is the onslaught of the modern world on their developing immune systems. Just as improved hygiene and nutrition began to make a real impact on reducing acute infections and deficiency diseases, so other conditions became worse, to the extent that a whole new range of chronic illness is now becoming increasingly widespread.

A child's vital organs and immune system are developing and growing all the time. For the first few months of her life, a baby relies on antibodies inherited from her mother to protect her from disease. This immunity is further enhanced if the baby is breastfed because there are antibodies and nutrients present in breast milk. This is why being breastfed is such an important factor in a child's health (see also Breastfeeding, on page 16).

A growing child will be less likely to develop a properly functioning immune system and good health if he or she is affected by such things as a poor physical inheritance (that is, unhealthy parents); a poor diet (for example, a diet of refined, additive-laden, processed foods); a polluted environment (perhaps living or going to school near a main road or polluted industrial site); polluted drinking water (containing toxic metals or an excess of chemicals such as nitrates); too much medication (most commonly in the form of antibiotics); and over-vaccination.

The damage done to a developing immune system by vaccination, in particular, is often underestimated. Viral elements injected into a child's body as vaccinations may persist and sometimes mutate in the system for years. Because of this, many people working in health care now believe that vaccinations may actually suppress and damage the immune response mechanism. Studies indicate that there is a direct link between the increased incidence of auto-immune diseases in recent decades and the increase in vaccination.

Furthermore, as a result of injecting a vaccine directly into the body only the antibody response is stimulated, as opposed to the general immune response that occurs during the normal process of illness and recovery. The inflammatory response to an infectious illness (for example a fever, rash or cough) represents the body's natural efforts to clear the virus from the system. In this way the entire immune system is profoundly stimulated, and not only will the child who recovers from the illness have a natural immunity to it, but he will also be able to respond rapidly and effectively to other infections. In fact, infectious diseases are necessary for the maturation of a healthy immune system (this is particularly true of the 'common' childhood illnesses such as chickenpox, measles and mumps).

Many medical professionals recommend vaccines, arguing that immunization has been responsible for the decline in infectious illnesses like diptheria. In fact, because of better sanitation and hygiene, most of these diseases – including diptheria, cholera and typhoid – were in rapid and continuous decline well before the introduction of immunization procedures.

It is not irresponsible to decide against vaccination for our children. A healthy diet – one sufficient in nutrients, based on unrefined foods and containing plenty of fresh fruit and vegetables – will help a child to resist disease, and when illness does occur her body will be in good shape to deal with it rapidly and effectively. Natural remedies will help a child to recover from an infectious illness by supporting his immune system, not suppressing it. It is a good idea to register your child with a practitioner of natural medicine, such as a homoeopath, so that if he does become ill, you can get professional advice quickly.

If you do opt to have your child vaccinated, be selective about it. If she gets a deep punctured wound, then consider the tetanus vaccine. If you must travel to an area where there is an outbreak of yellow fever, or other tropical diseases, then it may be necessary to consider some other immunizations. But if you keep vaccination to a minimum you will greatly increase your child's chances of becoming a healthy adult with a well-functioning immune system. Susan Curtis has written a book called *Homoeopathic Alternatives to Immunisation* (Winter Press, 2002), which is a useful guide for parents considering other options to vaccination.

See also the Immune System, page 61.

Bedwetting

Bedwetting is not usually considered a problem until a child reaches school age. Many children go through a phase of bedwetting and there is nearly always a psychological factor to take into account. Prolonged bedwetting often causes considerable stress to both child and parents, and great care and understanding are necessary to solve the problem.

Bedwetting may be caused by an organic problem, such as a kidney defect, so if it persists, it is advisable to take the child to a physician for an examination.

A child's tendency to wet her bed will be aggravated by fizzy drinks, refined sugar and food additives (especially food colourings), so these should be avoided. It sometimes helps if you avoid giving her a drink too late in the evening and wake her up to urinate when you go to bed.

If the problem persists, try consulting a practitioner of natural medicine. Homoeopathy is often particularly good at treating bedwetting. Homoeopathic remedies to consider include CALC CARB, CAUSTICUM, EQUISE-TUM and KREOSOTUM. A herbal infusion that may be given to strengthen the urinary system and gently help to relieve any stress can be made from CATNIP, CHAMOMILE, HORSETAIL and ST JOHN'S WORT. This infusion may be sweetened with buckwheat honey and drunk twice a day.

⚘ Chickenpox

Chickenpox is one of the most contagious of all the childhood illnesses and it provides a great opportunity for the vitality of the child to assert itself and throw off inherited or acquired toxicity. Any distressing or uncomfortable symptoms can be effectively treated using natural remedies, but seek professional advice if the symptoms seem particularly severe, or if the spots become seriously infected.

The contagious period for chickenpox lasts from 24 hours before the rash starts to the time the spots scab over. A rash is often the first sign of chickenpox, but it may begin with a temperature or general malaise. The rash will appear on different parts of the body and will be extremely itchy. At first, the spots are like dark red pimples, and within a few hours these will develop a small blister on top; this will eventually form a scab and drop off.

A herbal infusion may be drunk every few hours to soothe the child and encourage a rapid recovery. Consider the herbs BALM, BURDOCK, CHAMOMILE, ELDERFLOWER and HEARTSEASE. Also, sponge the child down with a soothing lotion made by infusing the herbs CHICKWEED, LAVENDER, MARIGOLD and ST JOHN'S WORT and then waiting for the infusion to cool. Diluted WITCH HAZEL also has a pleasantly cooling and soothing effect.

Consult the *Materia Medica* section of this book to see which of the following homoeopathic remedies are best for your child's particular symptoms: ANT CRUD, ARS ALB, BELLADONNA, PULSATILLA and RHUS TOX. Of these, the most commonly indicated homoeopathic remedy for chickenpox symptoms is RHUS TOX.

Essential oils may be diluted into a vegetable-base oil and then gently rubbed onto the skin for a soothing and healing effect. Try a combination of CHAMOMILE, LAVENDER and TEA TREE. COMFREY ointment may be massaged into the skin once the scabs have fallen off to prevent scarring.

⚘ Colic

Colic is experienced as a spasmodic pain in the abdomen. It usually comes on after feeding in a baby and causes the infant to cry in pain and pass wind. Most babies outgrow colic at around three to four months, but it can be very distressing to deal with at the time. If the symptoms are very severe or persistent, or if there is any doubt about the diagnosis, then professional advice should be sought. For older children, a warm hot-water bottle hugged to the stomach will often bring relief. An infusion of the herbs CHAMOMILE and DILL SEEDS will be soothing and ease griping pains in children or babies. This infusion may be given in a bottle or beaker while it is still warm.

The homoeopathic remedies that are most often used to relieve colic are CHAMOMILLA, COLOCYNTH, LYCOPODIUM, MAG PHOS and NUX VOMICA. You can blend a couple of drops of the essential oils of CHAMOMILE or MELISSA with almond oil to gently massage into the abdomen to relieve colic in children. Do not use essential oils to treat very young babies.

Croup

Croup is a harsh cough accompanied by loud, laboured breathing. It generally occurs at night. You need to seek emergency care if the symptoms persist for more than half an hour, or in any case where the child appears to have severe breathing difficulties.

A traditional remedy is to make a steamy atmosphere by boiling a kettle in a room and this helps the child to breathe. EUCALYPTUS leaves, or a few drops of the essential oil, can be added to a basin of boiling water and placed near the child so that he can inhale the vapour. CHAMOMILE essential oil also relaxes the respiratory system. LAVENDER essential oil may be applied to the child's head and chest as a soothing compress.

A mixture of herbs to drink as an infusion to relieve croup can be made from ANISEED, CATNIP, CHAMOMILE and WHITE HOREHOUND. Homoeopathic remedies to treat croup include ACONITE, HEPAR SULPH and SPONGIA. Compare these in the *Materia Medica* to see which is the best for your child.

Earache

Ear infection is one of the most common childhood illnesses and almost every child will experience at least one before he or she is seven years old. Unfortunately, for many children, ear infections are a frequently recurring problem.

Not all earaches are due to infection – catarrh and inflammation during a cold will often cause ear pains or impaired hearing. These symptoms are generally less dramatic than when there is infection.

Ear infections develop when germ-laden fluids from the nose and throat enter the middle ear. This may happen as a result of a cold or allergy, or because the Eustachian tube is so small and short in young children. As the infection develops, white blood cells and antibodies are secreted into the tissues of the middle ear area where they attack and kill infecting bacteria. As dead bacteria and white blood cells accumulate, pus forms and puts pressure on the ear drum; as the thin membrane bulges outward from the pressure, the pain increases. Sometimes the membrane bursts, allowing pus to drain out of the ear; this is the body's way of expelling the pus. The torn eardrum will usually heal rapidly in children, although take care to prevent water, soap or shampoo getting into the ear until the membrane is fully healed.

The orthodox treatment for an ear infection is with antibiotics. However, recent studies have revealed that children who are given antibiotics are significantly more likely to have recurrent ear infections than children who do without.

If your child develops an ear infection, you could consider treating her yourself with natural remedies. But if the symptoms are severe or persistent contact a practitioner, such as a homoeopath, for advice. And if the child has other symptoms, such as a severe headache, a stiff neck or swelling or tenderness of the bony area around the ear, then seek medical advice immediately.

If ear infections keep coming back, you should also seek constitutional treatment by a qualified practitioner of natural medicine, such as a homoeopath, in order to prevent or treat any hearing loss, and to improve the child's health and resistance.

Anti-inflammatory and antimicrobial herbs can be used to treat a child suffering from an ear infection. Consider especially CHAMOMILE, ECHINACEA, GOLDEN ROD, GOLDENSEAL and PLANTAIN. An oil macerated with the herb MULLEIN is a traditional herbal treatment for earache: put a few drops of the oil on a piece of cotton wool and gently place it inside the outer ear. Earache can be greatly relieved by making a bag from clean cotton, filling it with salt, heating it in a pan until it is thoroughly warm but not too hot, then holding it against the ear. This method is useful if you do not have any other remedies to hand.

The essential oils of CHAMOMILE and LAVENDER can both be effective in treating an ear infection: put a few drops on a piece of cotton wool and place it gently inside the outer ear. Alternatively, use it as a compress over the ear area.

Homoeopathic remedies can work quickly and effectively if you find the right remedy. Consider the following by looking them up in the *Materia*

Medica: ACONITE, BELLADONNA, CHAMOMILLA, HEPAR SULPH, KALI MUR, MERC SOL, PULSATILLA and SILICEA.

German Measles (Rubella)

German measles is a harmless disease in children. It is shorter and less severe than regular measles and usually lasts three days or less. An infected child will often be slightly feverish, have a nasal discharge and develop a rash of small, lightly raised spots that tends to move down the body. If any uncomfortable symptoms do arise, use the remedies suggested for the treatment of measles *(see below).*

German measles is a potential threat to pregnant women, since those who contract it during the first three months of pregnancy have a 10 per cent risk of having a baby with birth defects, including blindness, deafness, a heart condition, cleft palate and mental problems. The natural immunity from having had German measles offers more protection than a vaccination, so try to ensure that your daughter catches it as a child.

It makes more sense to restrict vaccinations to those young women who have not managed to contract German measles by the time they get to childbearing age rather than vaccinating all children against it. There is a test that can be carried out for a natural immunity to the disease if there is any doubt. This would prevent unnecessarily vaccinating entire generations of children.

Measles

Measles used to be another classic childhood illness. The early symptoms of measles are a sore throat, cold symptoms, inflamed eyes, a cough and feverishness. On about the fourth day a rash appears on the child's neck and behind his ears, which gradually moves downwards to cover the rest of the body. Most children will recover without treatment after seven to ten days.

The incubation period for measles is 10 to 12 days, and the most infectious period is the few days before the rash appears.

Measles is not usually a dangerous disease and, like scarlet fever, it has tended to become milder in the last 20 years or so. Complications do develop very occasionally. These are usually caused by dehydration from a high fever or breathing difficulties because of a secondary chest infection. Contrary to the popular myth, there is no danger of permanent eye damage resulting from measles, although if the child is sensitive to bright light during the illness you should keep her in a darkened room to help her rest and heal quickly.

A more serious complication involving inflammation of the brain tissues (encephalitis) may develop very rarely. Look out for any unusual drowsiness, a severe headache or marked irritability, and seek urgent treatment if any of these symptoms becomes apparent. Encephalitis is most likely to result from 'atypical measles', which is in fact more common in those children who have received the measles vaccine. Classic measles is rare these days because of the high incidence of immunization.

A Danish study has shown that the measles vaccine leads to a predisposition to arthritis, dermatitis and bone diseases later in life. Dr Wakefield has provided evidence that the measles component of the MMR vaccine has been linked to a particular bowel disease that causes autism in children. The British medical establishment has attempted to discredit the work of Dr Wakefield, but his ongoing research in the US does appear to support his theory.

Chinese medicine believes that measles is a chance for the child to eliminate those poisons that accumulated during pregnancy. If the child is immunized, they cannot be eliminated and this will make the child vulnerable to other disorders later in life.

The measles rash can be very itchy and this is the most likely cause of your child's discomfort. Antibiotics do not have any effect on the measles virus, so they should not be considered unless a secondary infection has developed. General home care should involve bed rest, sponging down with tepid water during the fever, and responding to any uncomfortable symptoms as they arise with natural remedies.

You can give an infusion made from the herbs BURDOCK LEAVES, CHAMOMILE and ELDERFLOWER to soothe the child, bring down the fever and promote healing. If her eyes are sore and inflamed then add the herb EYEBRIGHT to the mixture (this may also be bought in tincture form to dilute and bathe the eyes). An infusion made from the herbs CHAMOMILE, CHICKWEED, MARIGOLD and MARSHMALLOW and used when cool to sponge down the child will help to relieve feverishness and itching. Alternatively, add a few drops of the essential oils of CHAMOMILE, EUCALYPTUS or LAVENDER to tepid water and use this to sponge the child.

The most commonly indicated homoeopathic remedy for measles symptoms is PULSATILLA. Other homoeopathic remedies to consider include ACONITE, BELLADONNA, BRYONIA, EUPHRASIA, KALI BICH and RHUS TOX.

⚘ Mumps

Mumps is a highly infectious but usually harmless childhood disease. The virus causes one or both salivary glands (parotids), located just below and in front of the ears, to swell. Other symptoms of mumps include feverishness and a sore throat. The gland-swelling usually begins to diminish after two or three days, although one gland may become affected first and the other several days later.

These days many infants are immunized against mumps, along with measles and rubella, in the MMR vaccine. This vaccination is promoted on the basis that although mumps is not a serious childhood disease, it may lead to orchitis (a complication affecting the testicles) in the adult male. Orchitis can cause sterility, although this is rare because usually only one testicle is affected.

If you have mumps as a child it nearly always leads to a life-long immunity. It is now thought the mumps vaccination confers an immunity only into puberty. Consequently, there is the possibility that if a child is immunized against mumps in childhood he may suffer more serious consequences if he catches it as an adult. The side-effects of the mumps vaccine can be severe, ranging from allergic reactions to, more rarely, febrile seizures, nerve deafness and encephalitis.

A child who has mumps needs plenty of rest and lots of fluids. Try a soothing drink made from an infusion of BALM, BORAGE and CHAMOMILE. If the illness lasts for more than a couple of days, add ECHINACEA and YARROW to the mixture.

A compress can be very pleasant and will have a soothing and healing effect. Add a couple of drops of the essential oils of CHAMOMILE and LAVENDER to water and apply to the child's forehead and neck. The essential oils of EUCALYPTUS or THYME, added to a steam inhalation, will act as a decongestant and help the body fight the infection. You can also dilute these oils in water and spray them around the child's room with a plant spray.

The homoeopathic remedies that are most frequently indicated for treating the symptoms of mumps include ACONITE, APIS, BELLADONNA, MERC SOL, PHYTOLACCA and PULSATILLA.

⚘ Whooping Cough

Whooping cough (pertussis) is an infectious disease that affects the mucous membranes of the air passages and usually occurs in children. The initial symptoms are like those of a common cold but after about a week a violent, convulsive cough, often accompanied by vomiting, follows. At first the cough occurs only at night, but as the illness progresses it may appear during the day as well.

Whooping cough can be a very distressing and exhausting experience for the parents and the child. The child may cough a dozen times with each breath, and his face may darken to a bluish or purple hue. During a coughing bout you may hear the characteristic 'whoop' as the child struggles to inhale. This may not happen during a mild attack but you should always seek careful treatment and professional help with a case of whooping cough, especially in babies, in case they contract pneumonia or damage their lungs.

Although the vaccine against whooping cough has been used for decades, it is one of the most controversial of the immunizations. Doubts persist about its effectiveness, and many health care professionals are concerned that the potentially damaging side-effects of the vaccine, which include skin conditions and convulsions (in rare cases leading to permanent brain damage), may outweigh the alleged benefits.

Using natural remedies to treat whooping cough can reduce the risk of complications setting in and help to shorten the illness. However, the following suggestions should be used in addition to professional supervision, not as an alternative to it.

A herbal infusion to reduce the spasms, fight the infection and strengthen the lungs can be made from ANISEED, COLTSFOOT, HYSSOP, LIQUORICE, THYME and WHITE HOREHOUND. Add two teaspoons of herbs to a cup of boiling water (it may be sweetened with honey). The dosage for babies is one teaspoon of infusion every four hours; for children of six months to five years two teaspoons every four hours; and for children over five years one tablespoon every four hours.

Essential oils may be added to steaming water so that the child can inhale the vapour, or add a few drops to a vegetable-oil base and massage onto the chest. Those oils to consider are CYPRESS, LAVENDER, ROSEMARY, TEA TREE and THYME. They may be used in a combination.

You can get excellent results by treating whooping cough with homoeopathic remedies. However, finding the right remedy is not always easy and it is advisable to consult a qualified homoeopath for advice. The most frequently indicated homoeopathic remedies for whooping cough include BELLADONNA, BRYONIA, COCCUS CACTI, DROSERA and IPECAC.

5

The Circulatory System

The blood circulatory system is the transport system of the body. It carries oxygen from the lungs to the tissues, and carbon dioxide in the opposite direction. It transfers absorbed food substances from the gut to the liver and then throughout the body. It carries waste products from the tissues to the liver and kidneys for detoxication and excretion. The heart is the pump in this system, the blood vessels provide the route and the blood is the carrier.

Blood is the prime symbol of life and vitality for many cultures. Its ability to flow throughout the body and distribute nutrients is a symbol of the free circulation and sharing of resources throughout any system, personal or planetary. Diseases of the circulatory system are caused by and result in congestion, stagnation and decay; an appropriate image for this is a polluted river. Rivers should flow freely, carrying great life in their waters, but when they are polluted they become stagnant, poisonous and unable to support life.

Cardiovascular diseases are on the increase and are already the major cause of death among adults in the developed world. Considerable changes in attitude and lifestyle are necessary to revert this trend. The dictum 'Prevention is better than cure' is never more true than in the case of circulatory system diseases. Once the symptoms of heart disease are established, natural medicines have a lot to offer, but an individual case should be assessed by a suitably qualified practitioner.

Diet is a major factor to consider in the prevention of heart disease. It is well known that those people who eat foods that are high in animal fats are more prone to heart disease: food containing animal fats is slowly digested and is more likely to cause excessive cholesterol levels in the body. Cholesterol is a waxy substance that is produced naturally by the liver and adrenal glands; any excess can be considered a waste product. Its build-up in the bloodstream contributes to hardened arteries, and strokes and coronary disease are likely to

The Circulatory System

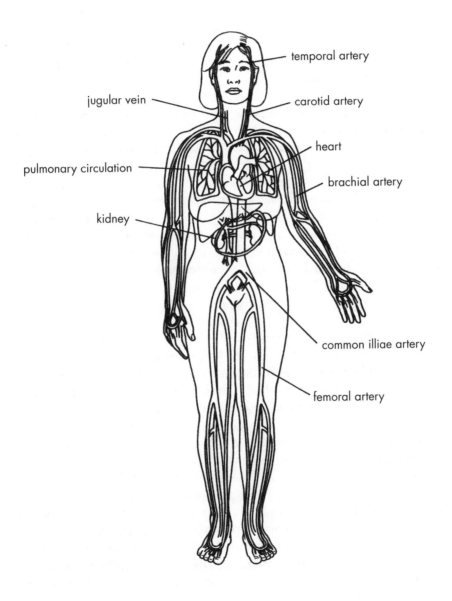

temporal artery

jugular vein

carotid artery

heart

pulmonary circulation

brachial artery

kidney

common illiae artery

femoral artery

result. Foods that are particularly high in cholesterol and should be kept to a minimum are: butter, cream, cheese, eggs and meat. Conversely, natural foods such as unprocessed fruits, vegetables, grains, legumes, nuts and seeds contribute towards the liver's production of lecithin, which acts as a fat-dissolving agent and protects the body from excess accumulations of fat within the arteries. Heat and other processes of extraction will destroy lecithin in foods. This shows how much better it is to use cold pressed vegetable oils, whole grains and unprocessed and unrefined foods.

It is advisable to stick to a low-salt diet to keep the risk of heart disease to a minimum. Smoking should definitely be avoided, and keep your alcohol intake to a moderate amount.

Exercise is important to keep the tone of the circulatory system in good order. Regular daily exercise which makes you feel warmed up and slightly short of breath is preferable to infrequent but excessive exertion.

Stress is widely acknowledged to be a major contributory factor to heart disease. Stress can become such a part of your lifestyle that it may be necessary to seek advice about trying to reduce it. There are many kinds of relaxation therapies available if you are aware that you do not relax easily. If you have been under a lot of emotional stress, some form of personal counselling can be a great help.

Anaemia

Anaemia may be the result of either a reduction in the number of red blood cells, or a lack of haemoglobin (the red pigment in blood that carries iron). Red blood cells carry oxygen from the lungs to the rest of the body, the oxygen combining with iron to form haemoglobin. Symptoms of anaemia include general weariness, debility, dizziness and headaches; a simple blood test will establish whether you are anaemic or not.

A common cause of anaemia is loss of blood, which may be sudden, as after an operation, an accident or childbirth, or sustained over some time, as with a heavy menstrual flow, bleeding from a peptic ulcer or haemorrhoids. Other causes are defective blood formation after or during severe or chronic infections, lack of iron in the diet, or inadequate absorption of iron from the digestive tract in disorders of the intestine. Pregnant women are more susceptible to anaemia due to the increased nutritional demands on the body. There are also a group of hereditary blood disorders, including sickle cell disease, that cause anaemia. Cure of anaemia must include the treatment of the condition causing it as well as increasing the intake of iron.

Calcium and copper, vitamin C and the B group vitamins must also be present for the body to be able to assimilate iron. A balanced diet of natural foods should supply sufficient quantities of these vitamins and minerals, otherwise food supplements may be taken; vegetarians in particular may need to take extra vitamin B12. Foods that are naturally rich in iron include meat, eggs, lentils, apricots, green-leaf vegetables, molasses and beetroot. The cruder forms of iron supplements, such as those usually recommended during pregnancy, often cause digestive upsets and constipation. FLORADIX is an excellent plant-based iron tonic which may be used to supplement the diet and can be taken during pregnancy.

The herbs ALFALFA, DANDELION ROOT, NETTLES, WATERCRESS and YELLOW DOCK are all rich in iron and may be taken regularly as an infusion. The homoeopathic tissue salt FERRUM PHOS can aid the assimilation of iron from the diet.

Artery Disease

The arteries are responsible for bringing oxygen and nourishment to the vital organs and other parts of the body. Without this they become diseased and die. Therefore the condition of the arteries is of prime importance to the overall health of the body. The most common cause of death in adults in Britain is insufficient circulation to the brain or heart because of disease of the arteries.

The arteries are tubes with muscular walls. When these walls become thickened and lose their elasticity, the condition is called arteriosclerosis. This is usually associated with high blood pressure. When the arteries become thickened by localized accumulations of fatty substances (atheroma), the condition is called atherosclerosis.

Atherosclerosis may begin early in life and often no symptoms are experienced for many years. Gradually the walls of the arteries become thicker and the flow of blood becomes restricted. Eventually atheroma may completely block a major artery with dramatic, maybe fatal, results – a heart attack or stroke. Atheroma also promotes the clotting of blood in arteries, and when these clots create a blockage in an artery supplying either the heart or the brain (a thrombosis), a similar crisis results.

A combination of arteriosclerosis and high blood pressure may result in angina which is caused by a reduction in the blood supply, and therefore oxygen, to the muscle of the heart. Angina pain is of a dull, gripping nature and is characteristically felt across the upper part of the chest, radiating down the left or sometimes right arm. The pain comes on during exertion; often it is most noticeable when going up a slope or climbing stairs. The pain is relieved by rest.

All the general advice about diet and lifestyle in the introductory section to the Circulatory System is relevant to diseases of the arteries *(see pages 36–8)*. The main causes of hardening of and deposits in the arteries are a high cholesterol diet, smoking, high alcohol consumption and a lack of exercise. It is only by changing these habits that this major disease of the modern world can be prevented. Natural medicines have a lot to offer, but obviously they will only be of long-term benefit if they are used alongside changes in diet and lifestyle.

The use of fresh GARLIC in your daily diet will help your body to break down any deposits of cholesterol that have built up. COD LIVER OIL and HALIBUT LIVER OIL also keep the arteries clean – they may be taken as capsules. Specific herbs for artery disease are GINKGO, HAWTHORN TOPS and its BERRIES and LIME BLOSSOM. For the treatment of angina MOTHERWORT should also be considered. A regular massage with the essential oils of JUNIPER and LEMON can also help to break down fatty deposits in the arteries.

Heart Weakness

Conventional medicine divides heart disease up into several different categories, but in natural medicine there are many remedies that can help to strengthen the heart and circulation generally. If there are symptoms of suspected heart disease, such as breathlessness when you exert yourself, pains in the chest or down the arms, or if you are already on medication, a professional therapist should be consulted.

The most important herbal heart and circulation tonic is HAWTHORN TOPS. This may safely be taken as an infusion or a tincture for several months. Other particularly useful herbal heart tonics are BALM, LIME BLOSSOM and MOTHERWORT. Among essential oils the main cardiac tonics are LAVENDER, MARJORAM, MELISSA, ROSE and ROSEMARY. These may be used singly or as a combination, and added to the bath or used for a massage.

⚛ High Blood Pressure (Hypertension)

Blood pressure depends on two main factors: first, the strength of the contraction of the heart; and second, the peripheral resistance to the blood flow which is determined by the size and condition of the smaller arteries. The more constricted these tiny arteries, the greater the resistance and the higher the blood pressure reading. As we get older, the arteries become thicker and less elastic; this leads to a rise in blood pressure and explains why it tends to be higher in older people.

There are two figures to a blood pressure recording: the higher number (systolic pressure) is written over the lower number (diastolic pressure). The systolic pressure, produced when the heart contracts, is more susceptible to changes induced by exercise and emotion, and more liable to fall when the subject is at rest. The diastolic pressure, the pressure maintained when the heart relaxes between beats, depends more on the state of the arteries and is less likely to be affected by outside events. Below the age of about 50 years, the diastolic pressure is normally less than 85.

There is usually no warning symptom of high blood pressure until a person suffers from one of its complications – most commonly a heart attack, stroke or kidney disease. The only way to discover the disease in advance is to have the blood pressure measured with a sphygmomanometer.

Some forms of kidney disease and certain gland disorders may lead to high blood pressure, but no obvious cause is found in the majority of people. Hypertension is equally common in women and men and it affects about 15 per cent of British adults. Sometimes the disease is hereditary. Mild cases of hypertension will often respond quickly to dietary changes, increased relaxation and natural medicines. Periods of trauma in people's lives can result in high blood pressure. In most people this will return to normal once the trauma is resolved. More severe cases of hypertension will need treatment over an indefinite period of time, in order to prevent strokes, kidney disease or heart failure.

Conventionally, hypertension is often treated with both a diuretic and a sympathetic nervous system depressant, which reduces the ability of the nervous system to constrict blood vessels. Increasingly, a type of drug called beta-blockers is prescribed. Sometimes vasodilators are used to relax the walls of the arteries. If you are receiving medication for high blood pressure, you must consult a qualified practitioner before trying any other remedies or cutting down on the drugs.

If you have high blood pressure, you must make changes to your diet and reappraise the amount of stress in your lifestyle. Smoking must be avoided. Your diet should be low in animal fats and you should not add any salt to food during or after cooking. Eat plenty of raw garlic.

The recognition and control of stress in your life is vital if you suffer from hypertension; this is probably the single factor that has the greatest effect in the long-term management of high blood pressure. It is often people who drive themselves very hard and have high standards who are most prone to high blood pressure. You need to reassess the amount of stress at work and within your personal relationships, possibly with the help of a professional counsellor. Consider some sort of relaxation therapy or meditation classes, too.

For a mild case of high blood pressure HAWTHORN BERRIES should be ground, infused and drunk on a regular basis (or use the tincture). CRAMPBARK can be used to encourage the arteries to dilate and other herbs to consider are LIME BLOSSOM and YARROW. Herbal medicine should not be used by someone already taking drugs for high blood pressure without consulting a professional herbalist, as we have already stated.

A regular massage by a skilled aromatherapist can really help to reduce high blood pressure. The oils with a particular role in the treatment of hypertension are LAVENDER, MARJORAM and YLANG-YLANG. These may be used in the bath or for a relaxing and therapeutic massage.

There are many examples of cases of hypertension that have responded well to acupuncture treatment, so it may be well worth consulting an acupuncturist from one of the acupuncture registers *(see page 425 for addresses)*.

Low Blood Pressure (Hypotension)

This problem is less common and has less serious implications than high blood pressure, but it can be distressing to the sufferer, causing fainting and weakness. It may be associated with a weak circulation or with general debility. Some teenagers experience a bout of low blood pressure, associated with periods of fainting, which then clears up of its own accord.

Herbs to consider are GINGER, HAWTHORN TOPS and ROSEMARY. If the low blood pressure is associated with general weakness and debility, you should consider nutritious herbs such as ALFALFA, NETTLES and PARSLEY. An invigorating massage with the stimulating oils of BLACK PEPPER, ROSEMARY or SAGE may also be of benefit.

Palpitations

Palpitations are experienced when the heart beats forcibly or irregularly and the individual becomes aware of its action. Although palpitations do occur with other symptoms of true heart disease, the vast majority of people experience them as a result of anxiety, and not as a direct result of heart disease at all. After a physical examination by your doctor to rule out organic heart disease, these remedies may be tried to relieve palpitations associated with stress or anxiety.

Look up the following herbs in the *Materia Medica* section to see which are the most suitable for you: LIMEFLOWERS, MOTHERWORT and VALERIAN. The essential oils which are particularly good for the treatment of palpitations include ANISEED, LAVENDER, MELISSA, NEROLI, PEPPERMINT, ROSEMARY and YLANG-YLANG. A regular visit to an aromatherapist for a relaxing massage will be of most benefit.

Many people find palpitations very frightening, which of course makes the palpitations worse. In this situation, the Bach FIVE FLOWER REMEDY can help to calm the feelings of panic and anxiety. If stress and anxiety are known to be the cause of palpitations then deep relaxation, as taught by relaxation therapists, can be a great help.

Poor Circulation and Chilblains

Poor circulation will cause cold extremities, and in a cold winter chilblains may develop. All the general advice at the beginning of this section is appropriate to tonify and improve the circulation. In addition, a mixture of the following herbs may be taken for several weeks: GINGER, GINKGO, HAWTHORN, PRICKLY ASH BARK and ROSEMARY. MUSTARD foot baths can also be very good for cold feet.

The essential oils of BLACK PEPPER, CYPRESS and MARJORAM will all help to stimulate the circulation, so try a regular, invigorating massage of these oils diluted in vegetable oil.

If you are prone to getting chilblains, you should wear warm socks and shoes and gloves when outdoors in cold weather. On returning indoors, you should warm your hands and feet slowly at room temperature. Do not expose them to direct heat, which will only aggravate the chilblains.

For the treatment of chilblains, compare the homoeopathic remedies of FERRUM PHOS and PULSATILLA. There is also a homoeopathic ointment made to relieve the itching called TAMUS OINTMENT. If the chilblains have caused the skin to break then use CALENDULA OINTMENT to promote healing. Essential oils that may be used to heal chilblains are CHAMOMILE and LAVENDER – these are both anti-inflammatory.

Varicose Veins

Blood is returned to the heart through the veins of the legs by the contraction of the leg muscles. Within the veins there are one-way valves which keep the blood flowing in the right direction. When the valves fail, the veins swell and the blood stagnates within them; this is the condition described as varicose veins.

Varicose veins are common in adults of both sexes, although they are about twice as common among women. They may be caused by constipation, pregnancy or other causes which partially block the veins in the pelvis, and by jobs which involve a great deal of standing without much movement, for example hairdressing and dentistry. There appears to be a hereditary factor involved, as the condition tends to run in families. High levels of oestrogen, such as occur during pregnancy and from some forms of the birth control pill, may also cause varicose veins. During pregnancy, they may appear in the early months but often disappear entirely after the delivery.

Varicose veins are usually just unsightly, but they may cause aching, heaviness of the legs and swelling of the ankles, especially at the end of the day. These symptoms are usually relieved if you rest with your feet up. When a clot occurs in the veins of the legs (the condition is called phlebitis), it causes local inflammation and pain, and must be urgently looked at by a practitioner to make sure that there is no danger of further complications.

Conventional treatment of varicose veins includes injecting them with a substance that will close off the affected part of the vein, or by surgically stripping the affected veins out of the leg. In both instances, the varicose veins often recur because the reasons why they developed in the first place have probably not been tackled.

It is difficult to cure varicose veins once they exist, but it is quite possible to prevent them from getting worse. It is important to avoid becoming constipated, so stick to a wholefood high-fibre diet. Do not drink strong tea or more than one or two cups of weak tea a day. Avoid becoming overweight. Make sure that you get plenty of regular leg exercise such as walking, cycling or swimming.

Avoid wearing tight boots, trousers or pants, and do not sit with your legs crossed. If varicose veins begin during pregnancy then elastic support tights can relieve any aching.

RUTIN helps to keep the vein walls in good shape, so eat plenty of buck-wheat (its natural source), or take RUTIN tablets. The homoeopathic tissue salt CALC FLUOR promotes the elasticity of vein walls and may be taken as a course for two or three weeks (this may be taken during pregnancy). HAMAMELIS, in homoeopathic form, will relieve varicose veins that are aching and causing a feeling of fullness in the leg.

Herbs to repair and tone the venous system are GINKGO, HAWTHORN BERRIES, HORSE CHESTNUT, PRICKLY ASH and YARROW; these should be infused and taken internally. An ointment made from MARIGOLD or WITCH HAZEL may be used externally if there is any irritation. The essential oils of CYPRESS, JUNIPER or LAVENDER may be diluted and massaged into the area around but not directly on the varicose vein, or add a couple of drops to a bath.

6

The Digestive System

Our health and energy are determined to a great extent by what we ingest into our bodies. Our digestive system is our prime contact with the produce of the earth. The food that we eat and feed to our families is one of the most important factors involved in caring for the physical body.

There is a great deal written about what we should and should not eat; in fact so much has been said that it can be quite overwhelming. We suggest a very common-sense approach to diet, with a few basic guidelines: eat food that is as fresh as possible; with as few additives and as little processing as possible, try to eat regular meals; eat a variety of foods for a well-balanced diet; and try not to overeat as this will put a strain on all your body's systems.

If the digestive system is already showing symptoms of disease and you suspect that your diet is not very good now, or has not been in the past, then it can be a great help to consult a dietary therapist or a naturopath. He or she should be able to isolate foods that aggravate your condition and guide you through a detoxification programme if that is considered advisable (or try the one on page 423). To help you find a naturopath or dietary therapist, *see* page 425 of this book. For general information on food and diet *see* pages 406–10.

Constipation

There are conflicting ideas about how frequent bowel movements should be. It is considered to be normal to open your bowels twice or more a day, or only two or three times a week; however, most women seem to feel better if they have a regular daily bowel movement.

While constipation is not a disease itself, there can be uncomfortable symptoms associated with it, such as bloatedness, abdominal pains or headaches.

The Digestive System

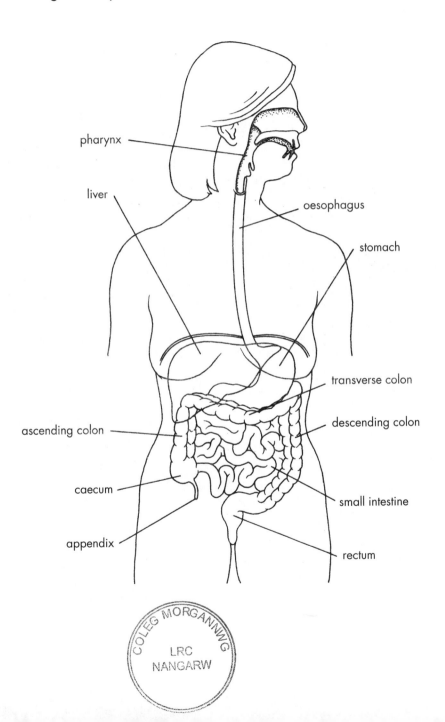

The factors that tend to lead to constipation are a diet that is rich in refined foods, stress and not putting the time aside for a bowel movement. Chronic constipation – a long-term tendency to infrequent bowel movements – can often only be treated by a radical change in diet. Even adding more fibre to the diet may not help sufficiently without first going on a cleansing programme to clear out the system and establish a more regular bowel habit.

It may be best to consult a naturopath or dietary therapist to get advice about a detoxification programme, or try the cleansing diet on page 423.

To help avoid constipation eat more foods that are high in fibre, fresh fruit and vegetables. The recent tendency to add bran to everything doesn't suit everyone; it can be rather drying in the bowel. Plain oats soaked in fruit juice can make a better alternative to bran or toast for breakfast. Linseed can also be a valuable addition to the diet; sprinkle a tablespoon of the seeds onto the oats at breakfast, or stir into a glass of water or juice. It can also be helpful to drink more water.

Avoid the frequent use of laxatives, as they can irritate the gut and weaken the tone of the bowel, thus making the constipation worse. The following suggestions will be good for the odd bout of constipation, but if you suffer from chronic constipation you should seek constitutional treatment from a practitioner of natural medicine.

For a herbal infusion that has a laxative effect, choose from FENNEL, LIQUORICE, MARSHMALLOW ROOT, RHUBARB ROOT and SENNA LEAVES. The main homoeopathic remedies to choose from are ALUMINA, BRYONIA, NAT MUR, NUX VOMICA and SEPIA. A pleasant way to relieve constipation is to massage a few drops of FENNEL, MARJORAM or ROSEMARY essential oils, diluted in vegetable oil, onto the abdomen. Look all these remedies up in the *Materia Medica* section of this book to help you choose the most appropriate ones for yourself.

Gastro-enteritis

Gastro-enteritis means an inflammation of the stomach, often causing nausea and vomiting, accompanied by inflammation of the small intestine, causing diarrhoea. Abdominal colic and sometimes fever may also be present.

The main causes of gastro-enteritis are food poisoning and any infection or virus that affects the small intestine. Food infected with the salmonella organism is responsible for many outbreaks of acute gastro-enteritis. There have also been some severe outbreaks of E. coli in recent years, even causing fatalaties. This is a problem usually associated with processed foods and especially processed meat.

If someone is vomiting or has diarrhoea, care must be taken to ensure that the person does not become dehydrated – this is particularly crucial with infants. Failure to hold down clear fluids, drowsiness, disinterest in fluids and decreased urination are all warning signs of the need for urgent medical advice in a young child.

Following the onset of gastro-enteritis, the stomach should be rested for the first eight hours with sips of water; after that plenty of fluids should be taken to prevent dehydration, possibly with a little honey added. After 24 hours plain, light food such as soup, plain crackers, ARROWROOT or SLIPPERY ELM may be introduced. If symptoms are not relieved after 24 hours of home care, or 12 hours in young children, seek immediate medical assistance.

The main herbs used in the treatment of gastro-enteritis are AGRIMONY, CHAMOMILE, MARSHMALLOW ROOT, MEADOWSWEET and SLIPPERY ELM. After comparing these herbs in the *Materia Medica* section, choose one or two of them to make into a drink, and take every four hours until symptoms are relieved. There are many homoeopathic remedies that may be indicated, so you will need to compare ARS ALB, CHAMOMILLA, COLOCYNTH, IPECAC, MAG PHOS, NUX VOMICA, PHOSPHORUS and PULSATILLA. The essential oils of CHAMOMILE or GERANIUM may be diluted and massaged into the abdomen to bring relief.

After a bout of gastro-enteritis a course of probiotics such as acidophilus can be very beneficial.

Gum Disease

Receding or bleeding gums are symptoms of gum disease. When the gum becomes loosened around the teeth, pockets tend to form and bacteria can accumulate; the gum margin and the underlying tissues can then become inflamed. This is called gingivitis. In more advanced cases, called pyorrhoea, the teeth become loose and may even fall out. One of the main causes of gum disease is a diet of soft, refined foods: the gums are stimulated by chewing crunchy and fibrous foods and this helps to keep them healthy.

The most important herbs to use to treat gum infections and gum disease are CALENDULA, ECHINACEA, MYRRH, RASPBERRY LEAF and SAGE; the best way to use them is to buy a selection of the tinctures and make up a mouthwash for regular use. The essential oils of FENNEL, LAVENDER and MYRRH are healing and antiseptic, and a couple of drops of one of them may be added to warm water to rinse around the gums. There are several brands of herbal toothpastes on the market these days that contain some of these herbs and oils.

❋ Haemorrhoids (Piles)

Haemorrhoids are varicose veins that develop either inside or just outside the anus. The main causes are being overweight, chronic constipation, straining during a bowel movement, the use of powerful laxatives, and pregnancy and labour. The symptoms are itching or pain at the anus, and if the pile ruptures, bleeding. Haemorrhoids are a common complaint that can be helped considerably by preventing constipation *(see pages 46–8)* and correct treatment, but other forms of rectal bleeding may mimic or co-exist with them, and a diagnosis should be established if this particular symptom is persistent.

RUTIN tablets may be taken as a dietary supplement to improve the strength of the capillary walls in the bowel. Internally, a course of the herbs DANDELION ROOT, GOLDENSEAL, HAWTHORN, HORSECHESTNUT and YARROW can be helpful. Externally, an infusion or the diluted tinctures of HORSECHESTNUT, PILEWORT or WITCH HAZEL may be applied. Homoeopathically, the main remedies to consider are ARNICA, CALC FLUOR, HAMAMELIS, NIT AC, NUX VOMICA, SEPIA and SULPHUR. A homoeopathic ointment containing AESCULUS, HAMAMELIS and PAEONIA is available from homoeopathic pharmacies for the treatment of haemorrhoids. A local compress of the essential oils of CYPRESS, FRANKINCENSE, LAVENDER or MYRRH will be very soothing and healing; these oils may also be added to a warm bath. Compare all these remedies in the *Materia Medica* section of this book to see which ones are most suitable for you.

❋ Indigestion

The stomach may be upset by diseases directly affecting the stomach and also by any general illness. In addition, nervous tension or anxiety frequently causes a digestive upset; most people experience loss of appetite, 'queasiness' and tension in the stomach when they are under emotional strain, or before an exam or interview. Other common causes of indigestion are eating rich food, drinking or smoking too much, eating too fast and eating at irregular times.

Symptoms of indigestion include heartburn, nausea, waterbrash, flatulence and general discomfort in the stomach region. Occasional symptoms of indigestion are felt by most people sometimes, but if the problem is more persistent or constitutes a marked change from a previously stable pattern, you should seek professional advice. Recurrent indigestion can be an early symptom of several different digestive diseases.

You can chew the seeds of ANISEED, CARDAMON or FENNEL after meals as an aid to digestion. An infusion of BALM, CHAMOMILE, MEADOWSWEET, PEPPERMINT or VERVAIN will be soothing and can be drunk in combination or singly as required. Compare the homoeopathic remedies of CARBO VEG, KALI MUR, NUX VOMICA and PULSATILLA to treat indigestion. Alternatively, the essential oils of CARDAMON, FENNEL or PEPPERMINT may be diluted and massaged into the stomach area. All these suggestions should be looked up in the *Materia Medica* section of this book before use.

Irritable Bowel Syndrome (IBS)

This used to be known as mucus colitis or spastic colon. It is a common condition where part of the large intestine (colon) is inflamed. The symptoms include a combination of colicky pains in the abdomen, diarrhoea, which may alternate with constipation, excess secretion of mucus from the bowel, flatulence and anxiety or depression.

The condition may have phases of active symptoms followed by periods of remission. It is not clear what causes it, but it is thought that a combination of physiological, dietary and psychological factors are involved. Because the causes are complex, a cure will most often require changes to diet, lifestyle and emotional habits. A diagnosis by a qualified therapist should be carried out to eliminate other possible causes of the symptoms, such as infections, ulcerative colitis, thyroid or other metabolic disorders and cancer.

Food intolerance should be considered as contributing to irritable bowel syndrome. The most common problem foods are dairy products, beef and gluten (especially wheat). It may be advisable to eliminate these and then reintroduce them one at a time to see if the symptoms return.

Many cases of IBS will improve with a change of diet. Try bland, easily digested foods, at least during its active bouts. Wheat bran products, highly spiced food, coffee and excess alcohol should all be avoided. Extra water-soluble fibre should be added to the diet in the form of vegetables, fruit and legumes. Oats are often a useful addition to the diet. They provide fibre but without the intolerance associated with wheat and wheat bran.

IBS appears to be increasingly common in our modern, high-stress lives, and dealing with stress and tension must be taken into account when it is treated. Avoiding coffee and building relaxation time into a busy day can be very helpful. Regular yoga or meditation can make a real difference. Also regular physical exercise, for example daily walking, has been shown to reduce symptoms in many sufferers.

There is a marked psychological component to IBS and it seems that sufferers hold on to their anxiety and frustration in their gastrointestinal tract. Many people suffer from IBS symptoms during a particularly stressful time of life, and long-term sufferers often find their symptoms are worse during stressful situations. Sufferers of chronic IBS may well benefit from counselling or psychotherapy as part of unlocking the cycle of stress and gastrointestinal symptoms.

Some herbal medicines have shown excellent results in the relief of IBS. Consider especially AGRIMONY, BALM, CHAMOMILE, GINGER and PEPPERMINT (*see* the *Materia Medica* section of this book). The essential oils of BERGAMOT, CHAMOMILE, LAVENDER or ORANGE may be diluted in vegetable oil and massaged over the abdomen for a soothing and healing effect. All these treatments are probably best administered by a qualified practitioner who can take the whole picture, both physiological and psychological, into account.

Mouth Abscess

A mouth or tooth abscess is a collection of pus that has gathered under a tooth. If this becomes inflamed, the site will become hot and red, and you will feel a throbbing pain. The fact that such an infection has developed shows that your gums are not healthy, and that your resistance to infection is probably low. A cleansing diet (try the one on page 423) or constitutional treatment by a natural health practitioner should be considered if your abscesses keep coming back.

The following herbs should be considered for mouth abscesses: BURDOCK ROOT, CLEAVERS, ECHINACEA, GOLDENSEAL and YELLOW DOCK. Make a decoction of these herbs, or buy them as tinctures, and take three times a day for three weeks. A compress of the essential oils of CHAMOMILE or LAVENDER may be applied externally. The homoeopathic remedies to consider are APIS, BELLADONNA, HEPAR SULPH and SILICEA. Compare all these remedies in the *Materia Medica* section of this book to see which are most suitable for you. Eat plenty of GARLIC to help fight the infection.

⚹ Mouth Ulcer

Mouth ulcers are small painful blisters that appear on the tongue, gums or lining of the mouth. They usually indicate a need to improve the general health of the sufferer, and a natural therapist should be consulted for constitutional treatment, especially if they are recurrent. The odd mouth ulcer can be treated at home using natural remedies.

An infusion of the herbs MARIGOLD, RASPBERRY LEAF, RED SAGE and THYME may be used as a mouthwash to heal mouth ulcers quickly. Alternatively you can dab either the tincture or the essential oil of MYRRH onto the ulcer. Compare the homoeopathic remedies BORAX, MERCURIUS and NAT PHOS.

⚹ Peptic Ulcer

Peptic ulcers are ulcers of the digestive system, they are usually either gastric (stomach) ulcers, or duodenal (small intestine) ulcers. Part of the mucous membrane of the stomach or duodenum becomes eaten away by the highly acidic digestive juices.

The main things that lead to a peptic ulcer are a faulty diet (too rich in fats and refined carbohydrates), smoking, an excessive intake of stimulants, such as coffee or highly-spiced food, and alcohol. Emotional stress tends to increase the secretion of digestive acids and this can also contribute to the formation of an ulcer.

The first symptom of a peptic ulcer is pain, this may be felt anywhere in the upper abdomen but usually under the sternum. The pain is often relieved for a short time after eating and by vomiting. Heartburn and nausea are other common symptoms. Most ulcers bleed at times and this may cause anaemia. Peptic ulcers are a very serious condition and complications include sudden and severe bleeding, perforation of the stomach or duodenum and a narrowing of the outlet of the stomach. Any persistent pain associated with the stomach should be referred to a medical practitioner for diagnosis, as other diseases may show similar symptoms.

The following suggestions will almost certainly bring relief to the painful symptoms of a peptic ulcer, but unless you are prepared to change your lifestyle, and particularly the level of stress in your life and your diet, home remedies will only temporarily alleviate the symptoms without really getting to the cause of the problem. We advise you to seek professional advice from a natural therapist, as this may well be a necessary part of the healing process.

The herbs to consider in the treatment of peptic ulcers are COMFREY, LIQUORICE, MARIGOLD, MARSHMALLOW ROOT, MEADOWSWEET and SLIPPERY ELM. Look all these remedies up in the *Materia Medica* section to see which ones are the best indicated for your particular symptoms.

It is known that a particular type of bacteria called heliobacteria can cause gastric ulcers. Clinical trials have shown that MANUKA HONEY and CRANBERRY JUICE both kill these bacteria. This reduces the symptoms of pain and also allows the ulcer to heal. MANUKA HONEY can be bought from a good health-food shop and needs to be taken daily. CRANBERRY JUICE can be bought as a drink from supermarkets and also needs to be taken every day until symptoms improve.

Threadworms

Threadworms (pinworms) are a very common complaint, especially in children of school age. The worms are passed on by taking the eggs into the mouth, usually after touching the anus, where the worms descend from the rectum to lay their eggs. The lifecycle from the egg to the threadworm is about ten days, so treatment must be aimed at breaking this cycle as well as alleviating the symptoms.

The sorts of symptoms to watch out for with threadworms are irritability, a desire to pick at the nose and, most markedly an itchy anus that will be worse in the evening when the worms come out to lay their eggs. Diagnosis may be confirmed by seeing the worms in the stools or around the anus in the evening.

The elimination of worms requires scrupulous hygiene. The hands should be washed with hot water and soap after every visit to the lavatory. Underwear, towels and bed linen must be changed regularly. Close-fitting underwear should be worn at night so that the anus cannot be scratched inadvertently.

Dietary control of threadworms involves eating plenty of the foods that the worms cannot thrive on, such as raw carrots, apples, onions, garlic and pumpkin seeds. All foods containing sugar, even natural sweeteners such as malt or honey, should be avoided because the worms live on sugar. ACIDOPHILUS tablets or capsules can be taken for several weeks to improve the general health of the bowel.

One very useful method of treatment is to add a few drops of EUCALYPTUS or LAVENDER essential oil to either CALENDULA OINTMENT or Vaseline and apply it to the anus every evening. This will help to stop the worms laying their eggs as well as relieve the itching. A mixture of the herbs LIQUORICE and WORMWOOD may be taken as an infusion or as an enema. One of the most useful homoeopathic remedies in the treatment of threadworms is CINA. Look all these remedies up in the *Materia Medica* section to check how suitable they are for you or your children.

Toothache

Persistent or severe toothache should be assessed by a dentist, but there are a few remedies that can be used to relieve the pain and inflammation temporarily, and that will help relieve transient tooth pains.

Biting on a couple of CLOVES will release the analgesic oil that they contain; alternatively, apply a few drops of CLOVE essential oil onto cotton wool and place over the area. A strong infusion of the herbs MARSHMALLOW, SAGE and THYME will have an antiseptic and soothing effect. Make an infusion to rinse around the mouth and then drink. The homoeopathic remedies of ARNICA, KALI PHOS, MAG PHOS and SILICEA should be compared in the *Materia Medica* section to see which is the most appropriate for your toothache symptoms.

7

The Eyes

Any eye or vision problem should be considered on a psychological level as well as a physical level so that you can gain insight into what the underlying problem really is. The eye enables us to see and build up information about the outside world; also, it tells other people about us. Other people 'look us in the eye' when they want to find out more about us. It is the eyes that break into tears, and they reveal to the outside world what is happening with our emotions inside. They are the 'mirrors of the soul' and they are the outward manifestation of the qualities of vision and insight in our life. If an eye problem arises we should consider what it is in our lives that we do not want to see and what it is in ourselves that we do not want to look at.

Conjunctivitis

The conjunctiva is the mucous membrane that covers the eyeball and lines the lids. Inflammation of this membrane is known as conjunctivitis, and the affected eye will water and look bloodshot. If the inflammation is a symptom of a cold then there will be a clear and watery discharge, allergic conjunctivitis is accompanied by itching, and bacterial infections result in a thick, yellow-green discharge.

If the symptoms of conjunctivitis persist for more than three days, if they are associated with any loss of vision or pain in the eye, or following an injury or possible exposure to flying fragments of metal or grit, then seek emergency medical advice.

When you treat the eyes take care to wash your hands and utensils carefully, and use only cool, boiled or distilled water on the eye.

The herbs that you can take to help conjunctivitis include ECHINACEA,

ELDERFLOWER, EYEBRIGHT, GOLDENSEAL and SAGE. Herbs that should be considered for infusions for external use include CHAMOMILE, ELDERFLOWER, EYEBRIGHT, GOLDENSEAL and MARIGOLD. Consult the *Materia Medica* section and make up a mixture of the best herbs for your own use. EYEBRIGHT may be bought as a tincture that can be diluted to make a soothing and healing eyewash.

The homoeopathic remedies that should be considered to treat these symptoms include APIS, ARS ALB, BELLADONNA, EUPHRASIA, HEPAR SULPH and PULSATILLA.

Eye Strain

Eye strain may develop after a long bout of focusing the eyes on one object or at one particular distance, for example, when you are sewing, reading, driving or working at a VDU screen. It can usually be avoided by taking a break every now and then, or at least by looking up from the work you are doing every few minutes and focusing further into the distance.

If your eyes feel very tired, try placing cold teabags or slices of cucumber over them – it can be very soothing. If they become sore or inflamed then a cool infusion of the herbs CHAMOMILE and EYEBRIGHT can be used to bathe them. You can also take EYEBRIGHT internally to strengthen the eyes. The homoeopathic remedy RUTA may be taken to relieve eye strain after reading or similar activities.

8

Fevers and Influenza

You will only 'catch' an illness when your body's resistance is weakened and you are susceptible to certain bacteria and viruses. The body's defences against disease can be diminished by many physical and psychological factors. When we treat an infection or other acute illness, it is important to reassess any inadequacies in our diet, environment and lifestyle, as well as relieving the immediate symptoms of the disease.

If an infection lingers, or if you regularly contract illnesses, you will need to concentrate on improving your immune system *(see* the Immune System, page 6). Any illness should be taken as a message from our body to slow down, or to look at what it is in our daily lives that is creating the conditions for disease to occur. Suppressing the symptoms of an acute infectious illness, for example with antibiotics or aspirin-type drugs, will tend to impair the immune system still further, and often means that we avoid investigating the underlying cause of the problem.

Fevers

A fever is part of the body's natural defence response to combat disease. A fever is marked by an increase in body temperature; as long as this does not rise too high, it is best to let the fever run its course and allow the body to heal itself. If you are caring for a child whose temperature rises above 40°C (104°F), then get emergency medical advice.

Mild fevers may be treated at home by drinking plenty of fluids, resting in bed and using natural remedies to promote healing and ease any discomfort. Sponging the body with tepid water will usually bring down the temperature effectively. If the fever is very high, or continues to rise despite attempts to bring it down, you should seek professional advice. It is especially important to keep a close watch on children because they can develop convulsions during a very high fever; emergency medical aid must be sought if there seems any likelihood of this occurring.

Herbal infusions can be an effective way of reducing a fever, promoting healing and increasing fluid intake. Consider especially BALM, CHAMOMILE, ECHINACEA, ELDERFLOWER and YARROW.

Essential oil of CHAMOMILE or LAVENDER may be added to tepid water to sponge down the body or applied as a compress to the forehead. The essential oils of CLOVE, EUCALYPTUS and THYME may be diluted in water and sprayed around the room in a plant spray to disinfect it.

The homoeopathic remedies most commonly indicated in the treatment of fever symptoms include ACONITE, ARS ALB, BELLADONNA, CHAMOMILLA, FERRUM PHOS, GELSEMIUM, MERC SOL and PULSATILLA. Compare these in the *Materia Medica* section of this book to find the most suitable, although by far the most common remedy is BELLADONNA and if you try this first you often have to look no further.

Glandular Fever

Glandular fever, also called infective mononucleosis, is caused by a virus, and is most common in teenagers. The symptoms are a very sore throat, fever, swollen lymph glands in the neck and often a general enlargement of the glands. There may be a red rash covering the body.

Glandular fever may drag on for weeks and the patient may feel 'run down' for months afterwards. The disease sometimes recurs after an apparently complete recovery. There is no orthodox cure for glandular fever, and antibiotics should not be given because they cannot kill the virus and they will impair the efforts of the immune system to fight the illness.

In severe cases of glandular fever there may be jaundice, in which case you should seek professional advice.

The herbal treatment for glandular fever in its initial stages will be the same as for fevers *(see page 58)* and sore throats *(see page 165)*. Once the acute symptoms are over, the most important herbs to use to promote healing and recovery will be the alteratives, including CLEAVERS, ECHINACEA and NETTLES. If depression and debility are part of the post-glandular fever picture, then also consider BALM, OATS and SKULLCAP.

Essential oils may be used in massage or in the bath. They will act as anti-microbials and will encourage the immune system to fight off the disease. Consider especially EUCALYPTUS, LAVENDER, NIAOULI, TEA TREE and THYME.

Homoeopathy can be really helpful in bringing a patient back to a full and rapid recovery following glandular fever. These remedies may be indicated in the initial stages or in a more mild attack; if the symptoms have dragged on for a long time you will get the best results by consulting a qualified practitioner. Look the following up in the *Materia Medica* section to see which is the most suitable: APIS, BELLADONNA, CALC PHOS, HEPAR SULPH, LAC CAN, LACHESIS, MERC SOL, PHYTOLACCA, PULSATILLA or SILICEA.

✳ Influenza

Influenza, commonly called 'flu, is an acute infection of the respiratory tract; it is often accompanied by symptoms of feverishness and aching. Different strains of influenza will produce different symptoms, such as sore throats, nausea and coughs, and these should be treated specifically.

Influenza normally lasts between two and five days, but more serious complications may develop, particularly in the elderly. People who do not respond well to home care should be referred to a practitioner. Increasingly, influenza tends to linger, leaving the person feeling debilitated and depressed afterwards. In order to strengthen the attempts of the body to fight off the disease, follow the general advice in the introduction to the immune system on page 6.

A general mixture of herbs to combat 'flu can be made from ELDERFLOWER, PEPPERMINT and YARROW. Add ECHINACEA if your resistance to illness is generally low. Add BALM or SKULLCAP if you feel depressed alongside your other symptoms.

Essential oils may be diluted in vegetable oil and massaged into aching limbs and onto the chest, used in a compress or bath, or the vapours may be inhaled in the form of a steam inhalation. The effect of essential oils will be antimicrobial, decongestant and stimulating to the immune response. Consider especially EUCALYPTUS, LAVENDER, ROSEMARY and TEA TREE. Essential oil of CLOVE may be combined with one or two of the others mentioned and diluted in water to spray around the room to disinfect and freshen it.

The main homoeopathic remedies to consider for 'flu symptoms include ACONITE, ARS ALB, BRYONIA, EUPATORIUM PERF, GELSEMIUM and RHUS TOX.

9

The Immune System

The immune system is the mechanism by which the body protects itself from infection and disease. In fact, several different organs and mechanisms are involved in the immune process.

Micro-organisms such as bacteria, fungi and viruses enter the body continuously, and some live there permanently without doing any harm. But infection will develop when the conditions are right for certain invading organisms to reproduce and multiply within the body. Once a threatening micro-organism enters the body, a chain of events involving a specialized group of cells known collectively as the white blood cells is set in motion. This is known as the immune response. White blood cells are transported by the bloodstream but are found in large numbers in the lymph nodes, spleen, thymus and tissue fluids.

The lymphatic system plays an active role in the immune response by forming some of the white blood cells that manufacture antibodies to suppress the growth and activity of bacteria and viruses. The lymphatic system also filters out and drains the body of bacteria and other unwanted substances. During an infection the activity of the lymphatic system is greatly stimulated, and the accumulation of cells and bacteria may cause the lymph nodes to become enlarged. This is experienced as swelling and possibly tenderness in the neck, armpits and groin. *See also* pages 72–3 for specific recommendations on how to improve the function of the lymphatic system.

The adrenal glands also play an important role in the immune response by secreting hormones that trigger off some of the necessary processes. The vitality of the adrenals is depleted by exhaustion and stress, which is one reason why we have less resistance to illness when we are over-tired or under stress.

In western society, an increasing number of health problems are the result of either an under-active immune system, as with ME or AIDS, or an immune system that has become deranged, as with allergies or rheumatoid arthritis. There are many reasons for this increasing prevalence of immune problems, including an unhealthy diet, exposure to pollution, over-medication and stressful lifestyles. By living in a society that allows pollution of the earth, air and water on a massive scale, we have undermined the health-sustaining capabilities of our environment, and as individuals we are becoming unable to defend ourselves against the levels of toxicity that we have created.

The best that most of us can hope for is an immune system which is effective in eliminating enough of the daily chemicals and pollutants that we are exposed to, to prevent an intolerable level of toxicity from building up in our bodies and causing disease. If the level of toxicity in our system does become too great, we will not be able to maintain a balance of health, our immune system will be unable to cope and illness will result.

In general, factors that tend to impede the body's attempts to eliminate what is not good for it and to increase the strain on the immune system include any foods containing additives, hormones, inorganic fertilizer or pesticide residues; refined sugar; polluted air and water; chemical drugs; vaccinations (for more information on vaccinations *see* page 32 in Children's Illnesses); constipation; smoking; anti-perspirants; and any creams, ointments or lotions that are put onto the skin and contain harsh chemicals or are suppressive. All these things should be avoided as far as possible.

There are some positive steps that we can take to minimize the impact that living in a polluted environment has on our bodies. We can eat fresh food, which is preferably organically produced, drink filtered or bottled spring water, use unleaded petrol, take regular exercise, use natural plant-based cosmetics and toiletries, and use natural remedies. Undertaking a cleansing diet for a period of time can be a good way of livening up the immune system: consult a dietary therapist or naturopath for advice, or follow the cleansing diet on page 423 of this book.

If your immune response is weak and your resistance to illness is low, there are some natural remedies which are known to generally strengthen and tone the immune system and encourage it to eliminate waste products. In herbal medicine these include plants known as adaptogens, such as GINSENG; alteratives, such as BURDOCK, CLEAVERS and RED CLOVER; antimicrobials, such as ECHINACEA, GARLIC, GOLDENSEAL and THYME; and general tonics, such as ELDERBERRIES, NETTLES and ROSEMARY. Certain essential oils are also known to strengthen the immune system: EUCALYPTUS, GINGER, LAVENDER, LEMONGRASS, NIAOULI, ROSEMARY, TEA TREE and THYME.

AIDS

The letters that make up the abbreviation AIDS stand for Acquired Immune Deficiency Syndrome. This indicates the collapse of the body's immune system and hence the body's ability to resist disease. People with AIDS become highly susceptible to a wide variety of infections and various forms of cancer.

Theories about the spread of AIDS are constantly being reviewed, but it is generally believed that it probably develops in those people who have previously contracted HIV (human immuno-deficiency virus). HIV can be transmitted via body fluids such as blood and semen, and it is most commonly contracted through sexual intercourse with an infected partner, from sharing a needle with an infected drug-user or from receiving contaminated blood products.

The virus probably needs to enter the body via the bloodstream to be contracted. This means that sexual intercourse with an infected male partner will not always lead to the woman contracting HIV, but she may do so if there are any small breaks or tears in her skin or the mucous membrane of her vagina. During anal intercourse, penetration frequently does cause a tear in the delicate membrane of the anus or rectum, which is why HIV is more common amongst sexually-active homosexual men. Using a condom during intercourse greatly reduces the risk of contracting HIV during vaginal or anal intercourse.

Not everyone who is known to be HIV positive actually develops AIDS. In order to prevent HIV multiplying and developing into AIDS, the immune system must be in peak condition. AIDS will develop in those people whose resistance to HIV is low, and so the virus can multiply and become destructive to the system as a whole. In order for this to happen the virus needs to invade its host cells, which are the white blood cells known as T-Helper cells. T-Helper cells stimulate and co-ordinate the activity of the other white blood cells active during the immune response mechanism. If these T-Helper cells are invaded and destroyed in large numbers by the virus, the body is unable to resist infection and disease, and AIDS has developed.

Therapists working with people who are HIV positive try to help them to strengthen their immune system. As well as the measures and remedies discussed in the introduction to the immune system on pages 61–2, many therapists of natural medicine have developed treatments which are particularly appropriate for people with HIV. Therapies that are popular, and have had notably good results, include herbalism, homoeopathy, nutritional therapy and naturopathy. Some people have found that creative visualization is greatly beneficial too, often in conjunction with other more physically-oriented therapies like herbalism or homoeopathy. Most counsellors or therapists will be able to guide you through an appropriate creative visualization programme.

The herbs and essential oils that are useful for treating people with HIV are those known as adaptogens, alteratives and tonics, for example BALM, BURDOCK, CLEAVERS, ECHINACEA, GARLIC, GINGER, GINSENG, GOLDENSEAL, LIQUORICE, NIAOULI (OIL), ROSEMARY and THYME (HERB AND OIL).

Once AIDS has developed, any treatment needs to be twofold: that is, it needs to attempt to rejuvenate the immune system while also treating symptoms of infection and disease as they arise. These symptoms are sometimes known as ARC (aids-related complex). Remedies to consider in addition to those mentioned above are those that combine the properties of strengthening the immune system with a marked antimicrobial effect: BERGAMOT OIL, EUCALYPTUS OIL, LAVENDER OIL, MYRRH, NIAOULI OIL, TEA TREE OIL and WILD INDIGO, for example. Obviously professional help will be required to maximize the potential of using these remedies.

Allergies

Our bodies react to the presence of foreign substances by bringing the immune response into action: this is the process designed to neutralize, kill and expel the invading substance. Part of the immune response involves the production of antibodies, which help to kill invading bacteria and assist the white blood cells in their job of removing any dead and dying foreign substances. The body remembers the particular substance (antigen) that produced those antibodies, and introduction of the same substance in the future can provoke a much quicker response to even a tiny amount of the antigen.

This process can sometimes become over-active, causing, in a susceptible person, an allergic reaction to a wide range of foreign protein substances. The reason for this is that a process similar to the antibody-antigen reaction is set off not only in the bloodstream, but also on the surface of the body cells. This antibody-allergen reaction damages the cell walls and liberates a substance known as histamine. Histamine produces two main effects: it allows the fluid part of the blood or serum to leak into tissues which results in swelling, blisters and irritation of the skin and mucous membranes; and it can bring about a spasm of the bronchial muscle, resulting in asthma attacks.

There is often a hereditary component to allergic sensitivity, particularly with what are known as the 'atopic' diseases – asthma, eczema and hayfever. Stress is also known to play a significant role in predisposing people to allergic reactions. The number of people suffering from allergies has increased enormously in recent years, and is particularly noticeable amongst children. This is because our immune systems are being undermined by over-medication and over-vaccination, and the proliferation of chemical pollutants and additives in food, air and water.

The term 'allergy' is now often used to describe reactions other than those caused directly by histamine production (such as itching, a runny nose, urticaria, wheezing and so on). These more recently recognized conditions have become known as 'sub-clinical' allergies, and include such symptoms as catarrh, cystitis, hyperactivity in children, migraine and a variety of skin disorders. It is increasingly acknowledged by people working in health care that certain foods and food additives are connected to these sub-clinical allergies. Special rotational diets, eliminating suspect foods for a week or more at a time, have been developed to try and establish which food substances are causing a particular problem. For more information, contact the relevant self-help group from the list of contacts on page 429.

While it can be useful to avoid specific allergens, such as milk or wheat, for a time, to give the body a chance to heal itself, the long-term aim of natural medicine must be to cure the individual, so that she or he no longer suffers from allergies. If you suffer from allergies, your immune system is no longer functioning smoothly and you will need to follow the general advice given in the introductory section to this section on pages 61–2. There are also a number of natural remedies that are particularly useful in the treatment of allergies. Herbs to consider are BALM, CHAMOMILE, ECHINACEA, ELDERFLOWER, EYEBRIGHT, LIQUORICE, RED CLOVER and YARROW. The most important essential oils are: CHAMOMILE, LAVENDER, MELISSA and YARROW. The homoeopathic remedies for first aid treatment of allergies, include APIS, ARSENICUM, RHUS TOX and URTICA. For constitutional treatment to cure the tendency to allergic reaction, you should consult a qualified herbalist or homoeopath.

See also Asthma on page 161, Eczema on page 169, Hayfever on page 163 and Urticaria page 172.

❋ ME or CFS

Myalgic encephalomyelitis (ME) is also called chronic fatigue syndrome (CFS), especially in the USA. The exact cause is not known, although the symptoms usually follow a viral infection such as 'flu or glandular fever. Instead of the usual recovery following the acute fever episode, the debility lingers and becomes ME. It is thought that the healthy function of the immune system somehow becomes impaired by the viral episode and begins to attack its own antibodies.

According to the Chronic Fatigue Syndrome Society, there is evidence that one potential trigger for ME is vaccination, particularly those immunizations against tetanus and hepatitis B. They strongly advise against these vaccinations for those who already have ME and also advise against any vaccination at the same time as you have an inflammatory illness such as 'flu.

An exact diagnosis of ME can be difficult because although specific viral elements are present in some people, they are not always detectable. This is one reason why the disease took a long time to become recognized by the orthodox medical profession. Diagnosis is usually based on an elevated antibody level plus the presence of several of the following symptoms: extreme fatigue, muscular pain, muscular weakness following exertion, recurrent sore throats, poor concentration, lymph node swelling, depression, headaches and digestive discomfort.

ME may typically last from several months to several years, and successful treatment programmes will need to include dietary and lifestyle changes, natural remedies and psychological support. There is no one magic remedy for ME and we would recommend that you seek advice from a qualified practitioner, but the following suggestions may be considered as part of an overall approach.

The first step must be to ensure that the body is able to eliminate any built-up toxins effectively and so support your vitality. A cleansing diet may be a good start. Also consider taking cleansing and liver-supporting herbs such as CLEAVERS, GOLDENSEAL, MILK THISTLE, POKE ROOT and WORMWOOD. Visiting a naturopath or herbalist can be very helpful. Avoiding all stimulants, caffeine, alcohol, refined foods and sugar and eating a wholefood, nutritious diet are essential.

To enable the body to heal itself it will be necessary to get sufficient rest. Most people with ME need to take time out from study or work commitments before recovery starts. Indeed, in many young people it seems to be a high pressure, 'rushing about' lifestyle that predisposes them to ME, hence one of its other names, 'yuppie 'flu'. In any case, slowing down and taking stock of real priorities in life may well be a necessary part of the healing process.

Following a detox, remedies to enhance the immune system and antivirals will be useful. Appropriate herbs include ASTRAGALUS, ECHINACEA, GARLIC and GINSENG. Other supplements that have proved useful are EVENING PRIMROSE OIL and SHITAKE MUSHROOMS. Essential oils that combine immuno-stimulant and antiviral properties include NIAOULI, TEA TREE and THYME. Regular aromatherapy massage can be very helpful for people with ME. Compare all the above remedies in the *Materia Medica* section to check how appropriate they are for you.

Food supplements that have proven especially helpful in the treatment of ME include BETA CAROTENE, B VITAMINS, VITAMIN C and ZINC. A good-quality multi-vitamin and mineral supplement may be a useful way to enhance your diet. Research also shows that probiotics can assist in recovery from ME. Supplements containing the probiotics acidophilus and bifidobacterium can be purchased from a good health food shop.

The Liver and Gall Bladder

The liver is the largest organ in the body and it carries out many important functions. It produces bile that is needed to emulsify fats; it stores glucose in the form of glycogen, which is one of the most important stores of energy in the body; it is needed for the metabolism of protein; it is active in the formation and storage of several vitamins; and it detoxifies the body of drugs and poisons. The liver also deactivates and eliminates a number of hormones when they are no longer needed, including oestrogen. A lot of women's hormonal problems, including breast tenderness, PMT, menopausal symptoms, etc., may be caused by the fact that the liver is not able to break down excess oestrogen efficiently.

The variety of these vital functions shows how important it is to have a healthy liver. Most people have experienced the effects of the liver working under pressure after a few drinks too many: the symptoms of a hangover (irritability, nausea, headache) all come on as it struggles to rid the system of the toxic effects of alcohol. These days, most livers are under even more strain as they detoxify and process the increasing quantity of chemicals and additives in modern foods.

A diet that is good for your liver includes plenty of fresh fruit and vegetables, preferably organically grown, whole cereals, such as brown rice, and proteins that are low in fat, such as white fish and chicken. Greasy and fatty foods should be avoided and so should foods which contain additives such as preservatives, flavour enhancers and colouring. Alcohol is particularly damaging to the liver and should not be taken by anyone with liver problems. Coffee is also bad.

Most cleansing diets are concerned with assisting the liver in the detoxification process; any dietary therapist or naturopath will be able to guide you through such a regime. Alternatively, follow the cleansing programme on page

423. Spring is a traditional time to undergo a liver cleansing diet, after the excesses of Christmas and the stodgy foods of winter.

There are several herbs that are considered liver tonics; these may be taken during a cleansing diet or when the liver is feeling sluggish. We recommend especially BARBERRY, DANDELION, MILK THISTLE, VERVAIN, WILD YAM and YELLOW DOCK. The most important essential oil to strengthen and cleanse the liver is ROSEMARY. Other oils that may be helpful and should be looked up in the *Materia Medica* section are CHAMOMILE, CYPRESS, GRAPEFRUIT, JUNIPER, LEMON and ORANGE.

The gall bladder is a pear-shaped sac attached to the liver. It acts as a reservoir for bile. Bile is used to break down large globules of fat into tiny globules so that they can be absorbed in the duodenum. Any diet prescribed for a condition of the gall bladder will involve cutting out fat.

Jaundice is the term given to the yellow discolouration of the skin and whites of the eyes caused by an excess of bile pigment in the bloodstream. This yellowness is a very common and marked sign of most diseases of the liver and gall bladder. Jaundice is a symptom rather than a disease – it is the underlying cause that needs to be treated and then the jaundice will clear.

In Chinese medicine the liver and gall bladder are known as the seat of anger. Anger causes certain tensions and also glandular secretions in the body that may in turn have an undesirable effect on the liver. Likewise, people often feel irritable and grumpy when they suffer from liver disorders. It may be that a two-way link develops between the emotions and the physical symptoms. It is worth considering whether people who develop liver disease are angry types, or if they have suffered a lot of frustration or suppressed anger in their lives. If this is the case, then as well as addressing the liver physically, a cure is going to be more permanent if these tendencies are also examined and dealt with as part of the treatment.

Gall-Bladder Inflammation

Inflammation of the gall bladder (cholecystitis) can be acute or chronic. It causes severe pain in the upper part of the abdomen under the ribs. This pain can radiate through to the back and be felt under the right shoulder-blade and even in the tip of the right shoulder. Nausea and vomiting can accompany the bouts of pain. The attack may come on after a long period during which you have experienced much indigestion and wind.

This condition appears more often in women than in men, and recurring attacks are usually treated by removing the gall bladder. This is a shame because the condition can often be successfully treated by natural medicine. It is much more common in women who have been on the birth control pill.

During an acute attack you should stay away from fats in your diet. The homoeopathic remedy MAG PHOS may be taken as often as you need to relieve the pain, or you can massage the diluted essential oils of LAVENDER and ROSEMARY over the painful area. Recurring attacks need to be cured with careful treatment by an experienced practitioner of natural medicine – a naturopath, herbalist, homoeopath or acupuncturist. A general herbal mixture that will relieve the pain and reduce the inflammation can be made from: BARBERRY, DANDELION LEAVES, MARSHMALLOW ROOT and MILK THISTLE. If infection is present add ECHINACEA.

Gallstones

Gallstones form when deposits from the bile concentrate in the gall bladder. They may consist of cholesterol or bile pigment, and sometimes calcium as well.

Many gallstones are 'silent' and there are no symptoms, or there may be flatulence, a feeling of fullness after meals and a sense of discomfort after fatty food. If a stone enters the bile duct it causes biliary colic; a severe colicky pain in the right upper abdomen which may make the sufferer roll about in agony.

Gallstones are more common in women than in men, and most common in women who are overweight. You should always reassess your diet if you have gallstones, and animal fats in particular should be excluded. Small stones may enter the duodenum and be passed with a bowel motion. A large stone may obstruct the bile duct and result in jaundice. This will require medical intervention.

It is well worth consulting a natural therapist to treat gallstones before resorting to the surgical removal of the gall bladder. For the acute pain of an attack, take the homoeopathic remedy MAG PHOS, although if you want to get rid of the stones and reduce inflammation permanently you must consult a qualified practitioner. The acute pain will also be relieved by massaging the diluted essential oils of LAVENDER and ROSEMARY over the area. Try the following herbal mixture to dissolve the stones, although this will need to be taken for some months to achieve a result: DANDELION LEAVES, MILK THISTLE and

STONE ROOT. Add CRAMPBARK for acute colicky pains. Check all these remedies in the *Materia Medica* section of this book to see if they are particularly suitable for you.

Hepatitis

Hepatitis is a term that is usually applied to an acute inflammation of the liver caused by a virus infection. Two main strains of virus have been identified: virus A and virus B (serum hepatitis), although hepatitis C is also now on the increase.

The symptoms of hepatitis are a marked loss of appetite, nausea at the sight of food, especially fats, and feeling off-colour generally. After a few days of these symptoms the urine becomes dark, owing to the presence of bile, and the bowel motions become pale. The yellow skin and eyes of jaundice will also become evident.

General treatment includes bedrest and a light, low-fat diet. You should not drink alcohol for some months after your recovery. Most people suffering from hepatitis get a mild attack, but in a small number of cases the attacks are severe, with a high fever. If you suspect that you have hepatitis you should consult a medical practitioner for a diagnosis and to assess the impact of the disease on your liver.

The majority of hepatitis sufferers make a complete recovery with no permanent damage to their liver. However, it can take several months to feel totally fit again, and it is not uncommon to feel low and depressed for some time following an acute attack. If this is the case, consult an alternative practitioner such as a herbalist, homoeopath or acupuncturist. Some of the general liver tonics mentioned on pages 68–9 will also assist recovery.

The Lymphatic System

The lymphatic system moves lymphatic fluids around the body through the action of muscles and the lungs via a one-way valve system, collecting waste products and toxins as it goes, and disposing of them through the bladder, bowels, lungs and skin. The lymphatic vessels are spread as a network throughout the body, but they are particularly concentrated in the groin, behind the knees, in the armpits, neck and upper chest.

Lymph fluid is involved in the absorption of fats from the intestines, as well as in the drainage and removal of toxic wastes from the body. Lymph fluid is also a reservoir for certain kinds of white blood cells that attack and ingest chemical and bacterial invaders, and clean out waste.

This system is one of the most important methods the body has of detoxifying itself and it is also a vital part of the immune response. If the lymphatic system is not functioning properly, a very wide range of illnesses can develop. General symptoms of the lymph system not working effectively include a tendency to oedema (swelling), swollen glands, a susceptibility to infections and viruses, recurrent tonsillitis or sore throats, and a tendency to constipation. The function of the lymphatic system will often remain impaired following a bout of glandular fever.

Regular exercise is necessary to maintain a healthy lymphatic system because vigorous motion stimulates the dumping of wastes, and the flow of lymphatic fluid. Skin brushing is also considered to be an effective way of moving the lymph fluid and freeing any impacted lymph mucus from the nodes. Use a brush made from natural fibres and brush towards the lymph nodes (up the arms and legs and inwards on the chest) in long, sweeping strokes. For best results, brush on dry skin for at least five minutes each morning. Skin brushing is particularly good for getting rid of cellulite.

A cleansing diet can be very effective for toning and clearing the lymphatic system. Consult a dietary therapist or naturopath for advice, or follow the cleansing diet on page 423. Foods that should be avoided are red meat, fatty food, dairy products, coffee, vinegar, alcohol, refined sugar and all artificial additives. All drugs, whether recreational or non-essential prescribed ones, should be avoided, as the lymphatic system has to clear chemicals and toxic residues out of the system.

Foods that are beneficial include fresh fruit and green vegetables, preferably organically grown. Also, drink filtered or bottled mineral water, as the lymphatic system has to struggle to remove the chemicals and metals that are present in high levels in our tap water from the body.

There are known to be some effective lymphatic cleansers amongst herbal remedies, including CLEAVERS, ECHINACEA, GOLDENSEAL, MARIGOLD, NETTLES and RED CLOVER. Consult the *Materia Medica* section to see which of these is most appropriate for you. Massage therapists have developed a specialized form of massage known as 'lymphatic drainage', and this can be particularly effective when essential oils are also used. The essential oils renowned for clearing the lymphatic system include FENNEL, GERANIUM, JUNIPER, LAVENDER, LEMON and ROSEMARY. You could also consider the homoeopathic tissue salt KALI MUR for symptoms resulting from a poorly functioning lymphatic system.

12

The Muscular and Skeletal System

The muscular and skeletal system allows us to stand upright, keep our shape and move around. It is a truly wonderful achievement of natural engineering. The key to the muscular and skeletal system lies in the balance between structure (rigidity) and flexibility (fluidity). It will stay healthy if we look after ourselves, avoid strain and injury where possible, eat a good diet, take moderate but not excessive amounts of exercise, know how to relax and let go of stress, and have a reasonable posture.

Emotional stress will affect our posture and well-being as much as physical abuse, and joint problems are particularly affected by unexpressed anger and prolonged feelings of guilt. Learning to express feelings of anger and aggression, rather than suppressing them so that they turn inwards, is an important part of the healing process for anyone with joint problems (and this is indeed a challenging task for many women).

Most problems that involve the muscular and skeletal system develop for a period of years before they result in physical symptoms. Diseases of the bones and joints are the end result of a combination of physical, emotional, dietary, hereditary and environmental factors. Helping yourself to unravel these various factors and to reverse the degenerative process into a process of healing will also take time, and a considerable commitment towards improving your health. Natural remedies will only be successful if they are part of an integrated approach aimed at healing the whole person.

Generally, people who suffer from muscular or bone and joint problems benefit from a diet based on wholefoods and plenty of fresh vegetables. You could try a detoxification diet for a limited period of time to help the body reverse the degenerative process: consult a naturopath or dietary therapist for advice, or follow the suggested cleansing diet on page 423. Many different therapies have played a part in helping to cure chronic diseases of the muscular

The Muscular and Skeletal System

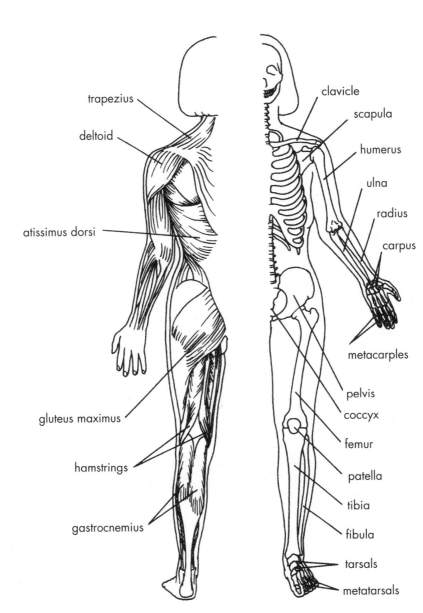

trapezius

deltoid

atissimus dorsi

gluteus maximus

hamstrings

gastrocnemius

clavicle

scapula

humerus

ulna

radius

carpus

metacarples

pelvis

coccyx

femur

patella

tibia

fibula

tarsals

metatarsals

and skeletal system, including acupuncture, homoeopathy, herbalism and naturopathy. Visiting a therapist who can also help you to understand the physical and psychological patterns underlying your disease may be the best way to get relief.

❧ Arthritis and Rheumatism

Rheumatism is an inflammation of the connective tissues covering the muscles and tendons; it is sometimes called myalgia, fibrositis and lumbago. The muscles in the affected area tighten as a defensive reaction and when this happens the nearby joint may become deformed. Once a joint becomes inflamed or painful, the condition is called arthritis; and thus the various forms of rheumatism and arthritis tend to overlap and become confused.

Although defining the exact type of rheumatism or arthritis that you have can be interesting, it isn't usually vital in terms of being helped by natural remedies. It will be more useful if you try and unravel the various factors in your particular lifestyle that are contributing towards your disease. Factors that need to be investigated include your diet, your genetic inheritance, physical stress or injury, environmental influences and your emotional patterns. While we can suggest some ideas and remedies here that will probably be of some help, to reverse a chronic degenerative process caused by arthritis or rheumatism you will probably need to try to improve your health on every level over a long period of time, and you may need professional help to unravel the underlying causes.

On a psychological level, joint problems are often the result of friction in your relationships with other people that is being ignored or suppressed rather than actively dealt with. Ignoring problems in personal relationships does not tend to make those problems go away, instead it leads to a build-up of anger, resentment and guilt. If these tendencies are not expressed they are carried around in our emotions, and eventually they can poison the whole person, including the physical body. Holding on to negative emotions causes a lack of flexibility, stiffness and pain.

Many women feel very guilty about feeling such so-called 'negative' emotions as anger, aggression and resentment. Guilt can lead to great restlessness and a tendency to overdo things to compensate; this overexertion may place a further strain on the muscular and skeletal system. If you recognize this pattern in your own life at all, it is worth considering some form of counselling or psychotherapy, or at least try talking about it to your natural therapist, so that you can work on trying to reverse the trends.

Changes in your diet can also be an important part of healing rheumatic and arthritic problems. An unhealthy diet will tend to lead to a build-up of toxins and waste products in the system. If the body cannot eliminate these waste products effectively, they may well be dumped in the joints, causing irritation, inflammation and pain. The foods that should be avoided are those that trigger an acidic reaction in the body, including red meat, dairy products, vinegar, wine, most spices, oranges, refined carbohydrates and refined sugar. Coffee, strong tea and salt should also be avoided, as they tend to add to the accumulation of toxins in the body.

Sticking to a cleansing diet for a limited period of time can be a great help, particularly if you use it to kick off a concerted effort to improve your general diet. Consult a naturopath or dietary therapist for advice on cleansing diets, or follow the one on page 423. Fresh, organically-grown vegetables, both raw and cooked, fruit (other than tomatoes and oranges) and brown rice are particularly good if you suffer from rheumatism or arthritis. Fish and white meat may usually be safely eaten. Try drinking plenty of mineral water (particularly the low-sodium varieties) and a drink made from a teaspoon of cider vinegar and a teaspoon of honey in a cup of hot water, taken every morning, helps many sufferers.

Food supplements that have been found to help people who suffer with arthritis are COD LIVER OIL capsules and EVENING PRIMROSE OIL capsules. Herbs that may be taken to heal rheumatism and arthritis include CELERY SEED, FEVERFEW, MEADOWSWEET and WHITE WILLOW. Look these up in the *Materia Medica* section of this book and make a mixture of the ones that look particularly appropriate in your case. A poultice to apply to the affected joints may be made from CAYENNE and SLIPPERY ELM.

To find a homoeopathic remedy to relieve symptoms of arthritis or rheumatism, compare APIS, ARNICA, BRYONIA, LEDUM, NAT PHOS and RHUS TOX. If the remedy only helps a little then it probably means that you require constitutional treatment by a qualified practitioner.

Essential oils help rheumatism and arthritis in a variety of ways. Detoxifying oils such as CYPRESS, JUNIPER and LEMON can be used in the bath and for massage to help the body to eliminate poisons from the joints and out of the body altogether. Anti-inflammatory and pain-relieving oils such as CHAMOMILE, LAVENDER and ROSEMARY may be used for local massage or compresses. Rubbing oils can be used to improve circulation in the area and relieve stiffness, try a combination of BENZOIN, BLACK PEPPER, EUCALYPTUS and MARJORAM, diluted in a vegetable-oil base.

Backache

Back pain is one of the most common ailments referred to medical practitioners. Its causes are very varied and the best method of treatment will vary accordingly. Pain caused by tensions arising out of bad posture can respond very well to the Alexander Technique. If the vertebrae or pelvis is out of alignment, then a manipulative therapy such as chiropractic or osteopathy can be of great help.

The most common cause of backache is overstraining or injury. In this situation, the remedies suggested here may well relieve the pain. If the problem does not clear up quickly, then consult an osteopath, chiropracter or other therapist of natural medicine. If the problem keeps coming back, then you will need to redress the physical weakness and look at any underlying pattern of stress that is contributing to the back symptoms.

Pain in the back at waist-level may be due to spinal disorders or kidney and bladder problems (toxins that should be eliminated by the kidneys and bladder can be deposited in surrounding tissue, causing inflammation and discomfort). In many women's cases, low-back pain can be caused by disorders of the reproductive organs. If there is any doubt about the cause of your back pain it is vital to get a diagnosis to rule out any serious causative factor.

One of the most pleasant ways to relieve backache is a massage with essential oils. The most effective essential oils for relieving pain due to fatigue or tension are GINGER, JUNIPER, LAVENDER, MARJORAM, PINE and ROSEMARY. Any one of these may be diluted in a massage-base oil and rubbed into the back, or a few drops may be added to a warm bath. You can rub macerated herbal oils into the back to relieve pain; the most useful will be made from COMFREY or ST JOHN'S WORT. Herbs may also be taken internally to reduce inflammation and relieve pain; try a combination of ST JOHN'S WORT, VALERIAN and WHITE WILLOW. The homoeopathic remedies that should be compared to find the most suitable one for you include ARNICA, BRYONIA, HYPERICUM and RHUS TOX.

Osteoporosis

Osteoporosis literally means 'porous bones', and it occurs when the mass of the bones becomes reduced. Bone tissue is constantly being worn out, resorbed into the bloodstream and excreted, and replaced by newly-formed bone. Usually bone mass reaches its peak when we are in our early thirties; thereafter there is a tendency for more bone tissue to be lost than replaced. As the density of the bones decreases, they become fragile and brittle, and break more easily.

A decrease in bone mass is part of the general ageing process but it tends to occur earlier in women than in men, although by about the age of 80 men have caught up. Osteoporosis occurs earlier in women partly because our bones tend to be less dense to begin with, because we exercise less than men (and exercise significantly slows down bone loss), and because the body is less able to absorb calcium from the diet and assimilate it into bones, as a result of the decline in the hormone oestrogen after menopause.

Advanced osteoporosis can lead to hip, forearm and wrist fractures, backache and loss of height (due to the vertebrae in the spine collapsing). The orthodox management of osteoporosis in women includes hormone replacement therapy (HRT) which boosts oestrogen levels and keeps the bones absorbing calcium. However, HRT does not cure osteoporosis, it merely delays it for as long as the medication is taken, and there are other risks associated with taking it *(see page 141)*.

The two most important things that we can do for ourselves to prevent osteoporosis is to take regular exercise and have a good diet. Exercising will actually slow down bone loss, but this has to be built into our lifestyle before the problem has had a chance to develop. We need to have an adequate supply of calcium in what we eat. Foods rich in calcium include dairy products, fish (especially sardines), watercress, soya bean flour, Brewer's yeast, eggs, nuts, sunflower and sesame seeds, chickpeas and lentils.

There is not much point in taking calcium supplements unless you eat a poor diet because it is the body's inability to use calcium properly that is the important factor. The homoeopathic tissue salt CALC PHOS may be taken from time to time to encourage the body to assimilate calcium well. Excessive amounts of phosphorous in the diet tend to disrupt the body's ability to use calcium, and foods which are particularly rich in phosphorous include red meat, fizzy drinks and many processed foods. Drinking coffee will also reduce bone density and should be avoided.

Nutritious herbs that encourage the assimilation of calcium and are beneficial for women prone to osteoporosis include ALFALFA, COMFREY LEAF and NETTLES.

If you have already developed osteoporosis it would help you to visit a practitioner of natural medicine who should be able to encourage your body to take in calcium more effectively. We particularly recommend that you visit either a herbalist or homoeopath so that she or he can deal with this problem properly.

13

The Nervous System

The nervous system is made up of the brain, the spinal cord and the nerves and sensory receptors distributed throughout the body. It is one of the great communication and transport systems of the body (the others are the bloodstream and the lymphatic system); in diagrams it looks rather like a tree, with smaller and smaller branches departing from a larger central trunk.

The nervous system is the link between mind and body. This link operates in two ways: physical experiences are conveyed via the nervous system to the brain, where they are registered or translated into information and experience; the reverse flow occurs when either there is an automatic response or the will to act is transmitted from the brain to the body via the nervous system. For this system to remain healthy there needs to be a balance between the ingoing tendency and the outgoing tendency – between the receptive and active sides of our nature.

A disease, such as sciatica or shingles, may seem to rise directly out of the physical components of the nervous system, or it may appear to arise from the realm of the mind, as anxiety and depression seem to. The truth is that here, more than in any other of the body's systems, the distinction between the physical and the psychological is always complex, and usually it is only partially understood. Most ailments associated with the physical nervous system will have an effect on the mind of the sufferer. For example, shingles is often accompanied by depression, and many so-called psychological disorders will result in physical complaints, just as stress causes migraine attacks.

If you suffer from a problem of the nervous system, you must be prepared to examine and work towards healing on every level – physical, emotional and mental – in order to bring about a cure. You need to reassess the amount of stress you live with at home and at work. You need to consider your ability to communicate thoughts and feelings, and also your capacity for putting ideas into action.

The Nervous System

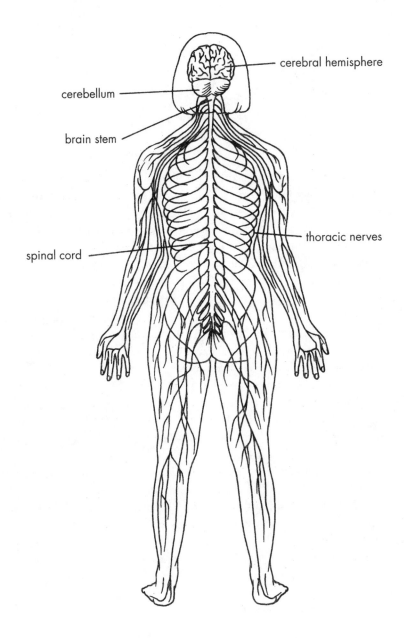

cerebral hemisphere

cerebellum

brain stem

thoracic nerves

spinal cord

For many people, modern life is stressful, and the barrage of stimuli and information that our nervous systems have to contend with is astounding (just think of the number of hours many people spend watching television). Driving a car, operating a computer or switchboard, even crossing a busy road, all require considerable powers of concentration and co-ordination. This creates extra stress for our nervous systems and increased stress may be one reason why people have suffered more from various diseases of the nervous system in recent years. A positive aspect of increased stress may be that all this stimulation is enlarging the capacity of this system (this is particularly noticeable in children), and this is one way that humanity may be continuing to evolve.

A fascinating book by Peter Fraser, *The Aids Miasm: Contemporary Disease and the New Remedies,* links the revolution of the communications age with the development of new nervous and immune system diseases such as AIDS, CJD and Alzheimer's. He also suggests that we may need a new range of natural medicines to treat these diseases. He discusses new homoeopathic remedies, but we can also see the massive rise in popularity of such nervous system herbs as GINKGO and ST JOHN'S WORT as indicative of an increasing emphasis on the nervous system.

Addiction

Addiction occurs when we allow our inner or spiritual purpose to be satisfied on a desire level. The impulse to search for purpose, love, fulfilment and creative expression is an ongoing process in everyone's life; if we allow this search to become a craving for a substance, object or particular way of being, for example power, sex, money, alcohol, drugs, cigarettes or food, then we are in danger of becoming addicted. None of these things will be ultimately satisfying because they are all only substitutes for the thing we really crave or seek.

Breaking an addiction, like breaking any habit, is extremely difficult because we have to confront the empty space in our life that we were attempting to fill with whatever we were addicted to. Every time that we feel dissatisfied or unfulfilled, we will automatically crave the same thing. In addition, most addictive substances contain chemical compounds that alter the body's biochemistry, and removing the substance will create a reaction that is uncomfortable, and at times dangerous.

It is a great challenge in life to break an addiction, and success brings benefits in terms of both an improvement in your health and self-esteem. It will always be a lonely task because it is only you that can put in the effort and only you that can reap the rewards, although the support of family and friends should always be gratefully received, and they no doubt will also enjoy your increased well-being. Self-help groups, like those for alcoholism, can provide a supportive environment to communicate feelings and to share ways of dealing with the difficulties that arise. Counselling and psychotherapy can also help us to understand and deal with the patterns that are underlying the addiction.

Breaking an addiction successfully depends on your will to succeed. The need to be free from the offending substance has to be greater than your desire for it. Once you have made the decision to break the addiction, and if you have the necessary support available, there are natural remedies that can help. These strengthen the nervous system and have an uplifting effect, supporting the body as it clears out the residual toxins. Acupuncture treatment has been shown to be particularly successful in treating certain forms of addiction, especially for alcohol, smoking and recreational drugs. The following suggestions may be used to support professional help, but they are not meant to replace it.

Amongst the herbal remedies used for treating addictions, the most useful is OATS, which is a nervine and is also said to help strengthen the will. HOPS, SKULLCAP and VALERIAN all calm the nervous system and can help to overcome the initial reactions to coming off an addictive substance. ANGELICA ROOT is said to create a distaste for alcohol. If alcoholism is associated with suspected liver problems then read the section on the liver and gall bladder on pages 68–7. A combination of COLTSFOOT and PLANTAIN may be taken to help strengthen and clear out the respiratory system after giving up smoking. ROSEMARY generally strengthens the nerves physically, and can be combined with BALM and SKULLCAP to calm the mind and lift depression. CRAMPBARK helps nervous tension and anxiety.

It will probably be necessary to have constitutional treatment for homoeopathy to be successful. However, many people have found that taking NUX VOMICA in low potency helps them to give up smoking. KALI PHOS is also a useful homoeopathic remedy for strengthening the nervous system and it is particularly useful to take each night if you are trying to come off tranquillizers for sleeping problems.

The Bach FIVE FLOWER REMEDY can be very helpful for the underlying emotional causes of addiction. Consult the chart on pages 199–206 and make up a mixture of the most appropriate ones.

All the antidepressant essential oils can help in breaking addiction, with BERGAMOT, CHAMOMILE, CLARY SAGE, JASMINE, ROSE and YLANG-YLANG being among the most useful. Detoxifying oils such as FENNEL and JUNIPER can also be helpful with clearing the toxic residues out of the body.

Use essential oils for massage or in the bath. But you will get the most benefit by visiting an aromatherapist for massage treatment combined with counselling and support.

Anxiety

All of us have experienced feelings of anxiety at certain times during our life, often as a response to stressful events such as exams, an illness or concern for a member of our family. If the anxiety becomes long term, remaining beyond a particular event, then some form of counselling may be necessary to help you break the habit that anxiety can become.

The symptoms of anxiety include feelings of uneasiness, apprehension and tension, and sometimes feelings of panic may also develop. You may experience tight breathing, palpitations, nausea, diarrhoea, perspiration and disturbed sleep. Continued anxiety may well result in physical disease, such as digestive disorders, headaches, backache or high blood pressure.

Tranquillizers and antidepressants are often prescribed for the orthodox treatment of anxiety. This is counterproductive because they rarely help in the long run. Drugs certainly don't cure the cause of the anxiety and, at best, they simply mask some of the symptoms; at worst, coming off the medication often aggravates all the initial symptoms, making it very difficult.

The following natural remedies will help to strengthen the nervous system and relieve the symptoms of anxiety, but if they are persistent you should seek constitutional treatment by a qualified practitioner. Curing anxiety should involve developing an understanding of the symptoms, redirecting the fears involved, strengthening the nervous system and dealing with any other contributory factors.

First, look at your diet to make certain that it contains sufficient sources of calcium, magnesium and vitamins B and C (consult the tables on pages 424–26 for rich food sources of these vitamins and minerals). Herbs that can be used to treat anxiety include BALM, CHAMOMILE, HOPS, LIMEFLOWERS, MOTHERWORT, OATS, ORANGE BLOSSOM, PASSIFLORA, SKULLCAP and VERVAIN. Consult the *Materia Medica* to see which herbs are the best indicated for you, and then make a mixture of the most suitable ones.

For chronic anxiety to be treated successfully by homoeopathy, constitutional treatment by a qualified practitioner is necessary. For more transient symptoms, the following homoeopathic remedies may be considered: ACONITE, ARG NIT, ARSENICUM, GELSEMIUM, IGNATIA, KALI PHOS and PHOSPHORUS. Bach flower remedies can be a very helpful way of treating anxiety – consult the table on pages 199–206 and make a mixture of the most suitable.

The essential oils that are most useful for treating anxiety include BASIL, CLARY SAGE, GERANIUM, LAVENDER, MELISSA, NEROLI and ROSE. You will probably get most benefit from visiting an aromatherapist and having a regular consultation and massage. Any of the oils may be diluted in a vegetable-oil base and used in massage, or add a couple of drops of the oil of your choice to a warm bath.

Depression

The word 'depression' means 'to be pushed down', and there are times when all of us have felt like this – 'low' and unhappy with ourselves and with life. Depression can develop after a stressful event like losing your job, a bereavement or housing difficulties, or it can be brought on by a physical condition such as an illness or from taking drugs. For some people, depression is chronic and it is a pattern that affects their whole life, and the immediate cause is not easily identified.

Symptoms of depression include an inability to feel pleasure, loss of appetite, sleep disturbances, fatigue, anxiety, poor libido, pessimism, thoughts of death, feelings of hopelessness and low self-esteem. The orthodox treatment of depression is to prescribe antidepressant drugs. This is counterproductive because the drugs don't cure the depression or help you to come to an understanding of it. Furthermore, it can be extremely difficult to stop taking the drugs because all the symptoms they have masked will reassert themselves.

Although there are many natural remedies that can help to relieve depression, no single remedy, in isolation, will cure it, because overcoming it is a learning process. Much depression springs from an attitude that is common in our society in which we tend to lose touch with our purpose for existence and our inner sense of creativity and self-esteem.

Difficult circumstances and various incidents may be the trigger for depression, but we only become its victim when we are unable to communicate our inner needs and feelings, and we are out of touch with our initial emotional impulses. Failure or inability to recognize and express these early primary emotions leads to suppression; this develops into a confusion and complication of emotions and we lose touch with our sense of self-worth and purpose. We call this depression.

A consultation with a practitioner of natural medicine, psychotherapist or counsellor may well be one of the steps necessary to help an individual investigate and come to terms with the life patterns that are contributing to his or her depression. A professional practitioner should assess the severity of the depression, particularly if it is persistent or if the depressed person is suicidal. Severe depression may need more intensive intervention, possibly including 24-hour care under professional supervision.

Mild symptoms of depression may be relieved by questioning yourself about what is going on and by treating yourself with natural remedies (such as those mentioned here) to strengthen the nervous system and relieve some of the more distressing symptoms.

The best antidepressant and nervine herbs include BALM, BORAGE, DAMIANA, LIMEFLOWERS, OATS, ROSEMARY, SKULLCAP, ST JOHN'S WORT and VERVAIN. Make a mixture of the most suitable herbs after looking them up in the *Materia Medica* section of this book.

There are many homoeopathic remedies that can be used to treat depression, but because the particular symptoms tend to be so individual, a visit to a qualified practitioner may be necessary to find the remedy or remedies that will be of most value to you. You may find it interesting to look up the following remedies in the *Materia Medica* and then try one if it appears to be particularly appropriate: AURUM, IGNATIA, NATRUM MUR, SEPIA and STAPHYSAGRIA.

The Bach flower remedies or Bach flower essences can be very helpful in the treatment of depression. Consult the list on pages 199–206, and make up a mixture of those that look the most appropriate.

The essential oils that are used to treat depression tend to be divided into two categories: those that are mainly sedating, and those that are mainly uplifting. Overall, most of the oils have a balancing effect and should help to strengthen the nervous system, as well as relieving particular symptoms. The mainly sedating antidepressant essential oils are CHAMOMILE, CLARY SAGE, LAVENDER, NEROLI and SANDALWOOD. The mainly uplifting antidepressant essential oils are BASIL, BERGAMOT, GERANIUM, JASMINE, MELISSA and ROSE. Oils from the two groups can be combined if that seems appropriate. Consult the *Materia Medica* and choose two or three of the oils that look the most suitable, and that you enjoy using, and use those oils on a regular basis. The oils that you choose can be made up into a massage oil, or added to a warm bath.

Headaches

Nearly everyone gets a headache at one time or another. There are many possible causes. For example, a headache may be caused by stress, exposure to strong sun, a cold or 'flu, pre-menstrual tension, overindulging in alcohol or drugs, or poor posture. If a headache is very severe or persistent, or results from a head injury, then seek immediate medical advice.

If poor posture is causing your headaches then consider consulting an Alexander Technique practitioner or chiropractic therapist. If headaches are recurrent, then constitutional treatment by a qualified therapist will be necessary to help discover the underlying factors contributing to them. With tension headaches, it may be useful to reassess the balance between the head and the heart (or the rational thought versus the feeling element) in your life. Relaxation techniques including meditation and yoga can teach us to let go of tension and relax more effectively. For the occasional headache with an obvious, non-serious cause, the following remedies will be helpful.

Look up these herbs in the *Materia Medica* section, depending on the cause of your headache: CHAMOMILE, GINKGO, LAVENDER, ROSEMARY, SKULLCAP, WHITE WILLOW and VERVAIN. Make an infusion to drink from the most appropriate ones.

The most effective essential oils for treating headaches include EUCALYPTUS, LAVENDER, NEROLI, PEPPERMINT and ROSEMARY. Add a few drops of one to a warm bath or make up a massage oil and massage the feet. It is generally not advisable to massage the head or neck when you actually have a headache, as this can intensify the discomfort.

A homoeopathic remedy may be chosen from the following list by comparing them in the *Materia Medica* section: ARNICA, BELLADONNA, BRYONIA, GELSEMIUM, KALI PHOS, NUX VOMICA and PULSATILLA.

Insomnia

An inability to sleep may take various forms. You may not be able to 'drop off' to sleep or you may wake during the night or very early in the morning. Most people experience sleeplessness at some time in their lives, maybe before an exam, during emotional trauma or because of discomfort or pain. Usually this will pass after the obvious cause has gone, but if a pattern of sleeplessness becomes established it can be difficult to break.

The amount of sleep an individual needs varies. Some people are convinced that they can only operate effectively with ten hours a night; others appear to manage perfectly well on only a couple of hours. If you worry about not having enough sleep you have the double problem of making it more difficult to actually get to sleep and the anxiety.

Where there is a clear reason for your insomnia – if you are in pain or discomfort or you are anxious – it is obviously best to deal with the causes, if this is possible. It is more appropriate to treat the pain, indigestion, depression and so on, than deal directly with sleeplessness. The specific remedies for insomnia suggested here are appropriate if you need to function in the short term, during a period of known stress such as during exams, interviews or emotional traumas. If sleep difficulties, particularly early-morning waking, are accompanied by dark moods, you should seek professional help to determine the possibility of underlying depression.

Most standard medications for insomnia are hypnotic sedatives that depress brain function. The principal 'sleeping pills' are benzodiazepines (tranquillizers), nonbarbiturates (bromides, chloral and so on) and antihistamines. All of them carry some risk of habituation and tolerance, so that the doses have to become ever larger to remain effective. Many people find also that they are drowsy or less able to concentrate during the day.

Insomnia is common during the later stages of pregnancy, when it can become difficult to find a comfortable sleeping position. Try a warm drink before going to bed and use extra pillows to find a more comfortable position. If all else fails, try and make the time to have a rest or nap during the day or after work.

It is worth bearing in mind that the body is basically a self-regulating organism and that given positive assistance, it will take the amount of sleep that is needed. Resting and relaxing generally will create the best conditions to encourage sleep and even if sleep is minimal, enable the body to cope better with that situation.

On a practical note, it is worth avoiding tea and coffee and other stimulants in the evening if you do suffer from sleeplessness. Similarly, try to avoid things that are intellectually stimulating or potentially stressful late at night. Physical exercise generally improves one's ability to sleep soundly, and for those of us who lead sedentary lives, a daily exercise routine can make a marked difference.

A great deal of sleeplessness is caused by an over-active brain, which will tend to dwell on worries and troubles and send them round in circles when you are tired. Meditation and visualization exercises can be used to distract the brain from such worries and encourage it to let go into sleep more easily. Try concentrating on relaxing the entire body, muscle by muscle, from the feet upwards, or running through the day backwards without becoming unduly attached to any one event.

There are many traditional herbal remedies to assist sleep. BALM, BORAGE (for low spirits), CHAMOMILE, HOPS, LIMEFLOWERS, ORANGE BLOSSOM, PASSI-FLORA, SKULLCAP, VALERIAN and VERVAIN can be made into an infusion, either as a combination or separately, and drunk in the evening. Essential oils can be a particularly pleasant method of assisting sleep and a few drops of CHAMOMILE, LAVENDER, MARJORAM or NEROLI either in an evening bath or dropped onto a tissue and placed on the pillow can be very effective. A useful homoeopathic remedy to try is KALI PHOS as a tissue salt, which is taken one each night on retiring, for up to a month. Homoeopathic COFFEA may also be indicated. The most frequently used remedy from Bach flower remedies for insomnia is WHITE CHESTNUT, which is indicated where there are persistent, unwanted thoughts or mental arguments preventing sleep.

Persistent insomnia may require psychological therapy if the cause is primarily emotional, or constitutional treatment, by an acupuncturist or homoeopath, if the body's energy is not readily able to establish a better sleep pattern to suit the individual.

Migraine

The pain experienced during a migraine is caused by a temporary spasm followed by considerable dilation of blood vessels in the brain. The symptoms are intense pain, usually only in one side of the head, nausea and visual distur-bances. The length of the attack varies from between a couple of hours to several days. A migraine attack is normally accompanied by the desire for soli-tude and to lie down in a quiet, dark room.

Factors known to contribute to migraines include stress, tension, hormonal changes during the menstrual cycle, congestive disorders, allergy, certain foods (commonly cheese, chocolate and red wine), and a hereditary predisposition. If your migraine attacks keep recurring, you should consider constitutional treat-ment or even psychotherapy to try and establish and change the more profound reasons for them. It is often necessary to help a migraine sufferer become more in touch with their physical body, particularly their sexuality, in order to bring about true healing.

For an infrequent or mild migraine attack, the following natural remedies may be of some benefit. Try an infusion made from the following herbs: BALM, HOPS, MEADOWSWEET, ROSEMARY and SKULLCAP. FEVERFEW capsules have also been proven to bring relief to some migraine sufferers. A warm or cold compress (whichever is preferred) may be applied to the back of the neck or forehead and temples, using one of the following essential oils: LAVENDER, MARJORAM or MELISSA. Consult the *Materia Medica* section of this book to see if any of the following homoeopathic remedies look particularly appropriate: BELLADONNA, BRYONIA, GELSEMIUM, KALI BICH, NUX VOMICA and PULSATILLA.

Neuralgia and Sciatica

Neuralgia is an acutely painful condition caused by the inflammation of a nerve. The trigeminal nerves in the face are the most common site of neuralgia. If the sciatic nerve in the spine is affected, then there is pain in the lower back and down the legs and the condition is called sciatica.

Neuralgia often seems to occur during a phase of life when there are a lot of worries and troubles around, particularly when communicating or the sharing of problems is difficult. If it seems possible that these are underlying factors in your case then you should consider some form of counselling. Sciatica often occurs in someone who has taken on a lot and is burdened by family, life or work, and this should be assessed and dealt with if necessary.

There are some natural remedies that can be of great benefit while you are confronting any underlying factors. First, however, make sure that you are getting the right nutrients in your diet, and particularly that you have a plentiful supply of B-complex vitamins (check the food source charts on pages 420–21 if you are unsure).

Herbs that have a nervine and pain-relieving effect include BLACK COHOSH, PASSIFLORA, SKULLCAP, ST JOHN'S WORT and VALERIAN. Look these up in the *Materia Medica* section and combine the most appropriate. The essential oils of CHAMOMILE, EUCALYPTUS, LAVENDER, MARJORAM, PEPPERMINT, ROSEMARY or SANDALWOOD may be applied in a compress, massage or bath. Look the following homoeopathic remedies up in the *Materia Medica* section to see if one of them looks particularly appropriate: CAUSTICUM, HYPERICUM, KALI CARB, KALI PHOS and RHUS TOX.

Shingles

Shingles, also called herpes zoster, is caused by a virus similar to the chickenpox virus. The distinguishing symptom of shingles is the very painful cluster of blisters on the skin at the site of the nerve endings, for example around the chest or on the thighs. The sufferer will feel generally unwell and may have a fever during the acute attack. The pain may persist even when the blisters have gone.

An attack of shingles is often a sign of general debility, and patients should reassess their diet and take plenty of rest. Particular attention should be made to an adequate supply of B-complex vitamins in the diet (check the chart on pages 420–21 for rich food sources of vitamins).

The following natural remedies will bring relief to shingles affecting the chest, back, thighs, buttocks and so on; shingles on the forehead or anywhere near the eyes should be treated only under the supervision of a qualified practitioner. Make a combination of the following nervine herbs and drink an infusion three times a day: PASSIFLORA, SKULLCAP, ST JOHN'S WORT and VERVAIN. Diluted tinctures or cool infusions of the following herbs may also be used to bathe the affected area: MARIGOLD, PLANTAIN and ST JOHN'S WORT. Essential oils can combine analgesics with antiviral properties, and may be applied as a compress or by diluting them in a base-massage oil to gently massage in. Try combining a couple of the following oils after looking them up in the *Materia Medica* section: BERGAMOT, CHAMOMILE, EUCALYPTUS, GERANIUM, LAVENDER, MELISSA and TEA TREE.

The homoeopathic remedies to consider for the treatment of shingles include ARSEN ALB, KALI PHOS and RHUS TOX.

Stress

Stress is not an illness in itself, but it is a response to any situation that puts us under pressure. Factors contributing to stress may be environmental, physical or mental. For example, environmental stress may be caused by pollution or poor housing; physical stress will result from an accident or injury; and mental stress may arise from pressure of work, or difficulties within a relationship.

We seem to be able to adapt to a certain amount of stress in our lives without showing symptoms of disease, but at some point, if the stress continues, or a new one is added, the balance is tipped and we begin to experience symptoms of one kind or another as a result. The amount of stress involved in everyday life in our society is considered to be unacceptably high by many people, and certainly therapists see a great many diseases these days which have a clear correlation with particular stress factors in the sufferer's life. Diseases that often have an obvious relationship with stress include allergies, asthma, eczema, headaches, migraine, digestive disorders, heart disease, insomnia and depression.

The only way that we are going to be able to reduce the amount of stress in our lives is to choose another way of doing things. For example, we must choose additive-free diets, reassess how hard we work, take steps where possible to improve our physical environment and develop our ability to communicate with others. Feeling helpless is in itself stressful, so it can be helpful to join an environmental pressure group or self-help group for the particular disease or problem that you have, in order to feel more empowered.

We need to be as healthy as possible so that our bodies can adapt efficiently to stresses. As well as dealing with any specific health problems, we must eat well, avoid excessive amounts of coffee and alcohol, avoid smoking or taking drugs, get enough sleep (which is the only time that the body can repair itself), and enjoy ourselves mentally and physically. There are a variety of different techniques that are known to help us deal with stress more effectively, such as yoga, meditation, music or art therapy, and certain exercises.

If we feel that we need some extra help during a particularly stressful phase of our lives, then there are some remedies that we can employ, but these should only be taken for a relatively short period of time before we really reassess the habits and activities in our lives that are causing the stress in the first place. It is useless to relieve the symptoms while maintaining the stressful lifestyle.

Our bodies use up the B group of vitamins particularly rapidly when we are under stress, so it is a good idea to check that our diet is rich in these vitamins (*see* the food source chart on pages 420–21), and consider taking a supplement. There are herbs that act as nervine tonics to feed and strengthen the nervous system, the best ones for treating stress in a general way are BALM, CHAMOMILE, LAVENDER, LIMEFLOWERS, OATS, ORANGE BLOSSOM, PASSIFLORA, SKULLCAP and VERVAIN. Any of these may be drunk as an infusion on a regular basis. BORAGE may be added for a short time.

GINSENG is known to be an adaptogen and it helps the body to deal with the effects of stress.

Essential oils that have an uplifting and relaxing effect can be helpful, for example BASIL, BERGAMOT, CHAMOMILE, GERANIUM, JASMINE, LAVENDER,

MARJORAM, NEROLI and ROSE. Essential oils that strengthen the adrenal system, which tends to be weakened by stress, may also be useful, for example GINGER, LEMONGRASS and ROSEMARY. All of these oils should be checked in the *Materia Medica* section and then they can be used in massage, baths or by burning them in a room.

14

Pregnancy and Childbirth

The experience of pregnancy and childbirth is one of the most exciting and challenging times in any woman's life. The experience of your own body creating another human being is one that is on the leading edge of nature at her most miraculous. Every pregnant woman, and every mother, is brought into an awareness of her inherent creative power.

Most healthy women become radiant during pregnancy; it is a shame that in our society we have fallen into the habit of looking upon pregnancy as an illness, and the pregnant woman as a patient in need of treatment. With reassurance, and practical advice where there is not the experience already built in, most women can enjoy pregnancy and labour without the need for medication and intervention.

In many ways, this is an exciting time for all those concerned with pregnancy and childbirth, because as well as the privilege that goes with being involved in this field, there have been many positive steps towards reclaiming the experience as the immensely creative, feminine, personal and natural process that it should be. The days when women are subject to all the intervention, restrictions and personal idiosyncrasies of the doctor or hospital concerned are hopefully numbered, as the numbers of women and midwives who demand the right to choose their treatment during pregnancy and the type of birth that they want grow.

Pre-natal classes in active birth and exercise are now increasingly easy to find. There is information available on how to arrange a home birth. More and more clinics and labour wards are responding to demands for facilities for an active labour, soft lighting in the delivery room and the desire of the mother to remain in contact with the baby as soon as she is born. However, in some areas, expressing your individual needs and wishes can still feel like a real struggle, at a time when what is needed is support and creative assistance.

The Baby in the Womb at Term

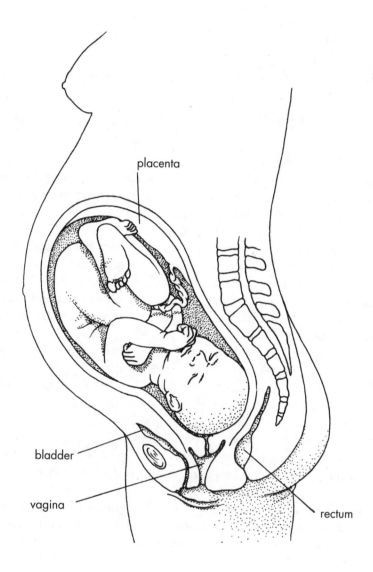

Potentially, we should have the best of both worlds: the wealth of technical expertise and knowledge gained by the medical profession over the last few decades, which is invaluable when necessary, and the growing awareness and support network available to help women get back in touch with what is natural and instinctually right for them. Unfortunately, choice can often result in confusion, and it can feel daunting to have to deal with all the changes occurring inside your body as well as having to try and run your pregnancy the way you want it and make arrangements for your own labour when you cannot really know how it is going to be. Probably the most useful thing to do is to talk to other women about their experiences, read books on natural childbirth, join an active birth class if there is one in your area and contact the National Childbirth Trust or other organizations dealing with childbirth for more information *(see page 425)*.

Diet

The importance of a good diet during pregnancy cannot be stressed enough. It is vital for the mother to be able to maintain her health and energy while nourishing the foetus, and to provide the growing baby with all the nutrients necessary for a healthy body. It is better to get nutrients from their natural food sources as opposed to supplements, because these are naturally in a form suitable for the body to absorb. If it proves difficult to establish a well-balanced, nutrient-rich diet, then some supplementation may be required.

Vitamin E aids the development of the reproductive system and is needed for a healthy and well-toned uterus. The daily requirement for this vitamin is doubled during pregnancy. Good natural sources of vitamin E are wheatgerm oil, wheatgerm, sesame seeds, oats, brown rice, sunflower seeds, cabbage and lettuce. The vitamin E content of foods is lost by most forms of processing, including freezing. Do not take a high-dose vitamin E supplement while you are pregnant because it can increase blood pressure in those women who are prone to high blood pressure anyway.

The growing baby will use up a lot of iron from the mother's supply, especially during the last two months of pregnancy. Unfortunately, most iron supplements are renowned for causing digestive upsets such as nausea, colic and diarrhoea or constipation, and they should be avoided. Foods rich in iron are liver, lean meat, treacle and molasses, lentils, haricot beans, dried fruit, eggs and green leafy vegetables. If you suspect that you may be anaemic, or a blood test indicates that you are, then follow the recommendations under Anaemia (*see page 38*).

Zinc is an extremely important mineral for the growing child in the womb; it is important for the development of healthy skin, bones and teeth. Good sources of zinc are shellfish, liver, cheese, lentils, haricot beans, sesame seeds, sunflower seeds, almonds, avocado and bananas. Herbal infusions that will provide a rich supply of zinc include ALFALFA and RASPBERRY LEAF, both of which are suitable for drinking during pregnancy.

The need for calcium increases greatly during the last three months as the baby takes what it needs to form healthy bones and teeth. A lack of it will cause leg and foot cramps in the mother and a susceptibility to tooth decay. Foods rich in calcium include dairy products, fish, watercress, wheatflour, oats, millet, soya beans and green leafy vegetables.

There are also things that should be avoided during pregnancy. Coffee reduces the availability and absorption of nutrients from your diet and should be avoided. Alcohol should be avoided or kept to a suitable minimum, such as half a glass of wine mixed with water. An excessive amount of alcohol during pregnancy has been shown to have a detrimental effect on the child. Smoking should be avoided for the sake of both the mother's and baby's health. Smoking greatly increases the risk of miscarriage, premature birth, stillbirth and neonatal death.

Medication and Remedies to Avoid during Pregnancy

Taking any medication in pregnancy is a matter of weighing up the benefits against possible damage to the foetus. For two-thirds of drugs commonly consumed by women, and for a third of those used in labour, there are no published reports showing that they do not carry any risk to the baby. Many other drugs that are taken regularly by women, for example some sleeping pills, tranquillizers, migraine pills and some antibiotics, are known to have a detrimental effect on the foetus

Basically, it is better to avoid taking any medication during pregnancy that is not absolutely vital to maintaining the health of the mother, such as for the treatment of diabetes and epilepsy. The foetus is particularly vulnerable to damage from medication during the first three months of pregnancy, when major organs of the body and the skeleton are forming. This is another argument for getting as healthy as possible before becoming pregnant so that there is no need for medication.

There are also a number of herbs that should be avoided during pregnancy. Basically this list includes those herbs that act as abortifacients, emmenagogues and strong laxatives. Any herb taken in therapeutic dosage should be specifically checked for safety and use during pregnancy; the list of those that should definitely be avoided (unless specifically recommended by a medical herbalist), includes ALOES, ANGELICA, BARBERRY, BETHROOT, BLACK COHOSH, BLOODROOT, BUCKTHORN, CASCARA SAGRADA, CATNIP, CELERY SEED, CINCHONA, COLTSFOOT, COTTONROOT, ELECAMPANE, FALSE UNICORN, FENUGREEK, FEVERFEW, GINSENG, GOTU KOLA, GOLDENSEAL, GREATER CELANDINE, HOLY THISTLE, HOPS, HORSETAIL, HYSSOP, JUNIPER, LADY'S MANTLE, LIFEROOT, LIQUORICE, MALE FERN, MANDRAKE, MARIGOLD, MILK THISTLE, MINT, MOTHERWORT, MYRRH, PENNYROYAL, PEPPERMINT, POKE ROOT, PRICKLY ASH, RED CLOVER, RHUBARB, ROSEMARY, RUE, SAFFRON, SAGE, SENNA, SHEPHERD'S PURSE, SOUTHERNWOOD, TANSY, THUJA, UVA URSI, VERVAIN, WHITE HOREHOUND, WILD INDIGO, WILD YAM, WORMWOOD, YARROW and YELLOW DOCK.

There are also some essential oils that should be avoided during pregnancy these include BASIL, CAMPHOR, NUTMEG, OREGANUM, PENNYROYAL, SAGE, SAVOURY, THUJA and WINTERGREEN.

Miscarriage

The first symptom of a miscarriage (medically referred to as a spontaneous abortion) is bleeding, sometimes accompanied by cramping pains. Slight bleeding, although alarming, does not necessarily mean that you will definitely miscarry, and some women lose small amounts of blood regularly throughout their otherwise healthy pregnancies. You should seek urgent medical advice for persistent or heavy bleeding. Bleeding accompanied by cramping pains nearly always indicates that a miscarriage is in process and you should seek urgent medical advice.

There is no concrete evidence that bed rest will prevent a miscarriage once it has started, but rest will probably help you to adjust and deal with the stress better.

The emotional trauma experienced after a miscarriage can be considerable, and the support of an experienced and caring practitioner can be a very helpful addition to that of friends and family.

An estimated 20 to 30 per cent of known pregnancies end in miscarriage in Great Britain, and this figure is much higher in Third World countries. The majority of miscarriages occur within the first three months of pregnancy. It is thought that many occur as the body's natural way of rejecting an unhealthy foetus. As a result, you should not take any form of treatment to prevent a miscarriage at any cost.

If you have a history of miscarriages, constitutional treatment by a qualified therapist of natural medicine should be sought from the beginning of the pregnancy, or preferably before. The following remedies may help, but should only be used in conjunction with treatment from a qualified therapist.

If a miscarriage is threatening, a herbalist may be able to suggest herbs that can help you maintain a healthy pregnancy. If you are suffering from a lot of stress and anxiety, SKULLCAP may be helpful.

The homoeopathic remedies that you should consider for a threatened miscarriage include ACONITE, ARNICA, BELLADONNA, CHAMOMILLA, IGNATIA, PULSATILLA and SEPIA. Compare these in the *Materia Medica* and select the most appropriate remedy for you. Remember that if the foetus is not viable, then the right remedy assists the mother through the miscarriage emotionally and physically, but will not save the baby.

The Bach FIVE FLOWER REMEDY can have a very calming influence during this stressful time. Take a few drops as often as required.

For remedies to help to restore health following a miscarriage, *see* Abortion below.

Abortion

Some people have attempted to use herbs and oils specifically to induce an abortion; this is an extremely dangerous and irresponsible way of terminating a pregnancy. In some cases it can cause haemorrhage, epileptic fits or an infection following a partial miscarriage; if the abortion is not successful, it can damage the growing foetus. If the decision is reached to terminate a pregnancy, it is far safer to have a mechanical abortion at a reputable clinic or hospital.

You should be aware that you will need ongoing emotional support and possibly counselling after an abortion. Be cautious about the possibility of an infection following an abortion. If there is an unusual smell to any discharge, pain or a general rise in temperature, seek immediate medical advice.

Herbs that may be used to rebalance the hormones and tone the uterus after an abortion (or miscarriage) include AGNUS CASTUS, BLUE COHOSH, FALSE UNICORN, HOLY THISTLE, LIQUORICE and RASPBERRY LEAF. Check the herbs in the *Materia Medica* section and take the most appropriate ones as an infusion or as tinctures for a month. If you are under a lot of emotional stress, consider adding BALM and SKULLCAP to the mixture.

The homoeopathic remedy ARNICA is useful to take following any physical trauma or operation. Other homoeopathic remedies to consider after an abortion are BELLIS PERENNIS, IGNATIA and STAPHYSAGRIA.

The essential oils of LAVENDER, NEROLI and ROSE can help to ease stress and promote healing after a miscarriage or abortion. Dilute to use in a massage or add a few drops to a warm bath.

Tests and Scans

There are a wide range of tests than can be carried out during pregnancy these days; some of these, although valuable in special circumstances, are now routine.

ULTRASOUND

Today, most pregnant women in the western world are subjected to one or more ultrasound scans. Ultrasound was invented during the Second World War and used to detect submarines at sea. It works on the principle that sound rays bounce off solid objects.

During an ultrasound scan, a probe that emits waves of sound too high for the ear to hear is passed over the uterus. The sound is translated into dots, which are used to build up an image on a screen. The ultrasound scan can provide doctors with a great deal of information about the placenta and the growing foetus. It can be used to locate the position of the placenta, to establish whether the heart is still beating after a threatened miscarriage, to reveal certain congenital handicaps and to date a pregnancy more accurately. But ultrasound also has many disadvantages. It often diagnoses conditions, such as a low-lying placenta, which may have righted itself by the time labour starts. Results are not always accurately interpreted, and many women have suffered terrible stress and anxiety because they were told that something was wrong with the unborn child when there was not. Between 16 and 24 weeks, ultrasound should be able to give an accurate dating of pregnancy; after that time it is very likely to be wrong.

At present there is no evidence that ultrasound is unsafe, but very little is known about its possible delayed and long-term risks. It has been suggested that ultrasound may produce changes in foetal cells which could lead to later health problems. It does also seem to affect the foetus in the womb, often by making it jump around wildly. It could be that while our ears cannot pick up the high-pitched sound waves, the sensitive ears of the developing foetus pick them up as intensely shrill and powerful noise. Because there is no evidence that the routine use of ultrasound benefits either mother or child, and because the possible long-term risks are not yet known, it seems wise to restrict its use to those cases where there are good reasons to suspect that all is not well.

AMNIOCENTESIS
Amniocentesis is a test carried out by inserting a needle through the mother's abdominal wall, into the uterus, and drawing off a sample of the amniotic fluid in which the baby floats. It cannot be done until you are 16 to 18 weeks pregnant because until then there is not enough fluid. Foetal cells from the fluid can be grown in a culture to reveal a range of abnormalities, including Down's syndrome, sickle cell anaemia, thalassaemia and spina bifida. Amniocentesis can also show the sex of the baby, which is important if there are sex-linked diseases, such as haemophilia or muscular dystrophy, in the family.

If the amniocentesis test does reveal that the foetus suffers from a congenital abnormality, the mother must decide whether or not to have an abortion. It is an unfortunate problem with amniocentesis that if the pregnancy is to be terminated, it results in a late abortion, after 20 weeks, which can be very distressing. Another drawback is that many results take three to four weeks or longer to come through, and this can be a very worrying time. If the mother has decided that she would not agree to an abortion there is no point in having the test.

Other risks involved with amniocentesis are a higher rate of miscarriage and an increased incidence of newborn babies who have difficulties with breathing. However, the medical authorities will always recommend amniocentesis if you are over 35 because of the link between older mothers and Down's syndrome babies. The test is also recommended for women from ethnic groups that are more at risk of a genetic disorder such as sickle cell disease, and for those women who are likely to pass on an inherited abnormality.

OTHER TESTS
Tests that should be carried out routinely when you are pregnant are measuring your weight; blood tests to ascertain your blood group and the possibility of

anaemia; blood pressure; urine tests to check for sugar and protein; and palpation of the abdomen to feel the size of the uterus and size and position of the baby. It is particularly important that weight and blood pressure are measured regularly throughout pregnancy.

Common Ailments of Pregnancy

We are going to discuss the issues and problems that may arise during pregnancy under three stages: the three trimesters (three-monthly periods) of a normal pregnancy. There may well be an overlap in many cases, for example, constipation may occur in any or all of the three trimesters, not just the second one as it is discussed here (although this is when it is most commonly experienced); in that case the information and suggestions given will still be relevant and can easily be applied to your stage of pregnancy.

THE FIRST TRIMESTER
The first three months of pregnancy can be the time when you experience some of its most distressing symptoms. After the initial excitement of discovering that you are pregnant, you can feel suddenly that you are out of control of your body and your life. Many women suffer with nausea in early pregnancy, and feeling exhausted is also common. If the pregnancy was unplanned, these symptoms can be even harder to accept. It is as if your body is expressing the turmoil of preparing itself for the enormously creative task ahead.

Some women sail through their whole pregnancy without experiencing any uncomfortable symptoms; indeed, they may feel healthier than they ever have before. However, most women experience some tiredness in the first three months. Fortunately these feelings of exhaustion do not usually get worse as the pregnancy progresses but improve considerably by the second trimester. If at all possible, the sensible thing to do if you do feel really tired is to assist your body at this time of adjustment and get plenty of rest.

The need to urinate more frequently usually starts in early pregnancy, once the uterus begins to swell and press on the bladder. Try to avoid drinking anything just before you go to bed to reduce the number of visits to the toilet during the night. Also cut out tea, coffee and alcohol, as these tend to stimulate urine production.

The one symptom that everyone associates with the early stages of pregnancy is morning sickness, and some morning sickness will be experienced by most women during the first few months of pregnancy. The symptoms include nausea, vomiting and a feeling of weakness. It seems to be caused by the massive upheaval of hormones occurring in the body, combined with low blood sugar. You generally feel it most in the morning, when the stomach is empty, although it may occur at any time of day. It is often helpful to get up slowly in the mornings, and try eating a dry biscuit before rising.

If you feel nauseous later in the day, try eating small snacks at frequent intervals. Your metabolism speeds up during early pregnancy, so you will probably find that your weight doesn't increase in the first two or three months even though you may be eating more. Foods that can aggravate feelings of nausea are fatty foods and milk, so try cutting these out.

The symptoms of morning sickness usually recede after the third month of pregnancy. In rare cases they persist throughout pregnancy, and you should seek professional help. You should also seek professional guidance if vomiting is persistent, or if you develop a prolonged aversion to eating. Herbs that can be safely used to alleviate the nausea of morning sickness include BALM, CHAMOMILE and MEADOWSWEET. Combine these, or use them separately, to make an infusion to drink three times a day. A little grated GINGER may also be added to hot water to relieve nausea.

The most commonly used homoeopathic remedies for relieving morning sickness are IPECAC, NUX VOMICA, PULSATILLA and SEPIA. Look these up in the *Materia Medica* section of this book to see which one is the most suitable for you.

THE SECOND TRIMESTER

The second trimester is a time for becoming attuned to the baby growing within. Around the fourth or fifth month you will feel the first movements of the baby. Actually, the foetus has been moving around for months, but the movements can only be felt from this stage. Most women feel very well during this time and the nausea and exhaustion of the early stages often recede.

Your pregnancy is also beginning to show at this stage. The foetus has begun to grow bulkier and your waist starts to thicken. The line from your naval to your pubic region becomes dark, as does the area around your nipples. Sometimes the facial pigment also becomes darker, but this will fade after the birth.

As your abdomen grows larger, the skin over it will stretch. If you do not have very supple skin, pink or reddish streaks may appear, called stretch marks. To reduce the likelihood of stretch marks developing, massage the abdomen regularly with the essential oils of FRANKINCENSE, LAVENDER or NEROLI, diluted in a base of combined almond and wheatgerm oils.

A homoeopathic tissue salt that is very useful to take during pregnancy is CALC FLUOR. This remedy will increase the suppleness of the skin to prevent stretch marks, give elasticity to vein walls, thus reducing the likelihood of varicose veins or haemorrhoids developing, and will also be good for the developing baby's teeth and bones. It is easily available in health food shops and many chemists and should be purchased in the 6X potency. Take one dose three times a day for ten days, then have a break for a few days and repeat the course once or twice more if required.

A herbal tea that has been taken by many thousands of women during pregnancy to tone the uterus is RASPBERRY LEAF. This is a pleasant-tasting herbal tea that can be taken by drinking a cupful at least once a day throughout the second half of pregnancy. SQUAW VINE is a Native American herb that is taken in the same way as RASPBERRY LEAF: to tone the uterus in preparation for labour. This may be taken as an alternative or take them together. Check the *Materia Medica* section for dosage and more information on its actions.

One unpleasant symptom that can develop once pregnancy is established is indigestion and heartburn. This may be due to progesterone and other hormones softening the valve at the top of the stomach and thus allowing digestive acids to rise into the oesophagus, or from the uterus pressing on the digestive organs later in pregnancy. To relieve this, eat small meals at more regular intervals, or eat slowly and chew everything well and avoid fatty and fried foods. It is also advisable not to eat late in the evening, and if the problem comes on at night, try sleeping well propped up on a number of pillows.

Remedies that will relieve symptoms of heartburn and indigestion include the homoeopathic remedies KALI MUR, NUX VOMICA and PULSATILLA. Check these in the *Materia Medica* section to see which is most suitable and take as required. An infusion of the herbs BALM, MEADOWSWEET or PEPPERMINT can also bring relief. Try sipping a cupful after each meal, or take SLIPPERY ELM half an hour before a meal.

Constipation is another symptom that can prove troublesome during pregnancy. This is sometimes due to hormone changes slowing down intestinal action and sometimes occurs when the uterus presses against the large intestine. Your diet is very important here and the problem can be solved by eating more fibre-rich foods such as oats, pulses, raw fruit and vegetables, and also more dried fruit, especially figs and prunes. Avoid all refined foods, particularly white flour and sugar. Do not take iron tablets. Constipation can be caused by the bowel absorbing more fluid during pregnancy, so try drinking more water (you should be drinking 6–8 glasses of fluid a day). One of the most effective remedies for constipation is by adding linseed to your diet. A dessertspoonful of linseed sprinkled over oats or muesli at breakfast will nearly always establish regular bowel movements after a couple of days.

If constipation becomes persistent, consult the *Materia Medica* to see if one of the following homoeopathic remedies looks appropriate: BRYONIA, NATRUM MUR, NUX VOMICA and SEPIA. The herbs FENNEL and MARSHMALLOW ROOT have a mild laxative action and may be taken as an infusion before bedtime. Do not take stronger laxative herbs during pregnancy.

Partly as a result of pelvic pressure, and partly due to the tissue-relaxing effect of progesterone and other hormones present in pregnancy, many pregnant women suffer from haemorrhoids and varicose veins. It is really important not to get constipated if you are trying to avoid haemorrhoids; if you do get them follow the advice under Haemorrhoids *(see page 50)*. Continuing to take exercise during pregnancy, combined with regular rest with the legs raised, should prevent varicose veins developing but if you do get them, *see* Varicose Veins, page 44.

THE THIRD TRIMESTER

The third trimester takes you from the twenty-ninth week of pregnancy to the birth. During this time your abdomen will be becoming very large as the baby puts on weight in preparation for the birth. Movements by the unborn child can be seen and felt from the outside by this stage. Many women begin to feel impatient to see and hold the child towards the end of pregnancy, and the last few weeks can seem like a very long time. The sheer extra weight that is being carried around by late pregnancy – as much as 11½–13½kg (25–30lbs) – can make a woman feel very tired and in need of plenty of rest and sleep.

Small irregular contractions will be felt across the uterus from the second half of pregnancy. These are called Braxton-Hicks contractions and are thought to prepare the uterus for labour.

Cramps in the legs are commonly experienced by pregnant women, particularly in the third trimester. It is thought the cramps are caused by metabolic changes that cause an imbalance of calcium and phosphorus. If you have had plenty of calcium in your diet throughout your pregnancy you are less likely to suffer with cramps. If you get a cramp, flex your foot upwards toward your knee and rub the calf. If cramps do become a problem, take the homoeopathic tissue salt MAG PHOS 6X one dose three times a day for ten days and repeat the course after a few days' break, if necessary.

It is not uncommon to experience shortness of breath in the last trimester, as the uterus can put pressure on your lungs, and your diaphragm may be pushed up. If the problem is worse when you lie down, try propping yourself up with several pillows. The pressure of the uterus upwards can also cramp the stomach and cause indigestion; in this case, try eating small meals at more regular intervals.

Usually sometime between six and two weeks before the birth, the baby's head drops or 'engages' into your pelvis. This usually eases any pressure on the lungs or stomach and some women say that they feel lighter, although it can then feel as if there is a large lump protruding between your legs. In mothers who have already had two or three children, engagement may not occur until labour starts, because the baby is not such a tight fit in a uterus that has already been stretched by childbirth. If a baby engages bottom down (breech), or any position other than head down, then ask an experienced midwife to suggest exercises to turn the baby, or to consider turning the baby by easing it round from the outside (external version).

Some water retention (oedema) is common in pregnant women, and often this will cause swollen ankles. Water retention can be reduced by cutting out salt from the diet. If oedema is associated with high blood pressure and protein in the urine, then a condition called pre-eclamptic toxaemia is developing. Mild pre-eclampsia in the last few weeks of pregnancy is common – around 25 per cent of all women get it – but pre-eclampsia that starts before 36 weeks, or that is severe, is very serious.

If the mother actually develops eclampsia and has fits, there is grave danger to both the mother and the baby. Some doctors advise all mothers with pre-eclampsia to agree to the baby's induction, but this should only be necessary for those women whose blood pressure is dangerously high. There is no evidence to suggest that diuretic drugs do relieve pre-eclampsia, although they are often prescribed; however, there is no harm in consulting a medical herbalist, acupuncturist, homoeopath or other natural therapist of your choice who may be able to prevent a serious situation developing.

Generally there is no reason why you can't continue to enjoy a regular sexual relationship throughout pregnancy, and sensitive lovemaking can be a good way of continuing to develop a loving relationship between your partner and yourself and the child. Most women find that being pregnant does affect their libido, but this varies in different women from having no desire at all for sex to an increased sex drive and heightened sexual response.

Many women find intercourse difficult during the last weeks because they feel bulky and tired, and find it difficult to get into a comfortable position anyway. With a gentle and patient partner it is often possible to find a position that enables intercourse to be enjoyable, probably by the women being on top, or by both partners lying on their sides with the man entering from behind. If you don't feel like having intercourse it is better to express this and try encouraging your partner to give you a massage and to stroke your abdomen if you both enjoy this.

Intercourse should not be attempted once the waters have broken, or for a few weeks after any bleeding, because it may increase the risk of an infection entering the uterus. If you are near term, or past the date when your baby is due, intercourse may help labour start, especially if it is combined with nipple stimulation.

❋ If the Baby Dies

A baby may die in the womb during the last few months of pregnancy. The mother will still need to give birth to the dead baby because this is the least hazardous way of delivery. Sadly, some babies also die during labour. While allowing yourself to experience the grief is the only way to emerge from such a life trauma, there are several things that can be done to assist the grieving process.

Mothers who have lived through the experience of their new babies dying say how helpful they found it to hold their dead baby for a few moments. Holding, or at least seeing the baby, gave them someone to remember, rather than an intangible, nightmarish experience. Be firm and build this requirement into your birth plan if you think it would help you in the same situation. Hospitals vary greatly in their ability to deal with a grieving mother sensitively, but you should have the right to insist on a room away from other mothers and babies, and to have your companion with you as much as possible, if that helps.

Your body will have to make all the physical and hormonal readjustments following any pregnancy. These can be particularly painful reminders of your loss. To help stop your breasts producing unneeded milk, you can drink an infusion of the herb SAGE three times a day. The homoeopathic remedy LAC

CANINUM will have a similar effect: try taking one dose of 200C and repeat after a couple of days only if necessary.

If you find it increasingly difficult to cope with your feelings of grief, or if you feel very depressed, then do seek professional counselling to help you at this time. It is better to avoid taking tranquillizers and sedatives if you can, because these only tend to delay the natural grieving process. Natural remedies can help you to feel stronger and calmer without the numbing and heavily-sedating effect of drugs.

Bach FIVE FLOWER REMEDY is a useful natural remedy that may be taken several times a day during an emotional crisis. The homoeopathic remedy IGNATIA is also likely to be helpful. Herbs that can be taken during this stressful time include BALM, CHAMOMILE, OATS, SKULLCAP and VERVAIN. These may be combined and an infusion drunk up to three times a day. Essential oils with a mildly sedative and antidepressant action include CLARY SAGE, LAVENDER, MELISSA, MYRRH and NEROLI. Choose one or two of these to burn in your room, add to a bath, or use in a massage. All these remedies may be looked up in the *Materia Medica* section of this book to help you find the most useful one for yourself.

Preparation for the Birth

The act of giving birth is for many women one of their most powerful life experiences. During childbirth the most amazing physical, emotional and spiritual processes occur in unison – and require a tremendous output of energy and effort by the mother. The overwhelming experience of delivery heralds the arrival of a new person who will affect the interrelationship of a whole family and the total life of the mother.

Preparation for birth means creating a context in which a new human can thrive physically, emotionally and spiritually. It is no wonder that so many of those involved in the birthing process today place more and more emphasis on improving the quality of the whole experience for all concerned, while at the same time doing everything possible to assist the mother and baby through it safely.

Interest in natural medicine has developed alongside an increasing awareness of the benefits of natural childbirth, a movement towards childbirth that is mother and baby-oriented, not doctor and technology centred. There is a growing number of midwives today who are reclaiming their traditional role of assisting at home births; there is a growing awareness of the benefits of active birth; and for those who choose or need a hospital environment for childbirth, there is an increasing tendency towards allowing the mother more choice about such things as who attends the birth, what position she adopts during labour and maintaining physical contact with the baby following delivery. However, there are still doctors who believe that all deliveries should be obstetrically controlled, and the rate of Caesarean sections is still alarmingly high, so it can require great determination and forward-planning on the part of the mother if she wants to be able to choose the course her labour will follow.

There are some excellent books on childbirth, and it is well worth reading several in advance to learn what options are available and to read about other women's experiences. Three particularly useful books are *New Active Birth* by Janet Balaskas (HarperCollins, 1991), *Spiritual Midwifery* by Ina May Gaskin (The Book Publishing Company, 1977), and *Pregnancy and Childbirth* by Sheila Kitzinger (Penguin, 1986).

Many women have benefitted from yoga classes or active birth classes during pregnancy. It is ideal if you can find a yoga class specifically for pregnant women; if not, do make sure that your yoga teacher knows that you are pregnant. Your teacher should concentrate on exercises that tone the pelvic-floor muscles. The exercises strengthen the muscles that support the weight of the uterus and baby, prepare the muscles for the delivery and make the muscles more elastic so that they spring back into shape more readily after the birth.

A good yoga or active birth class will also work on breathing techniques and special exercises and positions that can be used during labour. Ask at your local natural health centre or contact the Active Birth Centre *(see page 426)* for details about classes in your area.

Thinking ahead and making plans for your labour can mean that you have a lot more choice about how it will be. The basic things to consider well in advance are whether to employ an independent midwife *(addresses on page 425)* or use the NHS, whether to have a home or a hospital birth, who your birth companions will be, and whether or not you intend to have an active birth.

If you choose to have a home birth you will have a lot more control over such things as who your companions will be, soft lighting, music, your freedom to move around, the amount of contact with the baby following the birth, and so on. Hospitals do vary a lot in their approaches to childbirth these days. Some have special rooms with soft lighting, facilities for a companion to stay and an attitude which welcomes natural childbirth where possible. Others are very much stuck on the need for total obstetric control and it can end up like being in a ward for acutely sick people. If you are going to have your baby in hospital, do try and visit it beforehand, and if you are not happy with it ask your doctor or midwife to suggest another.

There are a relatively small number of women who are in one of the categories that make it advisable for them to have a hospital birth for health and safety reasons. Otherwise it really should be your choice, based on where you feel happiest and most relaxed. A hospital birth is advisable for those women who are under 16 or over 40, if the baby engages in a particularly difficult presentation, if there has been bleeding during the third trimester, and for those women who suffer with toxaemia or epilepsy or who have experienced severe postpartum haemorrhage previously.

One thing that many women find particularly important to establish in advance is their hospital's policy on allowing the mother to keep the baby with her. It should be possible to explain that you want to maintain physical contact with the baby immediately after the birth, and to allow the baby to suckle as soon as he or she wishes. Following the birth, some hospitals remove the baby to another room for several hours and only bring him in at set intervals to be fed. However, others have 'rooming in' facilities so that you can keep the baby with you and feed on demand. The first few days following the birth are now known to be crucial for the bonding of a loving relationship between mother and baby, and this can only develop with plenty of contact. Mothers who do have the chance to bond well with their babies are known to be less likely to suffer from postnatal depression.

It can be helpful to draw up a birth plan that covers all eventualities, when labour and birth go well and what you will choose if things get difficult. This means that you need to work out, ahead of time, whether you want the freedom to move around during labour, what, if any, forms of pain relief you find acceptable, under what circumstances you would opt for induction or a Caesarean, whether you want to deliver the placenta naturally or with Syntometrine, when you want to be discharged from hospital, and so on. You can give copies of the birth plan to your companion, midwife and doctor. For a detailed explanation on how to draw up a birth plan, the book *Pregnancy and Childbirth* by Sheila Kitzinger (Penguin, 1986) is very helpful.

It is worth bearing in mind that while planning and preparation are helpful and useful, no two births are ever the same, and that you cannot really know how your birth is going to be. Indeed, birth is about letting yourself go in the experience of bringing a new person into the world, and no amount of forward-planning can really prepare you for the reality of that experience.

Many women who carefully plan and organize a totally natural birth end up receiving a lot of obstetric assistance, and we should all be grateful that such technology is there when it is needed. If a birth does not go the way it was planned it is certainly not something that any woman should feel guilty about.

In addition to eating well, taking regular exercise and getting enough rest and relaxation during pregnancy, there are several natural remedies that have been used over the ages to facilitate an easier delivery. A herbal infusion taken traditionally to tone the uterus and help to make the labour easier is RASPBERRY LEAF: make an infusion with a teaspoon of herb to a cupful of boiling water, and drink two or three times a day throughout the last three months of pregnancy. SQUAW VINE is a Native American herb used for the same purpose: make a decoction and drink a cupful once a day throughout the last two months of pregnancy. Many women find that taking the homoeopathic remedy CAULO-PHYLLUM helps them to have an easier birth. Ask your homoeopath what she recommends, or try taking one dose of 30C a week during the last month of pregnancy. All these remedies may be looked up in the *Materia Medica* section of this book.

Massaging the perineum during the last couple of months of your pregnancy will help it to become more elastic and reduce the likelihood of a tear or the need for an episiotomy. Use either ALMOND OIL or WHEATGERM OIL and massage the area twice a day.

During Labour

Labour begins when contractions of the uterine muscles, aided by hormonal changes, cause the cervix to soften, thin out and dilate in order to allow the baby through. For medical purposes labour is divided into three stages: the first is the dilatation of the cervix, the second the expulsion of the baby and the third the delivery of the placenta. However, you may experience several different phases of mood and activity during each of these stages.

The average length of the first stage of labour with a first baby is about 12 hours, and with subsequent children about 7 hours. However, this stage may take anywhere from 2 to 24 hours or more, depending on the size of the baby, her position, the size of the mother's pelvic area and the behaviour of the uterus. First-stage labour is itself split into two categories: early and late.

During early first-stage labour, the cervix is drawn up and thinned out and dilates to 5–6 centimetres (2½ inches). There is no single sign that heralds the onset of labour, but occasional contractions become longer and stronger and more regular until they occur about every four or five minutes. You may have a 'show' if you have not already had one: this is the appearance of some blood-stained mucus, like the beginning of a period. The show is the mucous plug that was in the cervix to protect the uterus from any germs travelling up from the vagina. The waters of the amniotic sac may burst either with a slow leak, or so that water streams out. Once the bag of waters has burst there is usually an increase in contractions and your midwife or hospital should be contacted.

If labour starts fairly slowly this can be a useful time to have a light meal – perhaps soup and fruit. You should also be able to get some rest or sleep at this time, if you need it.

By the late first stage the contractions will be getting stronger, longer and closer together until they come every two or three minutes and last 60 seconds or more. You can use breathing techniques – welcoming a contraction by a slow breath out, then breathing more lightly over the peak of the contraction and giving another long breath out as the contraction finishes. The cervix will be dilating to 5–8 centimetres.

You may find it good to sip iced water, grape juice or honeyed water at this stage. If a mother becomes tense or anxious then sipping a glass of water with a few drops of Bach FIVE FLOWER REMEDY added to it can be very calming.

During this stage, the birth companion can be a great help: massaging, breathing with the mother, helping her into a more comfortable position when required and encouraging her to relax between contractions. A helpful massage oil can be made by blending the essential oils of CLARY SAGE, JASMINE and ROSE into a vegetable-oil base. This feels wonderful when it is massaged firmly into the lower back by your companion. Alternatively, a few drops of essential oil of BERGAMOT or LAVENDER added to some water in a plant spray can be sprayed around the birth room to freshen and disinfect the atmosphere.

The herb BLUE COHOSH may be taken throughout labour to tone the uterus and keep the contractions strong and regular. Make a decoction and drink a cupful every hour, or use the tincture. If labour becomes protracted and the strength of the contractions seems to be waning, then BLUE COHOSH may be safely used to strengthen and support the action of the uterus. The dosage should be one size 'O' capsule every half-hour.

There are many homoeopathic remedies that can be invaluable during labour. It is ideal if you can have a homoeopath present at the birth to prescribe for you when needed, so if you have previously consulted one, ask her if she will attend your labour. We can mention a few remedies that will be useful for you, your companion and preferably your midwife to know about here. If the mother becomes very fearful and anxious for any reason during labour, try ACONITE 30 or 200; if she becomes totally exhausted during a long labour then try CARBO VEG 30 or 200. When contractions are weak and irregular, or stop altogether, try CAULOPHYLLUM 30 or 200. If the mother becomes anxious and trembles, and the contractions are not productive, try GELSEMIUM 30 or 200. If she becomes irritable and weepy, and the labour pains are weak, try PULSATILLA 30 or 200.

Towards the end of the first stage of labour, just before the cervix dilates to its full 10 centimetres, the contractions become much more painful, longer and with less time to relax between them. This period is called transition and may be accompanied by nausea, vomiting, trembling and feelings of irritability. Fortunately, transition only lasts a short time – from between one contraction to half an hour, or, rarely, a couple of hours – and some women do not experience it at all. With positive encouragement all women who have made it this far can get through transition without pain-relieving drugs. This is important because drugs at this late stage in labour are likely to have a detrimental effect on the newborn baby's breathing. If the mother complains that the pain is unbearable and becomes very irritable, then the homoeopathic remedy CHAMOMILLA can be given in 30C or 200C to give some relief.

The second stage of labour begins with the complete dilatation of the cervix and ends with the delivery of the baby. During this stage, the baby descends as it is pushed downwards by the uterine muscles with the help of the abdominal muscles and the diaphragm. The amniotic membranes usually rupture during this stage if they have not done so already.

The urge to push gets stronger as the baby gets lower. The contractions may be further apart, and the degree and timing of the pushing urge may vary with each contraction. Advocates of natural childbirth now believe that once the cervix is fully dilated, the right time to push is when you want to, and that it is not helpful to encourage a mother to push when the urge is not there. The most helpful image at this stage is of opening up and breathing out the baby, not becoming tense by straining to push too hurriedly. Try BLACK COHOSH and MOTHERWORT after RASPBERRY LEAF and SQUAW VINE.

Different positions may be tried during this stage. Some women prefer squatting, kneeling or being supported from behind, and standing. The old-fashioned idea of making a woman lie flat on her back during second-stage labour was based on making it easier for the doctor to intervene, not on helping the mother to give birth.

Towards the end of the second stage you may begin to feel a hot, tingling sensation around the vagina; this occurs as the baby's head begins to press against and stretch the perineum. It means that his head is about to crown and that the birth is imminent. At this stage it is important to try and relax, not push too hard, and ease or breathe the baby out, otherwise you may tear the perineum before it has a chance to stretch fully. Trying to keep your mouth and lips loose can have a relaxing influence on the muscles of the vagina.

Your baby's head will emerge following a contraction, then the baby's whole body will slip out. The mother can reach out her arms and embrace and welcome the baby.

The third stage of labour is the delivery of the placenta. The placenta begins to separate naturally from the inner lining of the uterus as soon as the baby is born. Within about 45 minutes the placenta is expelled by the final contractions. If you want to deliver the placenta naturally it is important not to have the umbilical cord clamped until it has stopped pulsating, to remain in a squatting or kneeling position if necessary to allow gravity to assist the expulsion, and to push down if the midwife suggests you should.

In western countries, it has become the habit to clamp the umbilical cord as soon as the baby has been born and to give the mother an injection of Ergometrine or Syntometrine, which contracts the uterus and expels the placenta rapidly. However, this speeding up of the third stage tends to increase the incidence of retained placenta and maternal blood loss. It should be possible to reserve the use of Ergometrine or Syntometrine for those cases where the women is bleeding excessively and things need to be hurried up.

Clamping the umbilical cord before it stops pulsating has the disadvantages of depriving the baby of blood which is rightly its own, of cutting off the oxygen supply to the baby and throwing it onto its own resources, and prolonging the length of the third stage. However, if an injection of Ergometrine is given, it is important to have the umbilical cord clamped to prevent the baby receiving too much blood too quickly and then developing jaundice.

If you are hoping to deliver the placenta naturally and things do not seem to be happening fast enough, there are some herbs that can help the process. ANGELICA ROOT, RASPBERRY LEAF and SHEPHERD'S PURSE may be taken as a decoction; one cup is usually enough, although another may be taken after half an hour if necessary. You can also try BLACK or BLUE COHOSH: drink a cupful of the decoction, or take ten drops of the tincture.

❋ Haemorrhage

A postpartum haemorrhage is defined as blood loss of more than 500ml (just less than 1 pint) within 24 hours of delivery. The bleeding may come on very suddenly by gushing out or, more usually, it may be constant but moderate over a period of hours. The causes of postpartum haemorrhage may be when the uterus does not contract sufficiently after delivery of the placenta; failure to expel all of the placenta from the uterus; bleeding from lacerations in the cervix or lower segment of the uterus (for example, following the use of forceps); or a clotting disorder of the blood.

Postpartum haemorrhage is a very serious situation and can be life threatening if it is severe. The orthodox management of a haemorrhage like this is an injection of Syntometrine, and if it is severe, a blood transfusion.

There are natural remedies that have been used over the years to deal with postpartum haemorrhage, but you will probably need a midwife who is confident about the properties of natural medicine or a practitioner such as a herbalist or homoeopath present, in order to be given the chance to try these first. One effective herbal treatment that has been used to stop uterine haemorrhage is a combination of GOLDENSEAL, RASPBERRY LEAF and SHEPHERD'S PURSE: a decoction of these should be made in advance to drink if necessary, or take the tinctures.

Homoeopathic remedies that have been used successfully to treat postpartum haemorrhage include ARNICA, if the haemorrhage is due to lacerations or trauma; CAULOPHYLLUM, if the labour has been long and exhausting and the uterus is too weak to contract; IPECAC, if the bleeding is sudden and profuse, and especially if the mother feels nauseous; and SABINA, if the blood is dark and there are severe pains in the uterine area. These homoeopathic remedies need to be given in a fairly high potency, say 200C to work quickly and effectively.

❋ Caesarean Birth

During a Caesarean section, the act of delivery is taken over from the mother by the surgeon. An opening is cut into the abdomen of the mother and the baby is lifted out.

Despite many drawbacks to the mother and infant, the rate of Caesarean sections has risen dramatically in western countries since the 1970s. As with most methods of obstetric control, this intervention can be the wonderful use of life-saving technology but only too often it is performed routinely, for reasons such as the doctor's desire to control nature, fear and for the convenience of medical staff.

The most frequent situation that leads to a Caesarean section is when labour is slow (dystocia). Planning your labour ahead and thinking about such things as how you would cope with a long, tiring labour, whether you have the freedom to move about, have a bath or rest, and if you will be with a companion and midwife committed to natural birth can be really important in avoiding an unnecessary Caesarean delivery.

Other common reasons for Caesarean births are repeat Caesareans, breech births and foetal distress. A repeat Caesarean section is often performed because it is feared that the scar from the previous operation may rupture. If the labour is managed carefully, and oxytocin is avoided, many women can in fact go on to have a perfectly normal vaginal delivery. If you want to have a go at a normal birth following a Caesarean, you will have to press your doctor and midwife for a 'trial of labour'.

Caesarean sections are given for breech births on the basis that when the baby is born bottom-first there is a chance of a hold-up with the delivery of the head and then the baby will be starved of oxygen. However, studies have shown that the risk to the baby from a vaginal breech delivery is no greater than that from a Caesarean section. Certainly you should be able to opt for a trial of labour if you have a normal-sized pelvis, the baby is not very large, and if the baby is curled up with its head leaning forward onto its chest (frank breech).

Try to be well-nourished and rested when labour starts to avoid the likelihood of foetal distress. Decline induction, oxytocin stimulation and drugs during labour. Move about when you want to, lie down on your side rather than your back, rest and relax when possible, breathe deeply between contractions, and avoid prolonged breath-holding and over-straining.

The main disadvantages of a Caesarean section are that the risk of mortality to the mother increases by 400 per cent, it is more likely to result in an infection in the mother and it is more likely to result in breathing difficulties for the baby after delivery.

If it is necessary for you to have a Caesarean there are lots of natural remedies that you can use afterwards to lessen the impact of such a major operation. Herbs to take internally to promote healing and reduce the chance of an infection developing include COMFREY, ECHINACEA, MARIGOLD, MARSHMALLOW and RASPBERRY LEAF. These may be combined and taken as a decoction (or as tinctures) three times a day for up to a month after the birth. Taking homoeo-pathic ARNICA immediately after the Caesarean will help to prevent infection and promote healing. Take either a couple of doses of 200C or one 30C dose a day for five days. The homoeopathic remedy BELLIS PERENNIS is also very useful after a Caesarean to relieve discomfort and promote tissue healing. Try taking 30C each day for five days following the ARNICA. If, after two or three weeks, there is still a lot of abdominal discomfort, or the wound is slow to heal, try taking the homoeopathic remedy STAPHYSAGRIA. One dose of 200C should be sufficient.

Externally, compresses can be used to promote healing, soothe inflamma-tion and prevent an infection developing (but not on raw stitches). A suitable compress can be made from an infusion of the herbs COMFREY, MARIGOLD and ST JOHN'S WORT. This should be applied using clean lint when the infusion has cooled to blood temperature. Alternatively, a compress can be made using a few drops of the essential oils of LAVENDER, MYRRH and TEA TREE added to warm water. Once the wound has closed over then COMFREY ointment can be massaged in daily to reduce scarring.

After the Birth

Once the baby has been born, we begin the time of physical readjustment and healing, getting to know the baby and adjusting to our new role of being a mother. A few hours after the birth, your body will start to return to its normal, non-pregnant condition.

If this is your second or subsequent baby, you may feel afterpains, which occur as the uterus contracts back to its normal size (involution). Afterpains are not usually experienced with first babies because the uterus has not been stretched so much. These cramps may last several days, and can be quite strong, especially when breastfeeding. The homoeopathic tissue salt MAG PHOS 6X may be taken every few hours for up to five days to relieve the pain of the spasms. If they are very severe, and particularly if they make you feel irritable, then try the homoeopathic remedy CHAMOMILLA. A herbal combination that will relieve afterpains at the same time as helping the uterus to readjust can be made from BLACK COHOSH, BLUE COHOSH, CRAMPBARK and RASPBERRY LEAF. Make a decoction to drink three times a day for a few days, or use the tinctures. Alternatively, try adding a few drops of the antispasmodic essential oils of CHAMOMILE, LAVENDER or MARJORAM to a warm bath, or apply to the abdomen as a warm compress.

For a few weeks following the birth you can expect to have a vaginal discharge. It will change during this time from being bloody to pinkish-brown to yellowish-white. This discharge, called lochia, should not smell bad; if it does begin to smell bad at any time, seek urgent medical advice because this is a sign of infection. Also, seek advice if the lochia is still bloody after a few days because this may indicate that some placental tissue remains in the uterus. Other symptoms that should lead you to take urgent medical advice, are persistent abdominal pain, the inability to urinate, any feelings of feverishness or a temperature that rises above 38°C.

If you have been unfortunate enough to tear or have had an episiotomy during labour, there are several remedies that you can use to relieve the discomfort and promote healing. Internally, the homoeopathic remedies to compare are first ARNICA; if the stitches are very painful, HYPERICUM; if the wound is slow to heal, CALENDULA. Externally, take sitz baths containing an infusion of the healing herbs COMFREY, MARIGOLD and ST JOHN'S WORT. A poltice made of CHAMOMILE, GOLDENSEAL, MARIGOLD LEAF, MARSHMALLOW LEAF and SLIPPERY ELM in gauze and held against the perineum by a sanitary towel is very good. Alternatively, add a few drops of the essential oils of CHAMOMILE, CYPRESS and/or LAVENDER to the warm water in a sitz bath. Use a clean washing-up bowl or a baby bath (if you are small) for a sitz bath. Pour warm water into the bowl, then add the infusion of herbs or the essential oils and lower yourself into the water for several minutes. Dry yourself carefully when you get out. Ideally, you should take a sitz bath two or three times a day at first, less frequently as you begin to heal up.

Feeling tired after the birth of a child is very common and most women feel exhausted for a while at some point in the weeks after delivery. This is not surprising when you consider the tremendous hard work and emotional intensity of the birth, the sweeping hormonal changes that are occurring at this time and the irregular sleeping pattern that having a new baby involves. Having help around the house and with other children and getting plenty of rest after the birth are the first requirements in dealing with this.

There is an excellent Chinese herb that has been used by thousands of women over the centuries in China to restore energy and tonify the blood and generative organs following childbirth: CHINESE ANGELICA (DANG GUI). This is available as a tincture (take 5ml in water three times a day), or as a herb, so you will need to make a decoction *(see page 189 for details)*. Other herbs you can try at this time are ANGELICA, ELDERBERRY and LIQUORICE. If you are exhausted after losing a large amount of blood during labour, consider the homoeopathic remedy CHINA. If you are anaemic following childbirth, check the suggestions under Anaemia *(see page 38)*.

If your tiredness seems to be directly related to having your sleeping pattern disturbed, try taking the homoeopathic tissue salt KALI PHOS 6X three times a day for up to ten days. If you just feel generally weary and exhausted, then the Bach remedy OLIVE can help you to keep going. All these remedies should be compared in the *Materia Medica* section of this book to check that they are suitable.

Immediately after the birth you may feel excited and relieved about the arrival of your baby. It is not unusual for this to be followed after a couple of days by a sudden feeling of deflation when you feel exhausted and achy. The breast milk comes in around the third day and this is a common time for the 'baby blues', when you may feel depressed and tearful. This feeling of depression only lasts a day or two for most women, but if it becomes severe, or persists for more than a couple of days, then do talk to your doctor or natural therapist urgently, because postnatal depression can become a serious and ongoing problem if it is not dealt with properly in its early stages.

For mild postnatal blues, a herbal tonic to balance the hormones and nervous system may be made from BALM, BLACK COHOSH, BORAGE and OATS. Make a decoction to drink three times a day or take the tinctures. Essential oils that will have a good uplifting and antidepressant effect include GERANIUM, LAVENDER, MELISSA, NEROLI and ROSE. Choose one or two of these to be diluted in vegetable oil for a massage, or add a couple of drops of one to a warm bath.

15

The Reproductive System

It is the female reproductive system, more than any other sphere of bodily activity, that needs to be claimed back by the individual woman, away from the domain of male attitudes and invasive treatments. Attitudes and expectations about the processes of the woman's reproductive system have an enormous effect on the functioning of this system, and how these functions are experienced. The dominance of male attitudes over female processes has even led to certain natural functions being treated as illnesses or indispositions, as in the case of pregnancy and menstruation. It has become very difficult to have a positive attitude to certain natural and life-enriching experiences because of negative expectations around them. For example menstruation is treated as a 'curse' and 'proof' of a woman's changeability and unreliability.

The woman's sexual system connects her to the ever-changing rhythms of life. Just as everything in our universe is cyclic – the change from day to night, the yearly seasons, the cycle of life and death itself – so every aspect of a woman's reproductive system is cylic, from the menstrual cycle itself to the cycle of pre-pubescent non-fertiliy through the fertile phase and on to post-menopausal non-fertility. The importance of staying in touch with these cycles, and hence in touch with the processes of life itself, cannot be overstressed. Forms of control that take a woman out of her natural cycles, such as the birth control pill, HRT and other forms of hormonal intervention, are removing her from her individual contact with the rhythms of life.

The woman's reproductive system is particularly susceptible to disease. The probable causes of this are partly psychological and partly physical. A woman's relationship with her creativity and her sexuality is tied up within this one system. In our male-dominated society, negative attitudes towards a woman's creative role and sexuality abound. Things are changing, but any woman who is at odds with herself as a creative and sexual being is bound to develop

The Reproductive System

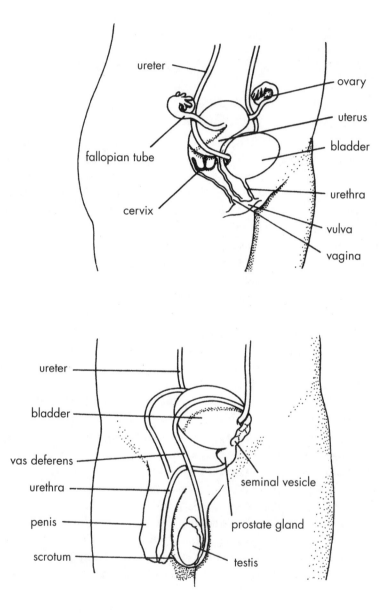

symptoms of disease to a greater or lesser extent, as tensions and negative patterns manifest themselves in her body. As these symptoms of disease develop and cause pain or irregularity, you can begin to feel less and less in control of your own processes, and out of touch with yourself as a naturally healthy woman. Breaking these negative patterns may well include consulting a professional practitioner, such as an acupuncturist who can redirect and unblock poor energy flows, or a skilled aromatherapist, herbalist or homoeopath.

Physical factors that influence the reproductive system include diet, hygiene and general lifestyle. Certain foods have been found to affect aspects of the reproductive system adversely. Caffeine has been found to contribute to fibroid and cyst formation, so it is wise to avoid coffee, coke, tea and other sources of caffeine. Mucus-producing foods such as dairy products and red meat generally reduce the ability of the uterus to clean itself out during menstruation and contribute to congestion. Alcohol is found to aggravate certain inflammatory complaints. Basically, a diet based primarily on fresh vegetables and whole-foods is going to reduce the amount of toxicity in the body generally, and symptoms of congestion and inflammation are less likely to develop in the reproductive system. A thorough cleansing diet has been found to be of great benefit in many reproductive system disorders, such as ovarian cysts, fibroids and endometriosis. A dietary therapist or naturopath will be able to guide you through a cleansing programme, or consult the one on page 423.

Hygiene is an important factor in the health of the reproductive system. The vagina is a delicately balanced mini-ecosystem. The vaginal walls are lined with a protective and self-cleansing mucous membrane. A healthy vagina contains numerous micro-organisms, among them lacto-bacilli, which help to create slightly acidic conditions that prevent infection by numerous disease-causing organisms. It is important not to introduce any substance into the vagina that may upset this pH balance. This includes most soaps and foaming bath products. If you use tampons they should be changed regularly, and if there is any dryness or irritation it is better to use sanitary towels.

Lifestyle may affect the reproductive system in many ways. Any form of stress or tension may cause you discomfort during the menstrual cycle, or you may feel more aware of discomfort. Anxiety and/or emotional trauma frequently disrupt the menstrual cycle. An irregular sleeping pattern or other lifecycle disturbances can also upset it. If the symptoms of discomfort or irregularity are prolonged, it is advisable to consult a professional practitioner to find out the causes of the problem.

⚘ Birth Control

A method of birth control that truly enhances a woman's overall health and well-being is not always easy to find. It often requires conscious commitment and sustained effort to employ the methods that are known not to harm your health. The positive side to this is that those unharmful methods tend to encourage us to be more aware of our bodies and to discuss and share responsibilities in our relationships.

The most simple-to-use and unharmful methods of contraception that are effective are the barrier methods: the condom (sheath) and the diaphragm (cap). Both these methods are very effective if they are used carefully and properly. The condom must be rolled onto the man's penis before there is any contact between it and the woman's genital area, as some sperm may come out with the drops of liquid that are emitted by the penis well before ejaculation (orgasm) occurs. Either partner may put the condom onto the penis as part of foreplay. Care should be taken not to tear the condom when rolling it onto the penis. When the man withdraws, one partner should hold the condom in place so that it does not fall off until withdrawal is complete.

In recent years condoms have escalated in popularity because they offer significant protection against the transmission of venereal infections, including AIDS, in addition to their use as a contraception. Used properly, a good-quality condom is 97 per cent effective as a method of contraception; in combination with a spermicidal jelly or cream, it offers close to 100 per cent protection. It may be advisable to use a condom in conjunction with a spermicide or diaphragm during the woman's fertile mid-cycle phase. Condoms are easily available in chemists and in many public lavatories, and they are free from family planning clinics.

The diaphragm is made of soft rubber and is shaped like a shallow dome that fits snugly over the cervix. It needs to be the right size and shape for each woman, so it should be fitted by someone with experience, such as a doctor or nurse at your local family planning clinic. It must always be used with a spermicidal cream or jelly to be effective, and must be inserted before there is any contact between the penis and the woman's genital area. If the diaphragm is used properly it is about 97 per cent effective, but if you are not very careful, its effectiveness drops to about 85–90 per cent. For extra protection, the man can wear a condom during his partner's fertile mid-cycle phase.

The disadvantages of the diaphragm and the condom are that you need to plan ahead or interrupt your lovemaking – which some people find off-putting. The added disadvantage of the diaphragm is that the spermicide is rather messy and it can cause irritation in a small number of women. The disadvantage of the condom is that some men say that it reduces the penis's sensitivity during intercourse.

Both the condom and the diaphragm may be used in conjunction with another, totally unharmful method of contraception called 'natural birth control'. In fact, there are several ways of working out this method, but the aim of them all is to establish when the woman is ovulating and to avoid intercourse at that time.

The most traditional form of natural birth control is that advocated by the Roman Catholic Church and known as the rhythm or calendar method. This is based on the fact that ovulation usually occurs about 14 days before the start of the next period, so if a woman has a fairly regular cycle she can use the length of past menstrual cycles to calculate the probable time of ovulation. This method has quite a high failure rate because it cannot take individual cycle fluctuation into account. In recent years, far more accurate methods of working out the time of ovulation have been developed, including the basal temperature chart and the cervical mucus chart. There are several good books on the market explaining how these methods work and how to draw up a chart for yourself; one of the clearest books is *Natural Birth Control* by Katia and Jonathan Drake (Thorsons, 1984).

In practice natural birth control methods mean that for just over half of the monthly cycle no extra contraceptive protection is needed, and for the rest of the time lovemaking which does not involve intercourse can be explored, or one of the barrier methods of contraception should be used. The success rate of natural birth control depends greatly on how carefully the cycle is worked out and followed, and the statistical success rate varies accordingly. It was found to be 98 per cent effective when the basal temperature chart method was carefully used, and around 90 per cent effective for women who stated that they intended to use this method to space the births of their children rather than to avoid pregnancy totally.

In contrast to the effective methods of birth control that are unharmful, there are those methods that are effective but carry a risk to the health of the woman using them. The intra-uterine device (IUD or coil) is a thin piece of bent plastic, metal or some other material that is inserted into the uterus for months or years to prevent pregnancy. It is not known exactly how the device works but it seems that it causes an inflammation of the endometrium (uterine lining), which probably prevents the fertilized egg from implanting itself in the lining.

An IUD must be fitted by a qualified nurse or doctor; it is effective against pregnancy immediately, although spontaneous expulsion from the uterus is not uncommon during the first few months after insertion. If the IUD remains in position, it is about 96 per cent effective in preventing pregnancy. For those women who do become pregnant with an IUD in place, the consequences are often serious: there is a 50 per cent chance of miscarriage. If a woman with an IUD does get pregnant it should be removed immediately to prevent infection.

There is also considerable risk of an ectopic pregnancy if you use an IUD (this is when the fertilized ovum implants itself in the Fallopian tube instead of the uterus). Ectopic pregnancies are far more common amongst IUD users; they usually mean the loss of the affected Fallopian tube and they can be life-threatening. Any woman who has an IUD and suspects that she may be pregnant should seek urgent medical advice.

Apart from pregnancy, the main complication of the IUD is a much higher incidence of pelvic infection. Such infections can be mild but if they are severe they can also become life-threatening. Any woman with signs of pelvic infection, such as abdominal pain or tenderness, fever or an unusual discharge, should seek urgent medical attention.

An IUD should never be used by women who have previously had an ectopic pregnancy, pelvic inflammatory disease, gonorrhoea, fibroids, endometriosis, endometrial hyperplasia, heavy periods, heart disease or diabetes. In addition, young women who have had no children should not be fitted with an IUD because of the greatly increased risk of pelvic infection which often leads to sterility.

Despite their disadvantages, about 50 million women throughout the world currently use an IUD, and for those who experience no complications it represents a reliable, convenient and reversible form of contraception.

The birth control pill (oral contraceptive) is a hormone preparation taken to prevent pregnancy that has been available since 1961. It was the first convenient method of contraception that offered nearly 100 per cent protection against pregnancy and it has been hailed as being responsible for the revolution in sexuality that has been occurring since its introduction. While the loosening up of old-fashioned and rigid attitudes to sex is arguably a good thing in many ways, unfortunately this has been at a cost to the health of a great many women.

The most common birth control pills combine the hormones oestrogen and progesterone, and are taken daily on a monthly cycle. The synthetic oestrogen released by the pill raises the woman's oestrogen levels enough to simulate pregnancy and checks the natural cyclic process that would normally result in an egg being released by the ovary. This means that during the time a woman is on the pill, her ovaries are relatively inactive and no egg is released to be fertilized by a sperm. The synthetic progesterone component of the pill provides two extra contraceptive criteria: it increases the viscosity of cervical mucus and alters the development of the uterine lining.

In theory the pill offers 99.5 per cent protection against pregnancy, but in practice it is more like 95 per cent. This is usually because women forget to take the pill for a day or the hormone content is lost before it can be absorbed because of vomiting or diarrhoea. The effects of the pill are supposed to be totally reversible: if a woman wants to become pregnant she simply stops taking the pills at the end of a packet. However, it is not uncommon to miss several periods when you stop taking the pill, and it can take several cycles before the ovaries function regularly again. The long-term incidence of infertility is higher for those women who have been on the pill, particularly for those women who have not had any children before taking it.

Much of the evidence about the risks and side-effects involved in taking the birth control pill appears to be contradictory, and sometimes it varies greatly according to the source of the information. Unfortunately, the medical profession does not receive ongoing training specifically in contraception, and most of the information that they do receive is given out by the drug companies that produce the pills, which can hardly be expected to be impartial. Some women feel that the Family Planning Association itself often plays down the risks involved in taking the pill, and this may be because they consider that their most important role is to advise women on how to avoid pregnancy, over and above any other factors.

The pill enters the bloodstream and travels around the body affecting many tissues, glands and organs as it goes, just as natural hormones do. It is not surprising then that the side-effects and complications of taking the pill are very varied. Some women experience side-effects, such as nausea, headaches and weight gain, immediately; others may not have any at all until a great deal of damage has already been done. The more serious side-effects are an increased risk of blood clots, high blood pressure and other circulatory diseases, cervical cancer, thrush, depression, increased susceptibility to venereal infections, gall bladder disease, epilepsy and liver tumours. It seems that women on the pill suffer from viral infections more than others, so there is evidence that the pill generally undermines the immune system.

In addition to the physical side-effects, all hormones, whether they are natural or taken in artificial form, have an effect on emotional balance (just as they do during pregnancy or with premenstrual tension), so we are also manipulating our emotional well-being by taking the pill.

When you come off the pill it can be good to take some herbs to help the body readjust its hormonal balance. Some useful herbs to consider are AGNUS CASTUS, BLACK COHOSH, BLUE COHOSH, FALSE UNICORN, SARSAPARILLA and WILD YAM. You can take a mixture of these herbs, but look them up in the *Materia Medica* section to check dosage and that they are particularly suitable for you.

Endometriosis

This is a condition where the kind of tissue that normally lines the uterus is also found growing in other places in the body. These are known as endometrial implants. Implants may be found on the ovaries and Fallopian tubes, on the peritoneum lining the pelvis, on and around the bowel and bladder, and unusually even outside the pelvic area.

The causes of endometriosis are not known, but it is a very common gynaecological problem, causing symptoms in an estimated 15 per cent of women. These range from mild discomfort in the abdominal area to severe pain. The severity of the pain is not necessarily linked to the severity of the disease, but probably depends more on the position of the implants. Pain can occur at any time during the menstrual cycle, for example linked to urinating or a bowel movement, but is most common for the week before and/or during menstruation. Endometriosis can be a cause of severely painful periods. Pain during intercourse (dyspareunia) is also not uncommon and is one of the symptoms that may lead to a possible diagnosis of the disease.

To understand why pain is caused you need to understand the nature of the endometrial implants. Uterine tissue is designed to respond to hormonal changes in the body during the menstrual cycle and it bleeds every time you have a period. The natural outlet for the uterus during menstruation is through the vagina and we experience that blood loss when we have a period. Endometrial implants will also be stimulated to bleed during menstruation, but there is no outlet for the blood, so it becomes trapped in the tissues, causing pain and inflammation and possibly leading to blood-filled cysts and scar tissue forming.

Endometriosis can seriously affect women's lives. The pain during menstruation can be so severe that women cannot work for a few days every month, or they plan all their activities and holidays to avoid the time of their period.

Intercourse can be painful, which may put strain on sexual relationships, and endometriosis can be a cause of infertility.

Nobody knows why endometrial implants grow outside the uterus, but there is evidently a strong link with the female hormones. The implants are particularly sensitive to oestrogen. Endometriosis is most common in women over 30 who have not had children, and this is why it is sometimes known as 'the career woman's disease'. This is probably because women who have lived a longer part of their life without breaks for pregnancy and breastfeeding have been exposed to more circulating oestrogen during their fertile years.

An estimated half of women with endometriosis will experience problems with fertility, and this is one reason why many women may find it more difficult to conceive during their thirties than they would earlier. Scar tissue can build up around the implants, damaging the Fallopian tubes or ovaries, and this may cause infertility.

Endometriosis can be difficult to diagnose and a definitive diagnosis is only possible by laparoscopy. Some surgeons say that you can find endometriosis in all women if you look hard enough, but obviously in some women the implants grow and cause problems and in other women they don't. On an energetic level, a woman affected by endometriosis needs to consider the blockages and flow of her creative energy.

The orthodox treatment of endometriosis is by hormonal drugs or by surgical removal. But unless the underlying causes are dealt with, the problem will tend to recur following treatment. Symptoms disappear during pregnancy, but they usually return after the birth. Fortunately, they do go completely after the menopause.

Because endometriosis is a chronic (long-term) disease, the best results with natural medicine will come from visiting a practitioner. Natural remedies combined with an enquiring approach into the energetic causes mentioned above can be very successful in both alleviating the symptoms and curing the disease. The following essential oils can be used in the bath or as a massage oil to bring relief to the symptoms of discomfort before and during the periods: CHAMOMILE, CYPRESS, LAVENDER, MARJORAM and ROSEMARY. Similarly, the homeopathic remedies of BELLADONNA, MAG PHOS and NUX VOM should be considered to help relieve painful periods. The chief herbal remedy used to balance the hormones and treat endometriosis is AGNUS CASTUS. The following herbs also relieve spasmodic pains before and during the period: CHAMOMILE, CRAMPBARK, GINGER, RASPBERRY LEAF and VALERIAN. Look them up in the *Materia Medica* section to see which are most appropriate for you.

✳ Fibroids

Fibroids are a type of benign (non-cancerous) tumour that grows in the womb. They consist of muscular and fibrous tissue enclosed in a capsule. They occur in an estimated 20 per cent of women over 35, and are more common in black women than in white.

Fibroids grow most commonly in the main part or body of the uterus, but they can also grow in the cervix or neck of the womb. Most fibroids of the body of the womb are multiple, while those of the cervix are often single. They may range in size from that of a small bean to a large grapefruit or even larger.

The symptoms of having fibroids arise from the effect of the swelling, which causes congestion of the womb or pressure on surrounding areas. Symptoms due to congestion include very heavy periods (menorrhagia) or bleeding in between the periods (metrorrhagia). The bleeding may be so heavy that some women also develop anaemia *(see Anaemia, page 38)*. The pressure on the abdominal veins may cause pain, retention of urine, varicose veins, swelling of the ankles and piles.

Some women have fibroids for many years but do not experience any adverse symptoms. Fibroids very rarely become malignant, so if they do not cause any distressing symptoms you can live with them for years without medical intervention. They usually shrink of their own accord and cause no further problems after the menopause.

The exact cause of fibroids is unknown, but increased levels of oestrogen will cause them to grow. For a few years prior to the menopause women often have a number of anovulatory cycles (without ovulating) and this causes a build-up of oestrogen which is not replaced by progesterone, so fibroids can become problematic just before the menopause. If present before conception, fibroids tend to grow during pregnancy when oestrogen levels are high. Despite such growth, they rarely interfere with the pregnancy, because they usually move up out of the way. If the fibroids do remain low in the pelvis, however, they may necessitate a Caesarean delivery. Very large fibroids may be a cause of infertility because they distort the uterus in such a way as to prevent conception.

The orthodox treatment of fibroids is by drugs to reduce heavy bleeding or by surgery. The drugs used to control bleeding do tend to produce side-effects and do not reduce the fibroids, thus the problem will return once the drugs are stopped. Surgery may attempt to just remove the fibroid (a myomectomy) or to remove the entire uterus (a hysterectomy).

Natural remedies for fibroids will work best if you also have an enquiring approach into what may be blocking the flow of creative energy in your life. The growth of fibroids indicates a blockage in your ability to express and manifest personal creativity.

Homoeopathy or acupuncture can be very helpful in the treatment of fibroids, but you will need to consult a qualified practitioner for ongoing treatment. Many women find that radically changing their diet can produce a huge improvement, particularly if they eliminate dairy produce, sugar, caffeine and wheat. Such a drastic change of eating habits may best be undertaken with the support of a naturopath or nutritional advisor. The following herbs may be considered to balance the hormones and reduce excessive bleeding, but again the best results will be obtained by consulting a qualified practitioner: AGNUS CASTUS, BETH ROOT, BLUE COHOSH, GOLDENSEAL, MOTHERWORT, SHEPHERD'S PURSE and YARROW.

Genital Herpes

Genital herpes is usually caused by the herpes simplex virus type II, although the herpes simplex virus type I that normally causes 'cold sores' around the mouth can also cause genital herpes. The symptoms of both types of virus are similar – the appearance of a group of small, painful, itchy blisters in the vaginal or anal area. The blisters are moist with red edges and when they burst they form a soft, acutely painful open sore. In addition to the local sores, there may also be the symptoms of feverishness, general malaise and swollen glands.

Genital herpes is one of the most common venereal diseases in Britain, particularly among women, who contract it far more often than men. Most women feel extremely angry and depressed when they first discover that they have contracted the disease, but although it is often a recurrent condition, the first attack is usually by far the worst, probably because no antibodies have built up in the body.

Untreated, the outbreak will usually clear up in two to three weeks. Individual outbreaks tend to be more likely during menstruation, pregnancy, emotional stress or when you are generally run down. Genital herpes can only be transmitted to someone else during an outbreak, so it is crucial to avoid sexual contact if there is any sign of a sore.

There appears to be a link between genital herpes and an increased risk of cervical cancer, so regular cervical smears are advised for herpes sufferers.

Pregnancy can be another complication for genital herpes sufferers. The baby is not normally affected before birth, but if the mother has a sore during labour the baby may become infected as he passes through the birth canal. The herpes virus can be dangerous for a baby, so if the mother has an attack at the time of the birth doctors normally advise her to have a Caesarean section.

All the medical prescriptions used to treat herpes are toxic to some degree, so natural remedies can be very helpful. Probably the best approach is to use remedies locally during an outbreak to relieve the symptoms, and boost the immune system with appropriate internal remedies and a cleansing diet to lessen the likelihood and/or severity of recurrent attacks.

To boost the immune system and help fight infection drink a decoction of CLEAVERS, ECHINACEA, GOTU KOLA and ST JOHN'S WORT (or take them as tinctures) three times a day for six weeks. Externally, dab on a strong dilution of the tinctures of GOLDENSEAL, MARIGOLD and MYRRH. Essential oils may also be applied locally; try dabbing on either BERGAMOT, LAVENDER or NIAOULI. The main homoeopathic remedies to consider are NAT MUR and RHUS TOX, although the best results will come from consulting a qualified homoeopath.

Infertility

When a woman finds out that she is not going to conceive easily it is often a devastating discovery. Most women assume that after a few months of unprotected intercourse the natural result is a pregnancy. When this does not happen, a woman often needs time for a profound and often prolonged reappraisal of her life's purpose and role as a woman.

A great deal of good can come out of such a reappraisal, whether or not the woman then goes on to have a baby. After all, to achieve a sense of fulfilment and satisfaction from one's own existence, without relying on one's children or the role of motherhood to provide it, is a very great achievement. This kind of self-reliance, however, is likely to be the very end result of learning to cope with a lot of disappointment, feelings of alienation and emotional realignment.

Some doctors state that infertility should be suspected after a couple have been having regular, unprotected intercourse for 12 months, although many others say that two years is a more realistic time-span. The age of the woman is a significant factor in terms of her fertility; in general, the older a woman is, the less fertile it is considered she will be. It seems that fertility usually declines throughout a woman's twenties, often to have an upsurge in her early thirties, and then declines more rapidly after the age of 35. With many women postponing starting a family until their late twenties or early thirties these days, infertility is becoming a common situation, affecting an estimated 15 per cent of couples.

Women over 30 who are anxious about not conceiving immediately can feel a lot of extra pressure because of the sense that they are running out of time. In fact, although many doctors and clinics start running tests and offering treatment to women in this age-group after only a year of unprotected intercourse, in one large study of women over 30 who became pregnant, three-quarters of them had not been using contraceptives for two to three years.

The orthodox treatment of infertility has rapidly become a highly technological and specialized branch of medicine based on a great deal of research and experimentation. The success rates of the most technologically-advanced techniques for establishing pregnancy – those involving in vitro fertilization (IVF) – are very poor (around 15–20 per cent). Unfortunately, the combination of many women's desperation to become pregnant and the prestige of genetic research within the field of science has led to a burgeoning of commercial clinics and drug-company interest to find highly-technological solutions to infertility. Another problem is that very often more than one egg is implanted in the woman and now IVF is responsible for a large increase in the number of multiple births. In very many cases, it is not primarily the overall well-being of the individual woman concerned that is considered before these methods are employed. This is especially surprising when you consider that it will be her body and hormonal system that will be controlled and manipulated by the processes involved, with only a slim chance of the result that she desires.

There are many natural methods of improving the chances of conception. Timing intercourse to coincide with ovulation is very important. Ovulation usually occurs about 14 days before the next menstrual period, so if your periods are fairly regular you can work out roughly which day of the cycle ovulation is likely. There are many books on the market on infertility or natural birth control that show how to draw up a fertility basal temperature chart, which can be used to determine on which day ovulation occurs, if you want to be more exact. If possible, it is ideal to make love on alternate days for the few days preceding and around ovulation. The temperature chart can also be used to establish whether or not you are ovulating and if not, then steps to stimulate ovulation should be considered.

The position you choose during lovemaking is also important to maximize the chances of conception. Generally, the best position is for the woman to be on her back, with her knees raised in the air, and for her partner to be on top, penetrating as deeply as is possible and comfortable for both of them. She should remain on her back, with her legs raised, for half an hour afterwards. A pillow placed under the woman's hips either during or just after intercourse encourages the sperm to come into contact with the cervix. If the woman has an orgasm after the man, the uterus acts like a vacuum during the contractions of her orgasm, and actually sucks up the sperm into the Fallopian tubes hundreds of times faster than they could swim there under their own steam.

Putting these suggestions into practice can make sex seem rather mechanical, but the important things are to be patient with your body and to remember that sex is a fun and sharing experience, just as it probably was before you started trying to get pregnant.

If, after a year or more of trying these methods, you are still not conceiving, it is time to consider visiting an infertility clinic to try and establish if there is anything preventing conception. If you are an established couple, it is important for both of you to attend the clinic from the outset, because the chances of a man having reduced fertility are about the same as for a woman. In about 40 per cent of cases infertility is attributed to the woman, and in about 40 per cent of cases it is attributed to the man; in the remaining 20 per cent of cases problems are found in both partners, or no cause is discovered at all.

The most common cause of infertility in men is a low sperm count. There may be several factors involved here. One of the main causes is an excess of alcohol: even two or three pints of beer a day is enough to affect a man's sperm. Obviously if a couple is trying to conceive it is advisable for both partners to drink small amounts of alcohol only occasionally. Another frequent cause of reduced fertility in men is that they wear underpants or trousers that are too tight: the testicles need to be a degree or two cooler than the rest of the body to be able to manufacture sperm efficiently, and if they are close up against the body they can become overheated.

Herbs that will increase the sperm count are HE SHOU WU (FLEECEFLOWER ROOT) and SAW PALMETTO BERRIES. These may be combined with known aphrodisiacs, if appropriate, such as DAMIANA and GINSENG. Consult the *Materia Medica* for individual suitability and dosage. To treat the more serious causes of male infertility such as obstruction of the sperm ducts or endocrine problems, professional advice by a qualified therapist of natural medicine should be sought.

Treating infertility in a woman by natural means should involve both the treatment of any specific problem inhibiting conception, and maximizing her general health. Improving her overall well-being will often increase her chances of conception because a generally toxic system reduces fertility.

A diet to improve fertility should include plenty of fresh fruit and vegetables, wholegrains and seeds to strengthen the conception vessel. If symptoms of toxicity are present (such as a dark, clotted menstrual flow, a tendency to colds and infections, constipation and so on) then a cleansing diet can be of great benefit: consult a dietary therapist or naturopath for guidance or turn to the one in this book on page 423. Foods containing chemicals and additives, excess salt, excess red meat and coffee should generally be avoided. Alcohol should be kept to a minimum, and smoking and the taking of any kind of drugs should be avoided. Sufficient vitamin E is particularly important for the reproductive organs, so eat lots of wholegrain cereals such as brown rice, oats and wheatgerm. It can also be helpful to take wheatgerm oil capsules which are a naturally rich source of vitamin E.

If there is a specific problem which is known to be inhibiting conception, such as endometriosis, blocked Fallopian tubes, fibroids, an absence of ovulation, or polycystic ovaries, then careful treatment by a qualified practitioner of natural medicine should be sought so that it can be overcome. Most practitioners of alternative medicine have had patients who came to them because they were infertile, often after many tests and treatments, and then went on to conceive after a course of treatment by homoeopathy, acupuncture, aromatherapy, naturopathy or herbalism, to name a few. Obviously, this depends on the severity of the factors inhibiting fertility, but most practitioners have had some seemingly miraculous results.

If there is no known specific cause of infertility, then consult the following remedies in the *Materia Medica* section of this book and try them out if they seem appropriate. The herb AGNUS CASTUS will promote fertility in cases where a hormonal imbalance is suspected. FALSE UNICORN ROOT helps to regulate the ovaries and strengthen the endometrium. MOTHERWORT is a good general tonic for the reproductive system. If a woman is suffering from stress, either generally or because she is not conceiving, BALM, PASSIFLORA and SKULLCAP should also be considered.

The main essential oils that are traditionally used to treat infertility are GERANIUM, MELISSA and ROSE. These may be combined and diluted in a vegetable-oil base and massaged over the abdomen on a daily basis, or add a couple of drops of the most appropriate oil or combined oils to a warm bath on a regular basis. It should be said, however, that the best results will probably come from a regular massage by a trained aromatherapist, who can choose specific oils on an individual basis, and combine the aromatherapy treatment with dietary advice and stress counselling.

⚘ Menopause

Growing older does not have to be just a process of losing our youth, looks and energy. There can be benefits, though they are not always obvious. Maybe these have almost been kept a secret for fear that they will be misunderstood. One problem is that we are so attached to the culture that promotes youth and energy that it is hard to recognize that the changes of ageing can start a time of becoming free from the demands of fashion, youthful looks and material success.

With ageing, our faces develop the lines and folds that reflect the maturing character. As we pass beyond the childbearing age, we change our sense of responsibility. We are free from the need to conceive or free from the fear of getting pregnant. Our focus shifts to appreciate that we can have a new and different role within society. Although this can be a painful process, as we start to reflect on what we have achieved, we can become truer to ourselves. In this way, we have the opportunity to become wiser as we are able to think for ourselves and speak more openly, and we realize that there is indeed a role for the elders in society.

Menopause is an initiation into the next phase of life. We enter a world where we can offer our experience and wisdom and act as guides to the following generations. In this phase we become aware of a world that has been balanced by the presence of older generations and their contributions to the family, the community and society. We can now become part of this new group, where we have the potential to become what is really needed in this society – real people, leaders and wise women.

How do we deal with this stage of transition? As with any time of change, it is not always easy and can throw up problems and symptoms that need to be dealt with before we can move on to the new phase in our lives. Just as puberty can be a time of stormy emotional upheavals as we make the transition from child to young woman, so menopause can throw up both emotional and physical symptoms as we adjust physically and emotionally from being someone who is probably younger-looking and fertile to being a more mature woman who is unable to bear children.

A woman's ability to adjust emotionally to life following the menopause will be greatly influenced by how much she values her life and role within society beyond being a mother. If she has identified herself only as a mother – in the valuable role of caring for and nurturing her children – and hasn't developed other abilities and interests sufficiently, then the menopause, which probably coincides with her children becoming independent, may seem to be a time when everything fulfilling in life disappears. Women who have managed to combine an interest in the world and society with their family life can look forward to life beyond the menopause as a time of greater freedom when they pursue their personal wants and needs.

How you cope with the menopause physically is determined by the body's ability to ride the huge hormonal changes that are sweeping through the system at this time. As hormones strongly affect our moods this can have a marked knock-on effect on our emotional well-being as well. Some women go through the menopause with few or no inconvenient symptoms. Many experience symptoms to the extent that they recognize the need for some assistance in helping their bodies to make the adjustments, or they put up with the bothersome symptoms and discomforts until they subside. But for a number of other women, the symptoms are severe enough to considerably disrupt their lives and pose a serious threat to their health. These women need careful and professional treatment to help them through this time.

The menopause usually occurs between the ages of 45 and 53, but it can happen quite normally several years earlier or later than that. Menopause beginning before the age of 40 is considered to be premature and requires investigation to rule out any underlying disease. A sudden menopause will occur if both of a woman's ovaries are removed (oophorectomy).

The symptoms that herald the onset of the menopause are often changes in the menstrual cycle. A variety of menstrual changes may be experienced: periods may become lighter and/or less frequent or heavier and/or more frequent. These irregularities are caused by the hormonal changes that are occurring. During menopause the pituitary gland signals to the ovaries to produce less oestrogen, ovulation also becomes less frequent and eventually menstruation tapers off. The menopause is usually complete when there has been no sign of menstruation for one year.

Although ovulation happens less frequently during the menopause, it is still possible to become pregnant. Birth control methods are necessary until you have not had a period for at least 12 months, to prevent an unwanted conception. There is a health risk involved in taking the birth control pill or using an IUD during the menopause, so it is advisable to use one of the safer barrier methods, such as a diaphragm or condom.

Some irregularity of the menstrual cycle is common during menopause. But if you experience extremely heavy bleeding, periods that are more frequent than every 21 days, prolonged staining between the periods or bleeding after there have been no periods for 12 months, you should get a medical diagnosis to rule out serious disease.

Obviously, the fitter a woman is generally, the better equipped she is to deal with menopausal changes. However, if you are experiencing specific symptoms that are distressing, or severe, or persist despite following the suggestions that we outline here, then professional treatment with a qualified therapist is necessary. One basic but crucial factor that can ease the passage through this time is sufficient rest. Giving yourself permission to rest more while your body is accommodating these massive hormonal changes can make the world of difference to your well-being. Regular although preferably not excessive exercise, such as walking, cycling or swimming, will help your body to remain fit and supple.

Diet is another part of your lifestyle that can help considerably during this time. Some foods actually contain hormone-like substances that can help to cushion the adjustment of the menopause. These foods include soya, pulses, wholegrains, seeds, carrots, ripe bananas, apples, royal jelly and bee pollen. Foods to be avoided are any containing chemicals, coffee and salt, and excessive alcohol.

We do not necessarily advise you to take synthetically-produced vitamins or minerals, because an individual's response to and requirement of these potent supplements is very variable. However, there are some food supplements that can be very beneficial during the menopause. Vitamin E helps to keep the reproductive organs healthy and also helps to keep the skin supple. KELP TABLETS are a useful source of iodine and a range of other minerals that can help improve your general vitality and help to prevent weight gain and depression. EVENING PRIMROSE OIL contains essential fatty acids that can help with menopausal symptoms and also help to keep nerves and skin healthy. ROYAL JELLY contains beneficial hormone-like substances and vitamin B complex, and can be taken as a tonic either in capsule form or preserved naturally in honey. The amount of vitamin B complex in your diet may need to be increased to help combat stress and depression. Foods naturally rich in the vitamin B complex are fish, free-range eggs, brown rice, wheatgerm, sesame seeds and Brewer's yeast.

Herbal remedies can prove to be very useful in assisting the body through the menopause. Useful herbs to help balance the hormones and tone the reproductive system are AGNUS CASTUS, BLACK COHOSH, FALSE UNICORN, MOTHERWORT, OATS, RED CLOVER, ST JOHN'S WORT and WILD YAM. Check all these suggestions in the *Materia Medica* section of this book to help select those that are particularly suitable for you. If anxiety or depression is present with other menopausal symptoms then consider adding SKULLCAP and VERVAIN to the above. Both acupuncture and homoeopathy have had excellent results in helping women to overcome problems associated with the menopause, but you really need constitutional treatment by a qualified practitioner to get the best results.

Some women have found natural progesterone cream based on WILD YAM to be very helpful to use during the menopause. This is a controversial product, however, with some sources saying it is unlikely to be effective. *(See* the Resources section at the back for suppliers.)

Essential oils can be a very pleasant way to ease menopausal symptoms. GERANIUM essential oil is said to be a hormonal balancer and should be used regularly, diluted in a vegetable-oil base as a massage oil or added to a warm bath. ROSE essential oil has useful tonifying and detoxifying effects on the reproductive system and will work well combined with GERANIUM. If you are particularly anxious or depressed then consider using CHAMOMILE or NEROLI. If you are in doubt about which oils are the best to use, then consult an experienced aromatherapist who will give you a wonderfully soothing massage, as well as helpful advice about diet and lifestyle. *(See also* Osteoporosis, page 79.)

HOT FLUSHES

One very common symptom of the menopause is hot flushes. These can be bothersome but easily tolerated, or they can become frequent, severe and very distressing. Hot flushes are caused by the body's struggle to adjust to the hormonal changes occurring at this time. The flushes usually cease once the body has adjusted to its lower oestrogen levels, but they may persist for several years.

The process of a hot flush usually begins when the body gets overheated. It seems that the brain overreacts to the fact that the body is warm and initiates a series of changes in the nervous system which cause the body to try to cool itself down. To do this the blood vessels near the surface of the skin dilate and blood pours through the vessels, bringing heat and redness to the skin. In this way, the heat radiates outwards, there is perspiration, and evaporation of the sweat cools the body down again. The experience feels like a sudden flush of heat, usually to the face, neck and chest, often followed immediately afterwards by perspiration, shivering and a chilled feeling.

The flushing process can occur even if a woman doesn't feel herself to be hot initially, but being overly warm, wearing tight clothing and emotional stress all tend to increase the likelihood of a hot flush coming on. Women who are prone to hot flushes often find it helpful to wear fairly loose-fitting clothes, preferably made from cotton, and to wear layers of clothes that may be discarded and then replaced after the flush. Alcohol, very hot drinks and spicy food can also trigger off the flushing process, and these are best avoided by anyone who finds hot flushes very uncomfortable or distressing. Hot flushes can also occur at night. A woman usually wakes because she is feeling very hot or because the sheets are soaked from the subsequent sweating.

There are many natural remedies that are excellent for relieving any tendency to hot flushes. If the flushes are not very severe, the following suggestions may be of help; if the flushing is severe or has continued for many years, you should consult a qualified alternative medicine practitioner for proper treatment. A helpful herbal mixture to relieve hot flushes can be made from BLACKCURRANT LEAVES, HAWTHORN TOPS and SAGE. Combine the herbs and make an infusion to drink three times a day for six weeks. This mixture may be even more beneficial if AGNUS CASTUS is added to balance the hormones. The essential oils of CLARY SAGE or CYPRESS may also be used to alleviate hot flushes. Add three or four drops of either diluted in a little base oil to a warm bath and repeat every other day for several weeks. The most commonly indicated homoeopathic remedies for hot flushes are LACHESIS and SEPIA. Compare all these remedies in the *Materia Medica* section of this book to check that they are suitable for your individual case.

GENITAL CHANGES

The decline in oestrogen and other hormonal changes during the menopause begin to affect the rate of cell growth in all our tissues and body organs. This means that there is a gradual thinning in the tissue of the vulva and the vagina. As the labia gradually lose some of their fatty layers, the clitoris begins to become more prominent.

Lower oestrogen levels also mean that there is less protective natural lubrication on the vaginal tissue and so some women are more vulnerable to vaginal infection and irritation. For specific remedy suggestions, *see* Vaginitis, page 156.

A woman's sex drive is not necessarily affected by the menopause and a healthy sex life can be enjoyed for many years afterwards. Indeed, many women enjoy sex even more after the menopause because they are free from the risk of getting pregnant. Genital changes may mean that physical sensitivity in that area slowly decreases, and lovemaking may need to become less vigorous to remain comfortable, as the vaginal tissues become less elastic and less moist. But many women adjust to these changes while maintaining a pleasurable physical relationship with their partner. The use of a lubricating agent such as K-Y Jelly (available over the counter at any chemist shop), can help to make penetration easier and more comfortable if vaginal dryness does become a problem.

The orthodox treatment for irritation or recurrent infection resulting from vaginal atrophy (the natural ageing process that affects the female genital area), is oestrogen creams. However, these are readily absorbed by the body and carry the possibility of serious side-effects, including an increased risk of cancer, and so we would not recommend this treatment. Some women have found natural progesterone cream (based on WILD YAM) to be very helpful, but orthodox medical sources say it is unlikely to be effective. (For suppliers, *see* the Resources section at the back of the book.)

HORMONE REPLACEMENT THERAPY (HRT)

A controversial orthodox treatment for menopausal symptoms is HRT (hormone replacement therapy). This treatment introduces synthetic hormones into the bloodstream to replace the oestrogen supplies that are waning naturally as part of the menopausal process. Sometimes the oestrogen comes from the urine of pregnant mares.

HRT comes in the form of creams, tablets or implants, all of which are absorbed into the bloodstream. While it does relieve certain menopausal symptoms, including hot flushes and vaginal atrophy, and it slows down osteoporosis *(see page 79)*, it does not prevent cardiovascular disease, arthritis or depression. Moreover, it only postpones menopausal symptoms and they will reassert themselves whenever HRT is stopped. Indeed, it can be argued that the adjustments that are occurring during the menopause are taking place at the natural time for the woman concerned, and postponing them with HRT could upset the delicate hormonal balance and rhythm completely by overriding the body's natural processes.

Another argument against the use of HRT is that there are serious side-effects associated with it. There is evidence that the use of oestrogen increases the risk of serious cardiovascular disease, especially potentially fatal blood clots. There is also a proven link between HRT and an increased risk of cancer, particularly cancer of the breast and uterus. Gallstones are also much more common among women who take HRT.

❋ Menstruation

AMENORRHOEA

Amenorrhoea, or the absence or cessation of menstrual periods at an age when regular menstruation is the norm, may have several causes. Many women will miss one or two periods during the fertile phase of their lives, perhaps during a time of emotional stress, and if periods then return to normal there is nothing to worry about. Obviously amenorrhoea is normal during pregnancy.

Primary amenorrhoea refers to the failure to begin menstruating by the age of 18. A physical examination should be carried out if a young woman has not begun to menstruate by this age to rule out the presence of a physical blockage or other obvious physiological reasons, preventing menstruation. If there is no physical blockage then constitutional treatment by a qualified practitioner of natural medicine should be considered to stimulate the sexual development and onset of menarche (the start of menstruation) of the young woman concerned.

Secondary amenorrhoea refers to when the menstrual periods disappear for more than three months after normal periods have been established, but before the onset of menopause. Missing periods during the several months following menarche is very common – it takes many young women months or even a couple of years to establish a regular cycle. This should be taken into account when secondary amenorrhoea is being considered, as should the possibility of pregnancy and the early onset of menopause. Other causes of secondary amenorrhoea include damage to the pituitary following post-partum haemorrhage or shock, ovarian cysts, drugs, extreme weight loss, very vigorous physical activity and severe stress. Obviously, to successfully treat the amenorrhoea the cause or causes need to be established. Any professionally-qualified practitioner should be able to diagnose the likely cause and suggest the appropriate treatment.

Occasionally you may miss a period because of a cold or a chill, in which case it may be brought on if you drink an infusion of ROSEMARY and YARROW. If periods are missed due to anorexia, weight loss or general debility, then nutritious herbs will help; try a mixture of ALFALFA, FENUGREEK and NETTLES. Compare all these remedies in the *Materia Medica* section of this book before you use them. If the symptoms persist for more than two months, consult a qualified practitioner.

One other common cause of amenorrhea is as an after-effect of coming off the birth control pill. As well as contributing to heart disease, thrombosis, vaginal infections and weight gain, the pill suppresses the natural glandular activities of the normal menstrual cycle and this can be difficult to re-establish. The following mixture of herbs may be taken three times a day for six weeks to help recover the hormonal balance after coming off the pill, but be certain that you are not pregnant first: AGNUS CASTUS, BLACK COHOSH, BLUE COHOSH, FALSE UNICORN and SARSAPARILLA. A regular massage with the diluted essential oil of ROSE may also help to re-establish the hormonal balance. If regular periods do not come back despite these remedies, consult a qualified practitioner.

HEAVY MENSTRUATION

Heavy menstrual flow, also called menorrhagia, is normally defined by the use of more than eight sanitary towels or tampons a day. Some women tend to have heavier periods than other women normally, so it is a marked change in a woman's own pattern that is considered more significant than a general tendency in this direction.

There are a number of causes behind heavy menstrual periods, including fibroids, polyps, pelvic inflammatory disease, cysts and thyroid disturbances. It is usually necessary to find out what the cause is before treatment is possible, so the best course of action is to get a medical diagnosis and then consult the relevant sections in this book.

It is not uncommon for heavy periods to result from the hormonal upheavals of menopause. In this case, you could try taking herbal astringents for a month or two, and if that does not work consult a qualified practitioner. Herbal astringents that may be taken for the odd heavy period include LADY'S MANTLE and SHEPHERD'S PURSE. They work best if they are taken as an infusion three times a day for six to eight weeks. If your heavy periods persist, consult a qualified therapist. Essential oils that can help to normalize heavy periods include CYPRESS, GERANIUM and ROSE. Add a few drops to a warm bath or dilute in vegetable oil and massage over the abdomen. All these remedies should be checked in the *Materia Medica*.

IRREGULAR MENSTRUATION

The average length of the menstrual cycle is 28 days, but for many women it is several days shorter or longer than this. The length of cycle does not matter, within reason (that is, between 23 days and 45 days), but if the cycle is widely varying, with some very short and some very long breaks between periods, this can indicate a hormone imbalance. Other possible causes of irregular periods are stress, crash dieting, anaemia and uterine growths (both benign and malignant).

Obviously, the cause should be established before treatment can begin.

It is not uncommon for periods to be irregular at the beginning and the end of a woman's fertile life, during the first couple of years of menstruating and during menopause – times of great hormonal upheaval. A useful herb that you can take during these times that acts as a hormonal balancer is AGNUS CASTUS. This may be taken three times a day for several weeks and may be combined with FALSE UNICORN ROOT, another hormonally toning and equalizing herb. An essential oil that has the ability to regulate hormones is ROSE. This may be used regularly in a warm bath or diluted in vegetable oil for a massage. All of these remedies should be looked up in the *Materia Medica* section of this book before use.

PAINFUL MENSTRUATION

A lot of women experience some discomfort during their periods at some time in their lives. If discomfort becomes real pain, especially if that pain is experienced month after month, it is an indication that there is a definite imbalance that should be dealt with. It really is not necessary to have painful periods on a regular basis because there is so much that natural remedies can do to help, both at the time of the period and to treat the causes of the pain.

If the painful periods (also called dysmenorrhoea) are due to some specific condition or disorder, such as endometriosis, fibroids or pelvic inflammatory disease, then appropriate treatment of the condition is necessary to clear that cause. Acupuncture, naturopathy, herbal medicine and homoeopathy can be excellent for treating these conditions. If painful periods are the result of having an IUD (intra-uterine device or coil) fitted, then the only cure may be to have it removed.

Repeatedly painful periods will occur if there is a lot of toxicity and congestion in the system as a whole. Many women find that their periods are less painful after a good cleansing diet; consult a naturopath or dietary therapist to assist you through a cleansing regime or use the one on page 423. A diet that is full of fresh fruit, vegetables and whole cereals and low in all meat, dairy products, sugar and processed foods will generally help to reduce the toxic burden on the uterus during its cleansing process. Caffeine tends to aggravate any muscle tension and increase sensitivity to pain, so it is best to avoid coffee, chocolate and cola drinks if you suffer from menstrual pain.

Women who are not very physically active do seem to suffer more than those who take regular exercise, so assist the flow of circulation and muscle tone with regular swimming, cycling or walking. Gentle exercise can also help to get the circulation moving and relax the muscles during your period. One of the best exercises is to lie flat on your back, bring your knees towards your chin and hold them there for a few minutes before lowering them again; repeat this several times.

There are lots of natural remedies to help with menstrual pain, and we suggest several here, but if the pain returns each month do consider consulting a practitioner to work at really improving your experience of your menstrual cycle and the quality of your life.

Herbs to take during the month to tone the uterus are BLACK COHOSH, CRAMPBARK, FALSE UNICORN ROOT, RASPBERRY LEAF and WHITE DEADNETTLE. Make an infusion of these to drink three times a day for two cycles, or take them as tinctures. Herbs to relieve the cramps during the period include CHAMOMILE, CRAMPBARK and VALERIAN. Make an infusion to drink three times a day when needed. All these remedies should be looked up in the *Materia Medica* section to check if they are suitable for you. The homoeopathic remedy MAG PHOS will help to relieve the cramping pains: dissolve a couple of the 6X potency in a little warm water and sip it at regular intervals. Other homoeopathic remedies that may be considered to relieve painful periods are BELLADONNA, CHAMOMILLA and NUX VOMICA.

Using essential oils can be a particularly pleasant way of relieving menstrual pain. You can add a few drops pre-diluted in base oil to a warm bath, or dilute one or two of the essential oils in a vegetable-oil base and gently massage the abdomen. Choose from the following essential oils by comparing them in the *Materia Medica:* CHAMOMILE, LAVENDER, MARJORAM, MELISSA and ROSEMARY.

Ovarian Cysts

A cyst is a small fluid-filled sac of tissue that can develop in various parts of the body. Many women develop cysts on their ovaries. These may be as small as a pea or as large as a grapefruit.

Often ovarian cysts do not cause any symptoms, exist quietly for years and are only discovered during a gynaecological examination, when one ovary is felt to be enlarged. Sometimes they may cause a sensation of fullness or swelling in the abdomen, pain during intercourse and possibly breakthrough bleeding (bleeding between the periods).

There are considered to be two main types of ovarian cyst: functional and abnormal. Functional ovarian cysts are so called because they arise out of the normal functions of the ovary during the menstrual cycle. A cyst can form when a follicle has grown in preparation for ovulation but fails to rupture and release an egg. This type is called a follicular cyst. Sometimes the structure formed from the follicle after ovulation, the *corpus luteum*, fails to shrink and forms a cyst. This type is called a luteal cyst. Functional cysts are often diagnosed by ultrasound. When diagnosed, the advised approach is often 'wait and see' because functional cysts often resolve themselves and disappear within a few menstrual cycles. If the cyst is not reabsorbed, it may be aspirated during a laparoscopy to drain off the fluid. It will then collapse.

Abnormal cysts are so called because they are the result of abnormal cell growth. Most are benign growths, although your doctor will usually advise a laparoscopy or a biopsy to rule out the possibility of the cyst being cancerous. The orthodox treatment of an abnormal cyst is surgical removal. This is to prevent them rupturing and causing internal bleeding, or becoming malignant. Some surgeons will be willing to do a cystectomy (removal of the cyst only) if possible. However, with a very large cyst, it may not be possible to save the ovary, and it too will be removed. Other surgeons strongly advise removing both the ovaries and the womb; this is rarely necessary. It is important that you feel involved in the decision-making process and confident about the treatment offered, so always seek a second opinion if you feel that your needs are not really being considered.

As we learn more about the amazing subtle and complex role of hormones in the body, we have realized that the ovaries continue to play a role in the balance of hormones even after the menopause. Previously it was thought that they served no purpose in the later years, but they not only continue to produce hormones that help to prevent osteoporosis, but energetically they are the seat of our inner creative impulse and have an increasingly important role in the intuitive process. Any woman with problems in this area will benefit from looking at her ability to be in touch with her intuition, and how well she follows it through into personal creativity. This may require some lifestyle changes so that space and time are created to allow those creative impulses the opportunity to come to fruition.

The natural approach to treating ovarian cysts will ideally include dietary changes and the use of natural remedies. It is essential that you give up smoking, caffeine and alcohol. Ovarian cysts are more common in women who smoke. Ovarian cysts are sensitive to oestrogen and the liver has to break down and eliminate hormones in the body, including oestrogen. If the liver is struggling then excess hormones and toxins will build up in the body. A cleansing diet can assist the liver, and avoiding caffeine and alcohol will also help. It may be helpful to visit a naturopath who can advise you on an appropriate cleansing diet, or you could follow the one on page 423.

Your diet should include a lot of fresh, leafy vegetables and fruit, foods that are rich in antioxidants. These help to mop up free radicals and prevent growths becoming cancerous. Foods rich in phytoestrogens should also be included; these will help to control how much oestrogen is circulating in your body and reduce the sensitivity of body tissue to oestrogen. Foods rich in phytoestrogens include soya products, lentils, pulses and garlic. FENNEL tea also has a phytoestrogen effect.

Ovarian cysts can respond well to homeopathic treatment, but you would need to see a qualified practitioner for best results. Other therapies to consider could be acupuncture and herbalism. Aromatherapy may be particularly appropriate if you do have surgery, to rebalance the hormones and help overcome the trauma of surgery, especially the essential oils of GERANIUM, LAVENDER and ROSE. The herbs that are most likely to be used in the treatment of functional ovarian cysts are AGNUS CASTUS and PULSATILLA. You could look these up in the *Materia Medica* section of this book and see if they are particularly appropriate.

Pelvic Inflammatory Disease (PID)

This is inflammation caused by a bacterial infection of the organs of the pelvis, including the Fallopian tubes, ovaries and uterus. Strictly speaking, inflammation of the Fallopian tubes is salpingitis, of the uterus endometritis and of the ovary oophoritis, but they are usually referred to by the umbrella term PID.

The bacteria causing PID usually enter the body through the vagina and work their way up into the pelvic cavity. The bacteria are thought to 'hitch a ride' from the vagina by attaching themselves to sperm, which of course are designed to travel through the cervix and up into the Fallopian tubes. Gonococcus, that causes gonorrhoea, and chlamydia are thought to be responsible for the majority of cases, thus PID is often classified as a sexually transmitted infection. The remaining cases are caused by other bacteria, such as E. coli, that normally resides in the rectum, or streptococci or staphylococci, which may enter through the cervix during childbirth, abortion, miscarriage or via an IUD. In the past the tubercle bacilli (that causes tuberculosis) used to be a significant cause, but this is rare nowadays.

PID can range from being mild to a very serious, even life-threatening disorder. It may be acute (a sudden severe infection) or chronic (a long-term inflammation with a low-grade infection).

The symptoms of acute PID include severe lower abdominal pain and tenderness, foul-smelling vaginal discharge, fever, breakthrough bleeding, back pain, painful intercourse, frequent or painful urination. If you suffer from any of these symptoms you must seek urgent medical advice for an accurate diagnosis. The same symptoms may also indicate an ectopic pregnancy or peritonitis, both of which are medical emergencies that can be fatal if not treated quickly.

Diagnosis will include pelvic examination, swabs of the cervical discharge and possibly laparoscopy and ultrasound scans. Treatment will be with broad-spectrum oral antibiotics, or in a severe case a stay in hospital and intravenous antibiotics.

Sometimes several courses of antibiotics are tried but fail to cure the symptoms; the disorder may then be called chronic PID. Chronic pelvic inflammatory disease may last for months. The symptoms are ongoing abdominal pain or discomfort, weakness, fatigue and heavy and painful periods. Chronic PID is a common cause of infertility because of scarring and adhesions that block the Fallopian tubes. It will also increase the likelihood of an ectopic pregnancy and may cause adhesions that cause long-term pain and discomfort. Thus any persistent abdominal pain should be checked out.

Chronic PID may be successfully treated using natural remedies, however the best results will come from visiting a qualified practitioner such as a herbalist or homoeopath to treat this serious condition.

The following herbs may relieve discomfort and help fight infection, and may be used in conjunction with professional treatment (check with your practitioner first): AGNUS CASTUS, CHAMOMILE, CRAMPBARK, ECHINACEA, GOLDENSEAL, WILD YAM. Look them up in the *Materia Medica* section to see which is appropriate for you. Essential oils used in a warm compress may also bring some relief. Consider LAVENDER, SANDALWOOD and THYME.

Polycystic Ovary Syndrome (PCOS)

Polycystic ovaries are ovaries that have multiple small cysts just below the surface. During each menstrual cycle hundreds of follicles grow on the ovaries. Eggs will develop within all of them, but one will reach maturity faster than the others and will be released into the Fallopian tubes (ovulation). The remaining follicles will then degenerate as part of the natural cycle of events. With poly-cystic ovaries, the follicles remain enlarged and appear as multiple small cysts in clumps on the ovary.

Polycystic ovaries are not always troublesome, and some women live with them and get pregnant without difficulty. However, sometimes the cysts inter-fere with the functioning of the ovaries and a complex hormonal imbalance is created. This is known as Polycystic Ovary Syndrome (PCOS).

The most obvious sign of the hormone imbalance is that the body produces too many androgens (the best known of which is testosterone). Androgens are produced naturally in men and women, but an excess of them in women tends to have a 'masculinizing' effect. Thus chronically high androgen levels have the tendency to produce the distressing symptom of excess bodily and facial hair (hirsuitsm). Other likely symptoms include acne and having very few or no periods (amenorrhoea). Women with PCOS also have the unfortunate tendency to develop diabetes and heart disease.

Chronically high androgen levels also block the development of eggs within the ovaries before they reach maturity and thus interfere with the normal cyclic egg development, leading to cysts developing from the unreleased eggs. So a negative cycle of hormone imbalance and polycystic ovaries is set up. In fact, it isn't really known whether the problem starts in the ovaries, in that they don't produce correct levels of hormones, or in the pituitary gland, which then affects the ovaries.

PCOS is also associated with obesity. But again it isn't really clear whether an excess of body fat makes women more prone to the disease or whether the hormone imbalance has a knock-on effect on insulin efficiency that tends to lead to obesity.

The orthodox treatment of PCOS is with hormonal drugs to reduce the symptoms. Birth control pills or progesterone hormones may be prescribed to induce artificial periods. Anti-androgen hormones may also be prescribed. None of these addresses the underlying imbalance and the symptoms will return when the medication is stopped. In the past, surgery was often carried out to remove part of each ovary; this was known as 'wedge resection'. Unfortunately this often caused scarring and adhesions on the ovary which resulted in infertility, and it is only very rarely carried out now.

Women with PCOS will not ovulate, because no eggs are being released, and thus they are infertile. The drug Clomid (Clomiphene citrate) may be prescribed to women with PCOS who are trying to conceive. Clomid will artificially induce ovulation, but unfortunately it also increases the chances of a miscarriage.

The natural treatment of PCOS will require an enquiring approach into the underlying causes of the disease combined with dietary changes and natural remedies. The symptoms of PCOS indicate an underlying lack of ease with the energy of the feminine. On a very profound level there is a denial of the power of being a woman. Causes for this may be themes such as sexual abuse as a child or an overly domineering mother, which makes developing into a woman unattractive to the girl. There will be a need to nurture all aspects of the feminine without fear of the darker, more intense energies, such as letting go and accepting chaos as part of life.

Dietary changes can be key to improving PCOS. If overweight women with PCOS begin to lose weight, their androgen levels fall and serum insulin levels go down, which can make a real difference to the symptoms. A number of studies have shown that overweight women with PCOS who have lost weight have begun to ovulate again and many have become pregnant without further treatment. The weight loss does not need to be dramatic – losing 10–15 per cent of body weight can be enough to improve hormone levels and reinstate ovulation. Eating a healthier wholefood diet with plenty of leafy vegetables can be more effective than calorie counting and buying special 'diet foods'.

Eating regular meals and never missing a meal is also important in helping to balance hormone levels. It will be far better to eat a small healthy meal or snack every three hours than to skip meals and then binge at the end of the day. Avoiding simple sugars is also important, as that will help insulin levels return to normal. Including foods rich in phytoestrogens (such as tofu and pulses) can also help to balance the sex hormones.

Herbal remedies to treat PCOS will include hormone-balancing herbs such as AGNUS CASTUS, BLACK COHOSH and FALSE UNICORN, also liver-cleansing herbs to help the body detoxify and remove excess androgens, such as DANDELION and MILK THISTLE. Look these herbs up in the *Materia Medica* section to find out more about how appropriate they are for you.

Pre-Menstrual Tension (PMT)

Pre-menstrual tension, also called congestive dysmenorrhoea, occurs as a result of the hormonal changes that take place between ovulation and the next menstrual period. The pre-menstrual symptoms most women commonly experience include bloatedness, nausea, headaches, swollen breasts, spots, fatigue and irritability. Many of these symptoms are a result of the increase in water retention in the body's tissues that occurs at this time, because of the higher levels of oestrogen and aldosterone hormones.

An individual woman's response to these hormonal changes will vary according to her physical and emotional health, and so the impact of pre-menstrual tension will also vary. Women who suffer distressing emotional symptoms before their periods should take this as an opportunity not to suppress these feelings and to reassess their well-being as a woman in our stress-filled society, perhaps with the help of a professional counsellor or therapist.

There are many natural remedies that can alleviate the symptoms of pre-menstrual tension, but if the condition persists after a couple of months of trying them, we suggest that you consult a professional practitioner of natural medicine. All the remedies that we suggest should be cross-checked in the *Materia Medica* section of this book to assess how suitable they are for you.

EVENING PRIMROSE OIL has helped many women with their pre-menstrual symptoms, particularly those who suffer with swollen and tender breasts. We suggest that you take 500mg a day for two months and then just for the ten days preceding each period. Vitamin B6 is also helpful for some women, this may be taken in conjunction with EVENING PRIMROSE OIL.

The herbs AGNUS CASTUS and FALSE UNICORN have a balancing effect on the hormones; these may be combined and infused (or taken as tinctures) three times a day for two or three months. Other herbs to use if there are symptoms of stress and anxiety present, are MOTHERWORT, OATS, PASSIFLORA and VERVAIN. If your water retention is marked and you feel bloated then make an infusion of COUCHGRASS and DANDELION to drink three times a day during the pre-menstrual phase.

The essential oils of GERANIUM and ROSEMARY can greatly relieve the physical symptoms of pre-menstrual tension, including the bloating and water retention. If you feel particularly irritable and depressed then consider CLARY SAGE, NEROLI and ROSE. These essential oils may be diluted in a suitable vegetable-oil base and massaged in, or add a couple of drops of the oil of your choice to a warm bath when required. A course of lymphatic drainage massages by an experienced aromatherapist may be particularly good for pre-menstrual tension *(see page 73)*.

In general, a poor diet can contribute to these symptoms by adding to congestion in the body, impairing the function of the liver and lowering your overall vitality. Women suffering from pre-menstrual tension should avoid food additives, caffeine (coffee, coke and so on), refined foods, salt, smoked foods and alcohol. One very important change to your diet that has been proven to have a beneficial effect on PMT for many women is to balance your blood sugar. The first step is to eliminate sugar from your diet. The second is to eat 'little and often'. Eat a small snack at least every two hours. Ideal snacks are made of complex carbohydrates, not refined foods. Try rice cakes or Ryvita, etc.

Prolapse

Prolapse means 'to fall', and it refers to an organ that slips or descends out of place. The bladder, rectum and vagina may all prolapse, but it most commonly refers to the womb, known as an uterine prolapse.

A prolapse occurs because the muscles that normally hold the organ in place have become weakened. A uterine prolapse is due to a weakening of the pelvic-floor muscles. This is usually the result of a prolonged labour or multiple labours (having lots of children), and it tends to be more common after the menopause. It is also more common after a hysterectomy, which may damage the pelvic muscles. Other causes may be being overweight, carrying heavy weights during pregnancy, an incorrectly performed episiotomy, chronic constipation, or a chronic cough such as asthma.

During a uterine prolapse the uterus protrudes down into the vagina, or in severe cases drops completely out of the vagina. There may be no symptoms at all, but usually there is a sensation of heaviness or 'dragging' in the vagina. It is quite common for a prolapse to cause constipation or urinary incontinence *(see also Stress Incontinence, page 178)*.

For a severe prolapse, surgery will be advised. There are also non-surgical measures available, which may be tried before resorting to surgery. A pessary device can be used that fits around the cervix and holds up the womb. This will not be curative, but it can alleviate the symptoms. Vaginal cones can be inserted into the vagina for several hours a day to help strengthen the pelvic-floor muscles. They should be available from your GP or a well-woman clinic.

Pelvic-floor exercises can remedy a mild prolapse and are a really good idea to do after childbirth and during and after the menopause. The best pelvic-floor exercise is to contract the muscles that you would use to stop urination in mid-stream. Do not actually do the exercise regularly whilst urinating, as it can lead to cystitis in some women, but if you do it once to learn where the muscles are then you can do the exercise every day. The best technique is to contract the muscles in several stages, like going up in a lift, then hold the contracted position for a few moments before releasing it, again in stages.

There are a number of natural remedies that can help tone the muscles and relieve a prolapse. The following should be referred to in the *Materia Medica* section for appropriate use in your case. The herbs of HORSETAIL, LADY'S MANTLE and SHEPHERD'S PURSE all act as astringents to tone tissues. The homoeopathic remedies NUX VOMICA and SEPIA are often indicated for prolapses. In more severe cases it will be advisable to see a qualified practitioner for best results.

Sexually Transmitted Infections

There are certain venereal diseases, such as gonorrhoea or chlamydia, that can cause vaginitis symptoms *(see page 156)* and if they are left untreated they may cause long-term problems. If you suspect that your symptoms may have been sexually transmitted, it is advisable to visit your local VD clinic to have a test. It is a legal requirement in Britain to have the main venereal infections (syphilis and gonorrhoea) treated by the orthodox medical profession. VD clinics tend to be better equipped to deal with these infections than your doctor, but both should be able to do tests and prescribe the appropriate treatment. Ask at your local health centre or look under 'Clinics' in the telephone directory to find your nearest VD clinic.

Suspicious signs of a venereal infection include an unusual discharge, soreness, redness, sores, itchiness or a foul smell in the genital area. There are many different infections that can be sexually transmitted, and a test will be necessary to establish which are present. Many women feel acutely embarrassed and humiliated when they suspect they may have contracted a venereal infection, but it is very important to have any infection treated as quickly as possible to prevent complications developing. Do get any suspicious symptoms checked as soon as they arise. Both syphilis and gonorrhoea can cause permanent damage, including sterility and heart disease, so it is particularly crucial to have these treated if there is any possibility that you may have one of them. The standard treatment for these diseases is high doses of antibiotics.

There are ways of reducing the risk of contracting a venereal disease. The most direct way is to sleep only with people that you already know and can ask in advance whether they have any infection. Failing that, condoms for both vaginal and anal intercourse greatly reduce the risk of contracting a venereal infection (and also of contracting AIDS, of course). The use of spermicidal cream, film, foam or jelly also reduces the risk, preferably with a diaphragm for added protection. No method is 100 per cent effective – if you do suspect that you have an infection, avoid sex until you have a test, and until the disease is cleared.

It is not uncommon for some symptoms to remain, for example dryness and a slight discharge, even when tests show that the disease had been cleared by antibiotics; this is particularly true of non-specific urethritis (NSU). In this case, constitutional treatment by a qualified practitioner of natural medicine can often clear the symptoms and get you back to feeling healthy again.

CHLAMYDIA

The sexually transmitted infection chlamydia has become increasingly common in recent years. It is caused by the organism *Chlamydia trachomatis*, which is also thought to be responsible for a number of cases of non-specific urethritis (NSU).

Chlamydia is often known as a 'silent disease', because a woman may have it for several years without any noticeable symptoms. In men it tends to cause burning during urination, so if your partner experiences this symptoms it is important that you are screened for the disease. In Sweden they screen women routinely for chlamydia, which has significantly reduced the number of cases.

Unfortunately, although chlamydia does not exhibit noticeable symptoms in the early stages, it may be causing damage to the reproductive organs. It seems the organism can travel up the cervix into the womb and Fallopian tubes. Once there, it may cause scarring and blockage of the Fallopian tubes. This may result in infertility and an increased risk of ectopic pregnancy.

If you have any reason to suspect that you may have contracted chlamydia it is a good idea to ask to be screened for it at a clinic. Orthodox treatment is with oral antibiotics and it may be advisable to take these and then use specific natural remedies to improve your immunity and repair any damage the infection may have caused. It will also be helpful to take a course of acidophilus following antibiotics, as antibiotics will kill the healthy bacteria as well as the unhealthy ones and you are more likely to get thrush following antibiotic treatment.

TRICHOMONAS

This is caused by a tiny parasite and is usually spread by sexual intercourse, although the organism can survive at room temperature on moist objects for several hours and so can be transmitted by using a contaminated towel, etc.

Trichomonas does cause symptoms in women, usually a thin or frothy yellow or greenish discharge and itching, soreness and inflammation of the vulva and the vagina. The discharge may have an unpleasant odour. Men may carry the parasite in their urinary tract but usually do not experience any symptoms.

If the organism invades the urinary tract in a woman, it may cause the symptoms of cystitis.

It is thought that trichomonas can encourage the growth of venereal warts and thrush, but it does not usually invade the uterus or affect fertility.

The main orthodox treatment for trichomonas is metronidazol (Flagyl), which unfortunately has a number of side-effects (including nausea, diarrhoea, headaches, alcohol intolerance and allergic reactions) and should not be used during pregnancy. It may be advisable to try natural remedies to treat trichomonas in the first instance and resort to orthodox treatment only if symptoms persist or are severe. Both partners will need to be treated, as otherwise the infection may be transmitted again. You will need to use a condom during intercourse while you are undergoing treatment.

Natural remedies for trichomonas include douching with diluted tinctures of GOLDENSEAL and MYRRH, or with TEA TREE essential oil. A clove of GARLIC may be peeled (taking care not to nick the surface), coated in olive oil and inserted overnight. Repeat for several days. Internally, the herbs AGNUS CASTUS, GARLIC and GOLDENSEAL should be considered. Compare all these remedies in the *Materia Medica* section and use the most appropriate.

Thrush

Thrush is caused by a yeast-like fungus called *Candida albicans.* This organism normally resides in the vagina of most women and does not produce symptoms unless it multiplies more than normal. Factors likely to result in the Candida organisms multiplying are taking the birth control pill, pregnancy and a course of antibiotics. Many women find also that making love after a period of abstinence can trigger off an attack of thrush if they are prone to it. The symptoms of the infection are vaginal itching and a thick white discharge.

A one-off attack of thrush is usually quite easily dealt with by using natural remedies. However, the problem can keep recurring and this will require constitutional treatment by a professional therapist. Women who suffer persistently with thrush symptoms may need to follow an anti-Candida diet which means avoiding all sugars and yeast, which the organism tends to thrive on. For advice on such a diet consult a naturopath or dietary therapist.

If you are sexually active with a male partner it is advisable for him to wear a condom during intercourse when you have thrush symptoms. The organism can live under the foreskin of the penis and be passed backwards and forwards between partners during intercourse.

An easy home remedy that has been found by many to relieve a bout of thrush is natural yoghurt. Eat plenty, and also apply it to the vaginal area either by dabbing it on and then using a sanitary towel to prevent too much mess, or with a vaginal applicator which can be bought in any major chemist.

To treat thrush with herbs it is advisable to take them internally to boost the immune system and use them externally to relieve discomfort and clear the infection. Drink an infusion or take the tinctures three times a day for up to six weeks of ECHINACEA, LADY'S MANTLE, MARIGOLD and WHITE DEADNETTLE. For external use, make an infusion to use as a douche or for bathing the area with cotton wool consisting of GOLDENSEAL, LAVENDER and MARIGOLD.

Essential oils may also be used as a douche, but make sure they are well diluted or they may irritate the delicate mucous membranes. Add four drops of LAVENDER or MYRRH essential oil and two drops of TEA TREE essential oil to one litre of boiled warm water for a douche. For a mild attack of thrush, just adding ten drops of LAVENDER essential oil to a warm bath once a day can bring great relief. It is also worth comparing the homoeopathic tissue salts of KALI MUR and NATRUM MUR to see if either of these seems appropriate, in which case take a course of one three times a day for ten days. The homoeopathic remedy PULSATILLA can also be well indicated.

Vaginitis and Vaginal Infections

Vaginitis is the term applied to vaginal irritation and inflammation; these symptoms may be found in association with a vaginal infection. The symptoms of a vaginal infection are an unusual discharge, an unpleasant smell from the genital area, a sensation of dryness and itching and/or burning of the vulva. All women secrete mucus and moisture from the vagina, it is only if this changes, becomes smelly, blood-streaked or irritating that it should be considered abnormal or unhealthy. Similarly, many useful bacteria live in the vagina of all women, and it is only if these multiply too rapidly, or other harmful bacteria are introduced, that the symptoms of an infection will develop.

There are many possible causes of vaginal irritation: using a diaphragm, an IUD string, spermicidal creams, tampons, deodorant sprays, bubble baths, douching or vigorous sexual intercourse can all cause inflammation and lead to an infection developing. Your resistance to infection can be undermined by stress, certain drugs or general ill health. Women who have passed the menopause or who have had their ovaries removed experience vaginitis more frequently because of the reduced supply of hormones needed to maintain healthy vaginal tissues. It is important to clear up any vaginal infections before you become pregnant, as they can cause a miscarriage.

There are several preventative measures that are helpful if you are prone to vaginitis: wash regularly and gently pat yourself dry; wear only cotton underwear and avoid clothes that fit closely against the crotch; avoid strongly-scented soaps and bubble baths; avoid all vaginal sprays and 'deodorant' tampons; and always wipe from front to back after bowel movements.

We recommend several natural remedies here to treat vaginitis, however, if the symptoms are very uncomfortable or persist for more than a few weeks, you should seek professional advice. Externally, herbs may be used as washes or douches. Try a mixture of COMFREY, GOLDENSEAL, LAVENDER, MARIGOLD and WHITE DEADNETTLE infused, and apply when cool. Internally, herbs can also be helpful to reduce inflammation and fight infection; try a decoction of ECHINACEA, ST JOHN'S WORT and WHITE DEADNETTLE. Drink this three times a day for up to six weeks. Many women have found that a whole clove of GARLIC, peeled without nicking the surface with your fingernail or knife, dipped in olive oil and then inserted into the vagina overnight, can help to clear the early signs of an infection.

Homoeopathically, there are three main remedies to choose from. If none of these seems appropriate, or if you have tried one and it hasn't worked, seek professional guidance. KREOSOTUM is the main remedy for vaginitis that has an irritating or corrosive discharge and a feeling of rawness in the vaginal area. PULSATILLA can be helpful where there is a thick, white or creamy-yellow discharge that is either bland or causes itching. SEPIA will be indicated when the discharge is yellow or greenish and has an offensive smell, and particularly when there is also an uncomfortable, heavy feeling in the lower abdomen. Try taking either the 6th homoeopathic potency once three times a day for ten days, or just two doses of the 30th potency eight hours apart. All these remedies should be looked up in the *Materia Medica* section of this book to check that they are generally well indicated.

A few drops of the essential oils of CHAMOMILE or LAVENDER in a warm bath can be very soothing for the symptoms of itching and irritation. If there are symptoms of infection present then SANDALWOOD, TEA TREE and THYME should also be considered (look them up in the *Materia Medica* to see which is most appropriate). These may be used as a douche, but make sure they are well diluted (two or three drops of essential oil dissolved in a teaspoon of vodka and diluted in one litre of water).

16

The Respiratory System

The function of the respiratory system is to take air into the lungs; it allows the absorption of oxygen into the blood, and the excretion of carbon dioxide from the blood into the alveoli and out through the nose and mouth. The respiratory tract can be divided into the upper and lower parts. The upper respiratory tract includes the nose, nasal cavity and pharynx and larynx; the lower respiratory tract includes the trachea, two bronchi, two lungs and pleura.

Our breath connects us to the earth's atmosphere, and symbolically as well as practically to the trees and forests, which have been called the 'lungs of the earth' because of their oxygen-creating capacity. As well as concentrating on healing a specific respiratory complaint, it is worthwhile considering our relationship to the air we breathe, and by its extension as the 'breath of life', to our enthusiasm for and positive attitude to life itself. There is nothing more likely to prolong a respiratory complaint than a negative and pessimistic attitude to life.

Air pollution is a problem that needs to be dealt with directly and urgently. There are two sides to the problem: what we are putting into the atmosphere and the decimation of rain forests that purify it. While those of us who are in good health are able to cope with a certain level of air pollution, at least in the short term, those of us who are very young or elderly or already suffer from a respiratory complaint such as asthma are at great risk from the increasing levels of air pollution. Smoking cigarettes does not only pollute your own lungs, it also pollutes the air of those around you to dangerous levels.

The Respiratory System

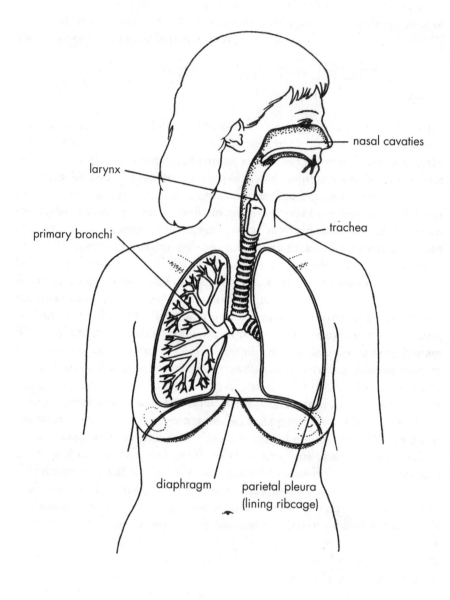

nasal cavaties

larynx

trachea

primary bronchi

diaphragm

parietal pleura
(lining ribcage)

❧ Asthma

Asthma is a disease of the respiratory system which makes it difficult to breathe out. It is caused by the spasm of the smaller air passages in the lung. The spasm makes it difficult to cough away mucus which collects in the small bronchi, which impedes the breathing further.

There is often a hereditary factor to asthma and attacks can be triggered by allergies, chest infections, stress and anxiety in different people. Like other allergic diseases, asthma seems to be very much on the increase in recent years, particularly amongst children. A diet eliminating all mucus-stimulating foods (particularly dairy products) may be of help.

Conventional treatment for asthma includes the use of drugs which dilate the air passages of the lungs (bronchodilators), usually given in the form of inhalers, such as salbutamol (Ventolin). Steroid inhalations may be given to relieve the congestion of the bronchial lining; these are also usually given in the form of inhalers such as beclamethasone (Becatide). The medicines are usually given to children as a syrup. For very severe asthma attacks corticosteroids, for example Prednisolone, may be given for a limited period of time. Increasingly, it is recommended that asthma sufferers should use their medication continually, instead of just during an acute attack, as a means of preventing them from coming on.

The main drawback with the conventional treatment of asthma is that it aims to 'control' the disease, or to relieve an acute attack, but not to cure the illness. It is for this reason that many sufferers and parents of children with asthma turn to alternative medicine for help.

The treatment of chronic or recurrent asthma is a difficult, complicated problem and should be handled by an experienced practitioner. Constitutional treatment by an alternative therapy can be very rewarding and a cure is possible, depending on the severity of the case and the amount of medication that has been used in the past. The switchover from orthodox inhalers and medication should not be attempted unless it is under the supervision of a suitably qualified practitioner.

Herbs that may help during a mild attack include COLTSFOOT, ELECAMPANE, MULLEIN, THYME and WHITE HOREHOUND. If there is stress and anxiety then MOTHERWORT and SKULLCAP should also be considered. TURMERIC has a bronchodilatory effect, and a teaspoonful stirred into a glass of warm water may be sipped at frequent intervals to help relieve an attack. The most commonly indicated homoeopathic remedies for an asthma attack are

ARSENICUM, IPECAC and NATRUM SULPH. MAG PHOS may be given as a tissue salt to relieve the spasm of an acute episode. Steam inhalations with essential oils can also be of benefit; try CHAMOMILE, EUCALYPTUS and LAVENDER. The Bach FIVE FLOWER REMEDY can be taken at frequent intervals to relieve anxiety and panic during an attack.

The general management of an asthma attack should involve rest, preferably propped up in bed, and plenty of liquids to prevent dehydration from increased perspiration.

Colds

The essential feature of a cold is an inflammation of the nasal passages, known as rhinitis, which produces a running nose and sneezing. Watering eyes are also common and the inflammation often spreads to the pharynx to cause a sore throat. The occasional cold is best looked at as an opportunity for the body to have a good clear out and, most importantly, a good rest. But frequently recurring colds are a sign that your resistance is very low, and that your diet and lifestyle are probably out of balance in some way.

When you have a cold it's sensible to make sure that you are getting enough vitamin C. Eat more fresh fruit and vegetables and avoid mucus-stimulating foods such as dairy produce and concentrated orange juice. GARLIC capsules, or eating plenty of fresh garlic, will assist the body to fight the infection; it can also help to relieve problems with catarrh.

Take regular baths with a few drops of GINGER essential oil in the water at the beginning of winter – it is said to increase the body's resistance to cold viruses. The essential oils of EUCALYPTUS, PEPPERMINT, PINE, ROSEMARY, TEA TREE and THYME will all help to fight the infection and reduce congestion. They will also help to relieve the catarrh that can often follow on from a cold. It is particularly useful to use essential oils as a steam inhalation for congestion, but they may also be diluted in vegetable oil and massaged onto the chest.

For an acute cold the most frequently used homoeopathic remedies are ACONITE, ALLIUM CEPA, EUPHRASIA, FERRUM PHOS, NATRUM MUR and PULSATILLA. If catarrh is persistent then KALI MUR or KALI SULPH can also be helpful.

Our favourite herbal mixture for colds is ELDERFLOWER, PEPPERMINT and YARROW. A course of ECHINACEA will help make those of us prone to recurrent colds more resistant to them.

❧ Coughs

The air passages of the lungs are lined with cells secreting mucus, which normally traps particles of dust. When the membranes are infected and inflamed, the secretion of mucus increases and the lining of the air passages is irritated; coughing is the reflex action by which excess mucus is driven out.

A cough may be due to a temporary external cause (for example, fumes), an allergy (such as asthma), an infection (bronchitis) or a chronic complaint (emphysema). These remedies will help to treat a mild cough, such as that following on from a cold or mild bronchitis; a more serious infection or a chronic complaint should be treated by a suitably qualified practitioner.

General care for a cough includes avoiding mucus-stimulating foods, such as dairy produce, and increasing the intake of foods and drinks which are rich in vitamin C. A soothing drink like hot lemon and honey can be very helpful.

For an unproductive, irritating cough, the herbs to try are ANISEED, COLTS-FOOT, MARSHMALLOW and MULLEIN. For a more productive cough, useful herbal expectorants include ELECAMPANE, LIQUORICE and WHITE HOREHOUND. If there are signs of an infection, as with bronchitis, then you should also use antimicrobials such as GOLDENSEAL, PLANTAIN and THYME. In this case take GARLIC capsules as well.

The best way to treat a cough with essential oils is by steam inhalation. EUCALYPTUS is particularly useful because it combines expectorant and antimicrobial properties. Other useful expectorant oils include BENZOIN, FENNEL, HYSSOP and SANDALWOOD. THYME is good where there are signs of infection.

The most commonly indicated homoeopathic remedies include ACONITE, ANT TART, BELLADONNA, BRYONIA, CAUSTICUM, IPECAC, PHOSPHORUS, PULSATILLA and SULPHUR. The tissue salt CALC PHOS is useful during the convalescent period after a cough.

❧ Hayfever

Hayfever seems to be becoming more common along with other allergic disorders, particularly amongst children. It is characterized by the irritation of the mucous membranes of the eyes, nose and air passages. This is caused by the pollen of various grasses and plants, so it is a seasonal allergy. Most cases of hayfever occur in spring and summer, when the antigen is grass pollen, but some occur in autumn when the pollen of ragweeds is usually the cause.

Conventional treatment consists of desensitization injections, which usually only last for one season, or antihistamine tablets or nasal sprays, which may temporarily relieve the symptoms. But these often cause side-effects, such as drowsiness, and also tend to deepen the imbalance in the natural defence system.

It is wise to eliminate all mucus-stimulating foods from the diet during the hayfever season, particularly dairy produce. You should also avoid sugar, as this seems to impair the effectiveness of the immune system. Food and drinks rich in vitamin C are helpful.

Constitutional treatment from a qualified practitioner is probably necessary to cure hayfever, but the following suggestions will relieve the symptoms. EYEBRIGHT is a particularly useful herb to use as a soothing eyewash or to drink internally. Other herbs to take internally for hayfever include ELDERFLOWER, GOLDENSEAL, HYSSOP, MULLEIN and NETTLE. The essential oils that will be of help are CHAMOMILE, EUCALYPTUS and LAVENDER; the vapours may be inhaled from a few drops placed on a handkerchief. The main homoeopathic remedies to choose from include ALLIUM CEPA, ARSENICUM, EUPHRASIA, NUX VOMICA and SABADILLA.

❊ Sinusitis

The sinuses are air spaces in the bones above the eyes and around the nose. Inflammation of the mucous membrane lining these cavities is called sinusitis. The symptoms of inflammation and infection in the sinuses are throbbing pains and tenderness over the area, and if the lower sinuses are involved, the teeth may also hurt. There is often an increase in mucus secretion which makes you feel stuffy and 'full'.

Home care will usually help a mild attack of sinusitis. But if the pain is severe or if you have a generalized fever you should go to a qualified practitioner. Home care should include rest, drinking plenty of liquids and avoiding mucus-stimulating foods like dairy products. GARLIC capsules or fresh garlic help fight any infection and relieve the build up of catarrh.

The main homoeopathic remedies to consider are BELLADONNA, BRYONIA, HEPAR SULPH, KALI BICH and SILICEA. Herbally, it is best to have a mixture that includes some herbs to fight the infection, such as ECHINACEA and GOLDENSEAL, anticatarrhals, such as ELDERFLOWER, EYEBRIGHT, GOLDEN ROD and PEPPERMINT, and an anti-inflammatory such as MARSHMALLOW.

Steam inhalations with essential oils can be very helpful in the treatment of sinusitis. The most useful oils are EUCALYPTUS, PINE and THYME.

✳ Sore Throats

These include pharyngitis, laryngitis and tonsillitis. Pharyngitis and laryngitis generally appear with the common cold virus, and infections affecting the throat can frequently recur in some people. As well as a slight feverishness, you may feel a general malaise and other cold symptoms with a sore throat, and have a hoarse, husky voice. If the fever is very high, or if the sore throat is very severe, then you should get professional medical advice. Laryngitis symptoms which last for a long time should also be professionally assessed.

Tonsillitis is another common type of sore throat, and often the bacteria Streptococcus is present. In this case, you are usually struck by a sudden fever, sore throat and difficulty in swallowing; the throat often feels very dry. A mild case of tonsillitis will clear up with home treatment. However, with young children, or if any of the symptoms mentioned are very severe, urgent professional advice should be sought.

Steam inhalations with essential oils are a useful anti-inflammatory and antiseptic method of treating sore throats. Amongst the most effective oils, you should try BENZOIN, LAVENDER, SANDALWOOD or THYME. The homoeopathic remedies of ACONITE or FERRUM PHOS are good for the first stages of a sore throat. Other homoeopathic remedies that may be useful are BELLADONNA, HEPAR SULPH, MERC SOL and PHYTOLACCA. One of the best herbs to use is SAGE; this may be taken as a gargle or as an infusion to drink several times a day while the symptoms last.

17

The Skin

Our skin helps to define us as individuals. As well as providing us with a primary physical boundary, it allows for tremendous individual variation in terms of texture, colour, smell, temperature and sensitivity.

The skin is both protective and semi-permeable. It acts as an interface between the interior and the exterior world, and it has the dual ability of absorbing some things and excreting others. We should be very careful about what we put onto the skin because it readily absorbs substances which then pass into the bloodstream to be transported around the whole body. Similarly, we should help our skin in its excretory function by keeping it clean, allowing it to 'breathe' by wearing natural fibres, and by not using substances such as anti-perspirants which hamper its efforts.

An enormous amount of money and effort goes into creating and advertising beauty products for the skin and hair each year. This is not really surprising because the skin is the part of us that we present to the outside world, and our society places great importance on external appearances. Even healthy skin is judged as beautiful or not according to the dictates of culture, fashion and taste. If we have a skin problem it can be very difficult not to feel self-conscious about it and not to let it affect our general confidence. Coping with a skin disease without suppressing it with strong medication is a real challenge for many people switching to natural medicine.

The actual causes of skin disease can be very difficult to unravel. They are often a complex combination of diet, environment, general health, hereditary factors, stress and individual susceptibility. The length of time it takes to cure a skin disease will largely depend on how long medicated ointments or drugs have been used to suppress the condition in the past and the state of health of your other bodily organs. The remedies that we suggest here will improve most skin conditions, but for deep-seated skin diseases finding a real cure can take time, and it may only be possible by working at it for several years with the help of a professional therapist.

Generally, maintaining healthy skin and hair starts with a good diet. This means a varied diet with plenty of fresh fruit and vegetables, and based on whole grains. Avoid too many fatty, greasy or refined foods and additives. Drink plenty of pure spring water to help to keep the skin clear. Too much alcohol and smoking has an extremely detrimental effect on the skin.

Clean, fresh air is a must for healthy skin, and this can be a real problem for anyone living in a city or by a busy road. Regular cleansing is very important to clear the pores of city grime. Apply a good plant-based moisturizer regularly to help to protect and nourish the skin.

Acne

Acne is a skin complaint that is characterized by blackheads and pustules that are usually found on the face and back. This problem is most commonly associated with adolescence and is linked with a hormonally-induced hyperactivity of the oil-producing glands.

There is a dietary factor in acne that is related to how well the body can metabolize fats and carbohydrates. The condition can often be helped considerably if you cut out fats, sweets and refined carbohydrates from what you eat, and eat more fresh fruit and vegetables.

A combination of alterative and antimicrobial herbs can be helpful to clear acne. Try drinking a decoction of the following herbs three times a day for several weeks: BURDOCK ROOT, CLEAVERS, ECHINACEA and YELLOW DOCK. Or look up the following remedies in the *Materia Medica* section to see if one of them looks appropriate: CALC SULPH, SILICEA and SULPHUR.

Skin cleansing is an important aspect of the treatment of acne, and regular facial steams are a good way of healing the skin and cleansing the pores without adding more grease to the skin. Make a facial steam with the herbs CHICKWEED, ELDERFLOWER and MARIGOLD. Alternatively, add a few drops of one of the following essential oils to hot water for a facial steam: BERGAMOT, CHAMOMILE, LAVENDER or LEMONGRASS. These essential oils may also be well-diluted in a vegetable-oil base to massage into the skin.

Once the acne has cleared up, massage COMFREY OINTMENT into the old sites of the spots to help to reduce any scarring.

❧ Boils

A boil is an infection of a sweat gland or hair follicle of the skin. They are most often found where clothes rub the skin – on the back of the neck, in the armpits or on the buttocks. Crops of boils may appear simultaneously or a succession of single boils may follow one another. They are more common among those people who suffer with diabetes.

A boil normally starts as a painful red lump which grows bigger and then breaks down in the middle for pus to collect. It is important not to squeeze a boil, or interfere with it other than to apply a compress or dressing, and keep the surrounding skin clean.

Boils usually indicate that you have a toxic condition. If you keep getting them you should consider a cleansing diet (try the one on page 423), and particularly eating more fresh fruit and vegetables. Add plenty of GARLIC to your diet or take GARLIC CAPSULES to help you to fight the infection.

A poultice of either powdered SLIPPERY ELM or chopped CABBAGE LEAVES will draw out the poison. Or apply a compress made by adding a few drops of one or two of the following essential oils to warm water: BERGAMOT, CHAMOMILE, LAVENDER, LEMON or THYME. Dip a clean cloth into the solution and apply over the boil.

You can take herbs internally to purify the blood and fight the infection. Make a decoction from BURDOCK and ECHINACEA, and drink a cupful three times a day for two weeks. The homoeopathic remedies that help to clear up a boil, include ARNICA, BELLADONNA, HEPAR SULPH, SILICEA and TARANTULA. Compare these in the *Materia Medica* section to see which one is the most appropriate.

❧ Cold Sores

Cold sores are caused by a virus that is retained in the body and produces a sore when the body's resistance is lowered. The cold sore will form around the mouth, or occasionally nose and eyes. It develops from a reddish lump into water-filled blisters which then form a scab. It is the watery discharge that is infectious, so you should prevent anyone else touching the cold sore at this stage.

If cold sores are recurrent you will need constitutional treatment to clear them up, but the odd cold sore may be treated yourself by using natural remedies.

BALM infusion has been proven to act against the herpes simplex virus. ECHINACEA is also a useful antiviral. Try dabbing on one of the following tinctures: CALENDULA, GOLDENSEAL, HYPERICUM and MYRRH (or make up a combination). Alternatively, the essential oils of LAVENDER or NIAOULI may be dabbed undiluted onto the sore. Homoeopathic remedies can be used to help a cold sore outbreak clear up more quickly; consult the *Materia Medica* section of this book to see which of the following is best indicated: ARSEN ALB, HEPAR SULPH, NATRUM MUR and RHUS TOX.

Dandruff

Dandruff is caused by dead skin cells flaking off the scalp. Strong detergents, including medicated dandruff shampoos, tend to irritate and dry out the scalp if they are used frequently, and may make the problem worse in the long run. Any hair, scalp or skin problem is generally an indication of poor health, so if you suspect an underlying cause you need to deal with that to find a cure.

Dandruff can be improved by applying an infusion of NETTLES, ROSEMARY and SAGE to the scalp and hair as the final rinse. It is also possible to buy mild shampoos that contain extracts of these herbs. The essential oils of CEDARWOOD, LAVENDER and ROSEMARY can be diluted in a suitable vegetable-oil base, such as ALMOND or COCONUT OIL, and massaged into the scalp to eliminate dandruff.

You can take a combination of the herbs BURDOCK, HEARTSEASE, KELP and NETTLE internally to improve the condition of the scalp. Alternatively, see if the homoeopathic remedies KALI MUR or KALI SULPH look appropriate.

Eczema

The symptoms of eczema include redness, flakiness and weeping skin. It may start as tiny blisters that burst and leave a red, raw surface. Eczema can cause intense itchiness during its dry and wet stages, and sufferers often scratch the affected areas until they bleed. Things can be made even worse if an infection starts up in skin damaged by eczema and scratching.

Unfortunately, the incidence of eczema has increased dramatically in recent years, especially amongst children. This is probably because the vitality and natural immunity of our children's health has been impaired by pollution, food additives, over-medicated parents and over-vaccination. Eczema often forms part of the inherited 'atopic' diseases, like hayfever and asthma. Different members of the same family will often display one or more of the illnesses in this group. It is particularly tragic that suppressing eczema with medicated ointments greatly increases the chances of asthma, hayfever or other respiratory problems developing later in life.

The standard treatment for eczema is steroidal ointments such as Betnovate or Hydrocortizone. These ointments will usually relieve the symptoms temporarily but continued use will actually damage the skin by 'thinning' it; at the same time they are absorbed into the bloodstream, potentially causing a wide range of side-effects which are common to all steroids (such as impaired adrenal function and a predisposition to infection). Steroidal ointments in no way cure eczema, and the condition will often return in an even worse form when they are discontinued.

Curing eczema using natural remedies is definitely possible. But it will take time, and in some cases even years, although some improvement should be obvious after several months of treatment. Basically, the length of time that it takes to cure eczema depends on how long you have had it, how many years you have been suppressing it by using medicated ointments, and on your general state of health. If a cure requires general detoxification, then the eczema may even get worse before it begins to clear up, as the body struggles to eliminate more through the skin and becomes generally healthier.

Many people find that certain foods aggravate their eczema. The most common foods that have this tendency are dairy and wheat products. The best way to find out if this is a factor for you or your child is to avoid all dairy products for three months and see if it makes a difference, then try the same with wheat products.

While we can recommend some natural remedies here that will help to relieve the symptoms, and may even cure a mild case, you will probably need constitutional treatment by a qualified natural therapist for long-standing cases of eczema.

A combination of herbs that combine alterative and anti-inflammatory properties will be most helpful. Consider BURDOCK, CHAMOMILE, GOTU KOLA, HEARTSEASE, MARIGOLD, RED CLOVER and YELLOW DOCK. You need to take the herbs three times a day for six weeks, then take a break for a couple of weeks before repeating. Check the herbs in the *Materia Medica* section of this book to see which are most suitable.

A soothing wash can be made by infusing the herbs CHICKWEED and

MARIGOLD in boiling water, and bathing the affected parts when the solution has cooled down. Alternatively, you can buy an ointment made from the same herbs. Essential oils can be added to the bath, diluted in a vegetable-oil base to apply to the skin, or used as a compress. The essential oils that are most suitable for treating eczema include CHAMOMILE, LAVENDER, MELISSA and YARROW.

Psoriasis

Psoriasis is a common skin disease in which red, scaly spots and patches appear on the skin of the bony areas of the body, such as the shins, elbows, eyebrows or scalp. The patches of psoriasis occur because the body is over-producing skin cells in those areas. The skin tends to flake off from the affected areas, and it can become itchy.

There is definitely a hereditary tendency with this disease, although the symptoms may not appear until adult life. Psoriasis can be triggered off by a shock or trauma, and flare-ups often occur during stressful times of life. The symptoms are often alleviated by sunshine and sea bathing.

The condition is notoriously difficult to treat by any method of medicine. However, more severe cases will often be considerably improved by natural remedies, and children tend to be easier to cure. We do mention some remedies here that may be a help, but if they don't seem to help after several weeks, we recommend that you consult a qualified practitioner who can take into account any other health problems that may be underlying the psoriasis, and also offer assistance if stress is a contributing factor.

Alterative herbs can help to clear psoriasis out of the system, try taking a decoction of BURDOCK ROOT, RED CLOVER, SARSAPARILLA and YELLOW DOCK ROOT three times a day for up to three months. An ointment made from COMFREY ROOT can be massaged into the patches to help reduce flaking. Essential oils can be diluted in a vegetable-oil base and massaged into the patches of psoriasis to improve the skin and reduce scaling. Try either a mixture of the essential oils of BERGAMOT, LAVENDER and SANDALWOOD.

When psoriasis occurs on the scalp it tends to be more itchy than elsewhere. An infusion of CHICKWEED, MARIGOLD and NETTLES, combined and used as a final hair and scalp rinse after washing, often helps to reduce flakiness and itching.

❄ Ringworm

Ringworm is a fungal infection of the skin that can occur on various parts of the body. The infection tends to spread outwards in a circle, the centre heals while the edges are still active, and a reddish ring-like eruption forms.

Scrupulous hygiene is required alongside local healing applications to eliminate ringworm. If the problem persists after following these suggestions, you should seek constitutional treatment from a qualified practitioner.

Combine the tinctures of ECHINACEA, MARIGOLD and MYRRH and dab the patches of ringworm twice a day. Add a few drops of the essential oils of LAVENDER, MYRRH or TEA TREE to your bath, and also dab on one of them undiluted to the patches of ringworm twice a day. Consult the *Materia Medica* section to see if the homoeopathic remedies of GRAPHITES, SEPIA or SULPHUR look appropriate.

❄ Urticaria

Urticaria (also called nettle-rash or hives) is an allergic reaction set off by being sensitive to various substances such as shellfish, sunlight or penicillin. The red raised lumps or weals that result are caused by the body releasing histamine into the skin and are often intensely itchy. Flare-ups can be associated with stress and this should be taken into account during treatment.

Herbs may be taken internally for a soothing and anti-inflammatory effect. Try drinking an infusion of BALM, CHAMOMILE and HEARTSEASE three times a day. An infusion of CHICKWEED and CHAMOMILE may be used to bathe the affected area. If the urticaria covers a large area of the body, a warm bath with a couple of drops of essential oil of CHAMOMILE or MELISSA will be very soothing to the skin, and will help relieve any associated stress. Alternatively, add a couple of drops of one of the oils to a bowl of warm water and bathe the affected part.

Homoeopathic remedies can be very helpful in relieving the symptoms of urticaria. Consult the following remedies in the *Materia Medica* section of this book to see which one is most suitable for your symptoms: APIS, RHUS TOX and URTICA URENS.

Warts

Warts are fleshy growths on the skin that are found in association with a virus. Only a person who is susceptible to the virus will produce a wart after coming into contact with one.

The most common sites for warts are the fingers, knees, face and genitals. Plantar warts, also called verrucae, are found on the soles of the feet. These usually have a visible dark core, and they may become painful.

External remedies will be successful where the warts are superficial in nature. If the warts do not disappear after several weeks of treatment you should seek constitutional treatment by a qualified practitioner. It is not a good idea to 'burn' off warts using acid and so on because this tends to thwart the body's attempt to express symptoms in a simple, direct way by using the skin as an outlet (anyway, they usually just return!)

A traditional way of eliminating a wart is to squeeze the milky sap from the stalk of fresh DANDELION onto it every day. Rubbing it every day with a slice cut from a clove of GARLIC can also be effective. The essential oils of LEMON and TEA TREE have marked antiviral properties. Try dabbing one of these on neat to the wart every day. For verrucae, make a footbath by adding a few drops of one of the essential oils to warm water and soak the foot every day (this will also help to soften corns or hardened skin on the feet).

18

The Urinary System

The urinary system consists of two kidneys which filter the blood to form urine, their ureters which propel the urine to the bladder, and the urinary bladder where urine is temporarily stored until it is discharged via the urethra.

The essential function of the kidney is to remove the waste products of metabolism from the body in the urine. In addition to this function, by excreting certain minerals and retaining others, the kidneys maintain the acid–alkali ratio of the blood at a constant level. The kidneys also regulate fluid balance. If a large amount of fluid goes into the body, the kidneys excrete more. In very hot weather, when a lot of fluid is lost in perspiration, the kidneys excrete less urine.

The urinary system as a whole is the physical expression of our relationship with fluids. This relationship is determined by our ability to deal with the 'water' aspect of our lives. Water is traditionally a symbol of the emotions, which may be expressed clearly and be a source of joy, or become negative and murky and a reflection of inner discontent. Symbolically, water represents our ability to 'go with the flow of life'. When we achieve this we feel purposeful and content, but when we feel at odds with the direction of our lives, resistance and tension can set in, which may become expressed in the body as symptoms of disease.

The role of the kidneys in detoxifying the body is like that of the running waters of a river that in normal conditions are self-purifying and support great life. But once the toxic overload of pollution becomes too great the waters become poisonous and nothing can thrive. The kidneys and urinary system cleanse and purify the body and keep it healthy, but once they become diseased and prone to infection the body as a whole becomes weakened and less healthy.

In Chinese medicine, the kidneys are considered to be the seat of the *chi* or vital energy of the body, and prolonged exhaustion or an excess of negative

The Urinary System

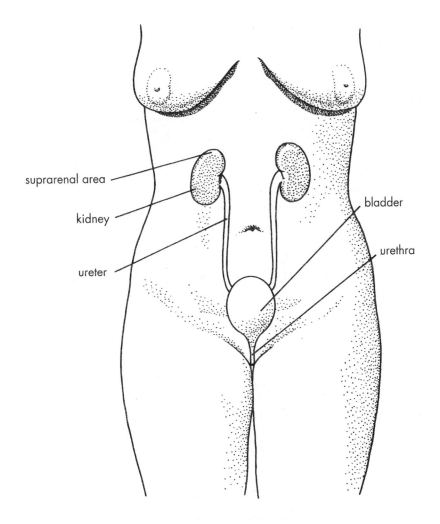

emotion, particularly fear, will weaken the kidney energy and thus the general vitality of the body.

In order to cultivate and maintain a healthy urinary system we should be confident about the quality of the liquids that we take into the body. Many people only drink stimulants, such as tea and coffee or sweet, fizzy drinks, and never pure water. The quality of the water that we drink is also important; it may be better to drink bottled spring water or filtered water because these days tap water is so often contaminated with chlorine, nitrates and unacceptably high levels of heavy metals. Food that is produced without an excess of chemicals and processing will be better for the body as a whole, and less likely to create high levels of toxins for the body's various systems to deal with. The use of salt in the diet tends to inhibit the action of the kidneys and so a low-salt diet will help to maintain a healthy urinary system.

If disease has already developed in the kidneys or urinary system, then professional advice should be sought as quickly as possible, before any further damage is done to this delicate and vital system.

Cystitis

Cystitis is an inflammation and/or infection of the bladder. It is one of the most common ailments in women; nearly every woman suffers from it at some time in her life. A woman's bladder is only about one inch from her urethra; in a man the distance is six or more inches and thus cystitis is much less common in men.

The symptoms of cystitis include feeling an urgent need to urinate, urinating frequently, pain (often burning) during urination and possibly the presence of blood or pus in the urine. Cystitis is not normally a serious condition and it will clear up quickly with the suggested remedies. However, if you have a fever or lower back pain, you should seek urgent medical advice as the kidneys may be involved. Also, get professional advice if the cystitis keeps coming back, so that the underlying causes are dealt with.

Sometimes cystitis or urethritis (inflammation of the urethra) is triggered off by having sex, particularly if it is with a new partner or after a period of abstinence. This is often referred to as 'honeymoon cystitis'. Urinating before and after intercourse and washing afterwards with cool water can help to prevent this. It can also be more frequent during pregnancy, when the foetus is pressing down on the bladder, preventing it from emptying.

The general treatment of cystitis includes drinking an increased amount of water and avoiding stimulants and irritants such as tea, coffee, alcohol and spicy food. Food additives, particularly food colourings, have been found to trigger cystitis symptoms in young girls.

Drinking home-made barley water can be very helpful in treating cystitis: boil pot barley in plenty of water for about 40 minutes, then strain off the liquid and drink several cupfuls a day, with lemon juice (and honey if desired) added. Another natural cure is to soak a tampon in natural yoghurt for an hour, then insert the tampon into the vagina and leave it in overnight. Clinical trials have shown that drinking cranberry juice can relieve cystitis. You can buy this as a drink from supermarkets and you will need to drink several glasses a day.

The herbs used to treat cystitis include urinary antiseptics and diuretics. Decide on a combination of the following herbs, after you have looked them up in the *Materia Medica* section, and make an infusion to drink every few hours: CORNSILK, COUCHGRASS, MARSHMALLOW LEAVES, UVA URSI and YARROW. Essential oils can also bring great relief to cystitis symptoms. Choose from BERGAMOT, LAVENDER and SANDALWOOD, or combine them and add a few drops to a warm bath for a soothing and antiseptic effect. The homoeopathic remedies to compare in the treatment of cystitis include APIS, BELLADONNA, CANTHARIS, MERC SOL and NUX VOM.

Kidney Stones

Kidney stones, also called renal calculi, are fairly common. They may remain silent in the kidney, without symptoms; however, if they move they may give rise to renal colic. Renal colic causes severe pain over the kidney area, with restlessness, sweating and maybe vomiting. If you have these symptoms consult a medical practitioner immediately for a diagnosis.

Kidney stones can respond well to natural remedies and they can be dissolved and passed out of the system during urination. For the best results, visit a professional practitioner, although the following remedies may be tried in a mild case or during a painful attack of renal colic.

It is important for anyone with kidney stones to drink plenty of water (about three litres a day) in order to flush the kidneys through regularly. The herbs that may be taken to dissolve the stones include CELERY SEED, MARSH-MALLOW, PARSLEY PIERT, STONE ROOT and PELLITORY OF THE WALL. A decoction (or tinctures) of these should be drunk twice a day for several months in order to obtain a result. During an acute attack of renal colic, try an infusion containing CORNSILK, COUCHGRASS, MARSHMALLOW LEAVES and YARROW. The essential oils that have been used to treat kidney stones include FENNEL, GERANIUM, JUNIPER and LEMON. Compare them in the *Materia Medica* section, then blend a chosen combination and dilute in vegetable oil to massage over the kidney area or use in the bath. You should consult a qualified homoeopath to rid the system of kidney stones by homoeopathy; if you want to treat the acute pain of renal colic, BERBERIS, CANTHARIS or MAG PHOS may be tried.

✤ Stress Incontinence

Urine may be lost involuntarily when coughing, sneezing, laughing or performing other motions causing abdominal pressure on the bladder. This is known as stress incontinence. The tendency to stress incontinence is the result of a weakening of the pelvic-floor muscles following childbirth. Long labours, large babies, multiple pregnancies and rapid deliveries may all weaken the pelvic-floor muscles and lead to stress incontinence. The problem may not show up until later in life, after the menopause, and it may be related to a prolapse *(see Prolapse, page 152).*

Mild stress incontinence may be improved by regular pelvic-floor exercises. Astringent herbs and other remedies may also be helpful. More severe cases may need surgery.

The best exercise is to contract the muscles that you would use to stop urination in mid-stream. Do not actually do the exercise regularly whilst urinating, as it can lead to cystitis, but if you do it once to learn where the muscles are then you can do the exercise every day. The technique is to contract the muscles in several stages, like going up in a lift, then hold the contracted position for a few moments before releasing in stages. (It is the same exercise as to correct a prolapse.)

The main herb used to treat stress incontinence is HORSETAIL. AGNUS CASTUS and ST JOHN'S WORT can also be useful, particularly if the problem becomes worse during the menopause. The most commonly indicated homeopathic remedies are CAUSTICUM, NATRUM MUR and SEPIA. Check all these in the *Materia Medica* section to see which is the most appropriate for you.

⚛ Water Retention

There are many causes of water retention, ranging from heart failure to premenstrual tension. It is noticeable when the tissue under the skin becomes swollen and puffy, usually around the feet and ankles, although it may occur in the abdomen or the hands. Obviously the treatment depends on what is causing the fluid retention and this must be established so that treatment can follow accordingly.

The intake of salt will tend to make water retention worse, whatever the cause, so a salt-free diet is advisable. If the cause of the water retention is of a serious nature, such as heart or kidney failure, then you must seek professional treatment. If the cause is not serious and the water retention is temporary, as it is with pre-menstrual tension, then there are several natural diuretics to try. Herbal diuretics include DANDELION, UVA URSI and YARROW. Make up an infusion of these to drink three times a day when required. The essential oils of CYPRESS and JUNIPER are effective diuretics that you can dilute and massage in where required, or add to your bath. Diuretics should not be taken during pregnancy without professional recommendation.

part II:

Materia Medica

Introduction to the
Materia Medica

This section contains the remedies that are described to help relieve the illnesses and problems mentioned within the systems. Remedies that have been suggested are outlined here so that you can become familiar with the remedy before a choice is made.

We are all individuals, with our own set of symptoms and with our own tendencies and personalities, so choose the remedy that is appropriate for you and your problems. We have selected the most common natural medicines, but there are a lot more: this selection is primarily a useful introduction. Also, the descriptions are not comprehensive – we have merely tried to present a picture that is wide enough for you to be able to use. They are intended to be a guide to some of the options available as opposed to a complete treatise on homoeopathy, herbalism or aromatherapy.

The therapies need to be understood and the remedies experienced. The best way of gaining knowledge is by deciding which one to use and seeing the results. The importance of making choices is discussed in the Lifestyle section. It is true here. Look up and read the remedy that you are interested in using and if it seems appropriate, try it. What are the results? By trying the remedies you will learn which ones work.

The choice may be quite easy. You scald yourself making a cup of tea but you don't have a handy tube of ointment or lavender oil. However, there is the aloe vera plant sitting in the window. Use it. Likewise, your child is hot, dry, flushed with a high temperature. You think she needs belladonna but you only have ferrum phos in the cupboard. Give this while you phone round for the right remedy. We also suggest that you combine remedies. Neuralgia, for example, may well be helped by mixing a couple of drops of lavender and chamomile essential oils into a macerated oil of hypericum, and gently rubbing the mixture onto the areas where the nerves are inflamed; it may also be a good idea to take repeated doses of kali phos or mag phos, which are known to help nerve tissue. Knowing these natural remedies will take a lifetime, but becoming familar with them is part of a process of involving yourself in your own well-being. Each remedy has its own secret – which we can start to discover through using them.

PLEASE NOTE: Throughout this section of the book, 1ml is equal to 25 drops. This is an approximation, as are the quantities given throughout the *Materia Medica*.

Herbal Medicine

Herbalism is part of the ancient art of healing. Traditionally, we used plants because they grew around us and we knew of their healing properties. They were part of our lives. We used plants for nourishment, for healing, for ritual. Nowadays, we are able to decipher a train timetable, road map or instructions to assemble a chest of drawers, but then we were familiar with our natural environment. We lived according to the changing seasons, we were skilled in healing, in collecting, drying and storing plants. Knowing plants was one of our skills and we knew which plants to use. In western industrialized society, our knowledge of herbs has been generally lost. But it is not just this knowledge that has disappeared, we no longer keep in contact with our natural environment and, in the same way, with our own bodies.

Over the centuries, the medical profession has became dominated by men, and the use of herbs has given way to developments that are less intuitive, are more scientific. Herbalism in many parts of Europe and the industrialized world has lost credibility. But now, as the awareness about our planet grows, so herbalism is returning. How many plant species are we destroying with the forests of South America, Indonesia and elsewhere? What healing potential is disappearing? How long is it before the indigenous people of these regions lose their skills? For example, as desertification increases, families are forced to move in search of livelihoods, so traditions in natural medicine are replaced by quicker solutions. Patterns of health change and treatments are based on the use of drugs and programmes of vaccination.

By entering the world of herbs we can discover a world network of knowledge and tradition. Even if the specific herbs used may be different, the language of use is similar. The various indigenous cultures across the planet will make use of the plants and other healing substances that they know. This use of their environment, the respect that they hold for it, seems to create a common language for world herbalism. In turn, every plant has adapted to its environment and so local diseases and needs reflect the territory and lifestyle of the local population. Arnica grows on high rocky mountains and is good for sprains, broken limbs, etc. The herbal systems of China have been established for centuries; similarly, in areas of the former Soviet Union, Africa, Australia, North and South America and elsewhere, they are part of the indigenous way of living. Throughout the world plants were or are used as medicines. What we all had in common was the knowledge that plants are effective healers and we shared the skills to use them.

For the last 25 years the tradition of herbalism has been returning to the West. Schools and courses have been established and herbalism, once again, provides a system of healing that is sympathetic with our natural environment and with the way our bodies work. There has been a considerable increase in research as herbs are the basis of many modern drugs and herbs are now seen as a commercial opportunity by several pharmaceutical companies. The active components are isolated and synthesized to respond to particular symptoms. This can create new problems of control and standardization. Debate about how herbs can best work and best be used continues. There are new issues too, as the popularity increases, regarding conservation and supply. Many species are in danger of extinction as people see herbs as a commercial opportunity. Individual knowledge of herbs and sensitive use and collection must be the way forward. Herbalism is not exempt from the effects of global commercialization and the media.

WORKING THE HERBS WITH THE BODY SYSTEMS
Herbs support the healing processes of the body and tend to be used to treat or rebalance a particular system of the body. They can be classified according to the function that the herb has on the body system.

THE CIRCULATION AND HEART
Herbs, e.g. ginkgo, hawthorn and rosemary, improve circulation to the head and act to normalize the blood pressure. Cayenne and prickly ash bark stimulate the flow of blood to the extremities. *Diaphoretics*, e.g. ginger and yarrow, help to promote sweating by encouraging the flow of blood to the skin. *Nerve sedatives*, e.g. borage, reduce heart rate and blood pressure. *Antispasmodics*, e.g. cayenne, help to relax the muscles and lower blood pressure.

THE DIGESTIVE SYSTEM

Anti-inflammatory herbs, e.g. chamomile, heartsease and meadowsweet, will assist in reducing inflammation of the gut. *Hepatics*, e.g. dandelion, will help detoxify the liver. *Demulcents*, e.g. marshmallow and slippery elm, will have a soothing effect due to their mucilaginous contents. *Bitter tonics*, e.g. milk thistle, will be protective to the liver and help the regeneration of cells. *Carminatives*, e.g. peppermint, will aid digestion and reduce flatulence. *Laxatives*, e.g. senna, will help the elimination from the bowels.

THE ENDOCRINE SYSTEM

Emmenagogues, e.g. black cohosh and sage, will stimulate or regulate menstruation. *Hormone regulators*, e.g. agnus castus, will stabilize hormones. *Styptics*, e.g. lady's mantle, will reduce blood flow.

THE IMMUNE SYSTEM

Immune stimulants, e.g. echinacea and thyme, help protect the body against disease.

THE MUSCULAR AND SKELETAL SYSTEM

Analgesic herbs, e.g. feverfew, St John's Wort, valerian and white willow, are pain-relievers. *Anti-inflammatory* herbs, e.g. chamomile, comfrey, marigold, meadowsweet and tumeric, reduce swelling. *Antispasmodic* herbs, e.g. balm, chamomile, cinchona and crampbark, relax or ease tension and cramps in the muscles.

THE NERVOUS SYSTEM

Nervines, e.g. lemon balm and oats, will have a strengthening and relaxing effect on the nervous system. Herbs serve as *antidepressives*, e.g. borage, and *nerve tonics*, e.g. nettles, rosemary and St John's Wort. *Sedatives*, e.g. limeflowers, passiflora and skullcap, will have a calming effect.

THE RESPIRATORY SYSTEM

Antiseptics, e.g. thyme, help to combat infections. *Lung tonics*, e.g. thyme, strengthen the lungs. *Diaphoretics*, e.g. elderflowers, help to reduce fever. *Expectorants* e.g. coltsfoot, heartsease and white horehound, stimulate the mucous membranes to eliminate phlegm and mucus.

THE SKIN
Herbs known as *alteratives* or *adaptogens*, e.g. burdock, cleavers, clover and nettles, assist the elimination and detoxification processes. They are known as blood cleansers. *Vulnerary* action promotes skin healing, e.g. comfrey, while other herbs are *anti-inflammatory*, e.g. chamomile and marigold.

THE URINARY SYSTEM
Diuretics, e.g. cornsilk, couchgrass, dandelion and nettles, stimulate the elimination of urine. *Antiseptics*, e.g. couchgrass and echinacea, are antimicrobials that disinfect the system of harmful bacteria. *Astringents*, e.g. agrimony, horsetail, raspberry leaves and witch hazel leaves, have a contracting effect on the blood vessels and mucous membranes.

HERBAL CONSTITUENTS
Herbs are made up of a huge number of constituents, many of which will affect the action of the herb. These components have been isolated recently and knowing a little about them can help you to understand how the plants work and will assist you in making the choice between one herb and another. Below are the main groups of constituents commonly found in herbs.

ALKALOIDS
Contain nitrogen and can have a direct action on the blood tissue. Examples are black cohosh and comfrey. Can be toxic.

ANTHRAQUINONES
Act as purgatives by causing contractions of the intestinal walls about 10 hours after taking. Examples are rhubarb, senna and yellow dock. Can be irritants.

BITTERS
This group is characterized by the bitter taste in the herbs. It will stimulate secretions of the salivary glands and digestive organs. This can improve the appetite and the function of the digestive system. Examples are chamomile, goldenseal and rosemary.

COUMARINS
A diverse group of chemical actions, used to prevent blood clotting. Meliot is an example. Can have strong adverse effects.

FLAVONOIDS

A wide group often characterized by their yellow-coloured plant constituents. Diuretic, *antispasmodic, antiseptic* actions. Need to be present to help absorption of vitamin C. Examples are coltsfoot, limeflowers and rutin.

MUCILAGE

Composed of polysaccharides that soak up water. Found in many plants, e.g. comfrey, slippery elm, mucilage lines the mucous membranes and protects against irritation and inflammation.

PHENOLS

This group of compounds includes salicylic acid. They are antiseptic and reduce inflammation when taken internally, but have an irritant effect on the skin. Take care when using essential oils that are part of this group. An example is white willow.

SAPONINS

These are glycosides that have a detergent effect and may resemble the body's own steroid hormones. Examples are liquorice and wild yam.

TANNINS

Most plants have tannins present, astringents that contract the body tissues. Examples are agrimony and witch hazel.

VITAMINS

Most plants contain some vitamins, which are necessary for vitality and growth. Plants especially high in vitamins include dandelions and nettles.

VOLATILE OILS

These constituents are the fragrant components of plants. When isolated from the plant they are known as Essential Oils (EO). They serve a wide range of functions.

USING HERBS

All the herbs mentioned in the *Materia Medica* are available from herbalist shops. A dried herb should look and smell fresh. Try to buy organically grown herbs that are certified by the Soil Association. These herbs will also be free of any fumigation processes or irradiation that imported herbs may be subjected to. Many of the herbs mentioned can be grown in your garden or are already there as weeds! It is best to gather them first thing in the morning. Herbs can be collected and used when needed. Herbs are best gathered from land away from pollution, traffic and domestic pets. Drying herbs need dry air circulating around them, so hanging bunches of herbs protected by paper bags in a ventilated spare room works quite well. Dried herbs should be stored away from light and in airtight jars.

Herbal preparations can be taken hot or cold. A hot infusion or decoction will encourage sweating, so use for treating 'flu, fevers, etc. Cold preparations tend to be more diuretic.

INFUSIONS
Make an infusion as you would tea. Pour 600ml (1 pint) of boiling water onto a heaped tablespoon (25g) of herb or herbal mixture, cover it and let it stand for 7–10 mins. If you want to make an individual cup the general rule is a teaspoonful per cup of boiling water. Use twice the quantity if you are using fresh herbs.

DECOCTIONS
When the herb being used is woody, such as barks, roots and berries, it is necessary to place the herb or mixture of herbs in a saucepan. Don't use an aluminium pan or a chipped enamel one. Add 600ml (1 pint) of water to each 30g (1oz) of herb and bring to the boil, allow to simmer for 10 mins. The mixture can be strained and stored in the fridge, as only a small wine glassful will be needed 2–3 times a day.

TINCTURES
A tincture is an extraction of the herb using water and alcohol. The quantities of liquid to plant material will vary as will the ratio of water to alcohol. Most tinctures use approximately 30 per cent alcohol to water, but calendula for example will use as much as 90 per cent. The herbs are left covered by liquid, shaken every other day and at the end of three weeks all the plant material is removed, leaving a tincture which should be stored in a cool dark place. This can be a much easier way to take a herbal treatment and is a way of preserving herbs out of season. The usual amount is between 1ml and a teaspoonful (5ml) in a glass of water taken three times a day.

MACERATED OILS

The main macerated oils available are St John's Wort oil, calendula oil, carrot oil and comfrey oil. It is quite possible to make your own macerated oil by covering the plant material with oil, such as sunflower or olive oil, leaving it in a warm place, such as a sunny window ledge, and shaking it from time to time. It will be ready to use when the oil has taken on the colour and smell of the herb. At this stage, take out the herb by passing the oil through a fine sieve. Another method of making macerates is to slowly heat the plant material covered by oil in a double boiler, maintain at a low heat for 20–30 minutes. Allow to cool before removing the plant material.

COMPRESSES AND POULTICES

When you are making a compress, use a clean cloth and soak it in the hot infusion or decoction of herbs that you require. Apply the cloth (as hot as you can bear it) to the area where it is needed. When it cools down, it can be changed. If it is appropriate, a sheet of plastic and a hot-water bottle may keep it warm for longer and enhance the action of the herb.

A poultice is similar, but you apply the fresh or dried herb directly onto the skin. Make a paste with hot water and apply as hot as possible. It may be a good idea to apply a little oil to the skin beforehand so that the poultice is easier to wash off afterwards.

HERBAL SALVE

An ointment or salve can be useful where you need a healing yet protective covering, and you can make it according to your needs. Use for cuts, blemishes, dry skin, rashes and other complaints. It can be a good barrier for a baby's nappy rash. One that we make is very easy and effective:

> 40g (1½oz) beeswax
> 104g (3½oz) soya oil
> 16g (½oz) apricot kernel oil
> 8g (¼oz) wheatgerm oil or oil of your choice

Melt together in a double boiler

> 8g (½oz) macerated oil (St John's Wort, comfrey, etc.) as required
> 3.5ml tincture (marshmallow, goldenseal, etc.) as required

Add 2g essential oil of your choice, macerate wax and tincture to the mixture and simmer until the liquid from the tincture has evaporated. Remove from heat and add up to 2g of an essential oil. Mix well and pour into sterilized jars.

DOUCHE

When there are local infections in the vagina, a douche may be used in conjunction with a course of remedies taken internally. Make an infusion of 15g (½oz) of herb, 570ml (1 pint) of water, or decoction, and sieve very carefully. Check that no bits are left before putting it into the container of the douche or drawing it up into the receptacle. Do check that it is the right temperature (36–37°C); if it is too hot or too cold it will be very uncomfortable. Insert the applicator into the vagina and let the liquid rinse the area. It is probably best to do this in the bath or on the toilet, as all the liquid will run out. Do not persist with douching if there is no improvement after a few days, and consult a qualified practitioner. Do not use a douche when you are pregnant.

USING HERBS IN THE BATH OR FOOTBATH

Herbal infusions can be absorbed through the skin. A pleasant way is to put them into the bath. A muslin or cotton bag can be made quite easily to hold either a herb or herbal mixture. Tie it tightly at the top and place under the running hot water. It can also be left in the bath while you lie there soaking up the benefits. 30g (1oz) will be needed to have a reasonable effect. This method is especially good for nervine tonics or anti-inflammatory herbs for the skin. A particularly good mixture for the skin is rose petals, lavender, chamomile, borage and cleavers, though of course put in the herbs that you feel are particularly appropriate for you. A relaxing herb bath can be made from orange blossom, chamomile, lavender, limeflowers and lemon balm.

A warming foot bath can be made by adding ginger and yarrow when you feel a cold coming on. Add peppermint, marigold and marshmallow when the feet are tired and aching.

Do not use herbs for a prolonged period of time unless otherwise indicated by a practitioner. Because a herbal remedy is a natural remedy it doesn't necessarily mean that it is safe to use on a continuous basis or in large quantities. Use care and common sense and always consult a herbal practitioner if you feel unsure about what you are doing.

Chinese Herbs

A number of Chinese herbs are mentioned in the book which we know to be beneficial in the ways mentioned. They should be seen within the context of the whole of the Chinese herbal system.

Essential Oils

Treatment using essential oils is generally known as aromatherapy. This term was first used by a French chemist, Gattefosse, in the 1920s, although the use of oils is recorded as far back as records go. It is the fragrance that is significant as well as the healing properties of the plant. Generally, smell is the least valued of all the senses, largely because it has escaped description. Perhaps because of our inability to categorize it, smell often has the power to evoke memories and associations more directly than other senses, and to affect us on a subconscious level. Different smells trigger different feelings and reactions. Essential oils can be very useful tools in healing, often because of this effect on our emotions. Research is now being done on various oils and they are coming to be recognized as valuable antibacterial and antiviral agents.

Oils are produced by distillation from plant material that contains volatile oils. This can come from roots such as orris (from the rhizome of the iris), barks such as cinnamon, seeds, berries and fruits such as cardamon, juniper and bergamot, leaves such as melissa, wood such as cedar, flowers such as ylang-ylang or gums and resins such as myrrh. It is only the oily part which is separated out. An essential oil is therefore a highly concentrated plant substance. An oil varies enormously according to the type of distillation process, the variety of plant used, the growing conditions, etc. Distillation is done by either water, steam or steam *and* water; different methods produce different results, and although generally it is known which type of distillation method is best for the particular plant, it can vary from country to country.

Other methods of extraction include the use of solvents in the flower oils (called absolutes), and cold pressing the rinds of the citrus fruit.

The variety of the plant can make a great difference to the oil. Eucalyptus oil is an obvious example, with over 700 known species. Be aware too of the difference in oils made from different parts of a plant. Clove oil can either be extracted from the bud, the stem or the leaf.

These are all ways in which the oils can vary. Until recently the market for which the oils were produced was almost exclusively for the perfumer and flavourist. Their particular sciences require their oils to be exact, predictable and often highly refined. Therefore the oils that are produced for them are not always appropriate for the aromatherapist, who needs a pure essential oil which is properly distilled from fresh and, if possible, organically-grown plant material.

These oils are often very expensive because of the small quantity of oil present in a leaf or flower. The collection of flowers such as neroli (orange blossom) is very labour intensive and it needs to be distilled quickly to prevent deterioration. Often a distillation of the neroli is followed by a distillation of the leaves to produce petitgrain. It is not surprising that a less expensive neroli oil can contain some petitgrain. Unfortunately, adulteration is common with many of the oils. The main problem is the lack of accurate information available which someone using essential oils for therapeutic purposes needs to know. Our advice, when purchasing an oil, is to ask for exact information. You need to know what you are getting: the variety of the plant, type of extraction, country of origin and part of plant used.

MASSAGE

One of the best ways of using essential oils is by diluting them in a base oil. There are a range of vegetable oils that are suitable to use. Sweet almond oil is easily obtainable, good for sensitive skin, light and with little or no smell. Apricot kernel oil is similar. Grapeseed oil is especially light and not quite so oily as almond oil. It is also very easily absorbed into the skin. Soya oil is inexpensive and makes a good base, although be careful to obtain an organic standard, guaranteed to be GM-free. It is good to use when you want to include a heavier oil such as avocado, wheatgerm or olive oil. These three oils are thicker, with their own fragrance, and are probably best included to make a richer base. Avocado is a thick, rich, green oil that is very nourishing to the skin. It is good to include when the skin is very dry and papery.

Wheatgerm oil is good to add where there is scarring and acne, etc. Being an antioxidant it can also help act as a preservative. It can be used on its own (rubbing it on the abdomen during pregnancy can help prevent stretch marks) but it is sticky and difficult to use, so it is generally mixed in with a lighter oil. Olive oil is another vitamin-rich oil and is excellent to keep the skin supple. Use it to prevent skin dehydrating in the summer or during a cold winter. It is good to mix with coconut oil as a base oil when the skin is exposed to the sun. It does have a strong smell and is less versatile when only a few drops of essential oils are required. Hazelnut oil has a beautiful rich, nutty fragrance and again is very nourishing. Evening primrose oil is excellent to add to mixtures for skin treatments because it is very healing. Care must be taken though, as it is one of the quickest oils to oxidize and will make the whole mixture go rancid if it is kept for some time. Jojoba oil is good to use when the skin is oily. It gives the skin a smooth, waxy feel.

Here are some suggested blends:

Soya	60%	
Almond	30%	An all-round base oil
Wheatgerm	10%	
Grapeseed	80%	
Macerated oil of calendula	10%	A very light oil where the
Evening Primrose	10%	skin needs healing
Olive	40%	
Coconut	50%	For dehydrated skin
Macerated oil of calendula	10%	exposed to sun
Olive	50%	
Calendula	25%	For sunburnt skin
St John's Wort	25%	
Macerated oil of comfrey	50%	A base oil for muscular
Calendula	25%	aches and stiffness
Grapeseed	25%	with bruising
Hazelnut	35%	
Avocado or wheatgerm	15%	For ageing, dehydrated skin
Almond	50%	

Adding essential oils to your base will vary according to the base, the oil and the person, but generally the proportion of essential oil to base should be 1–3 per cent. This roughly means that 20–60 drops of essential oil (or combined oils) should be added to 100ml of base oil. For one massage, pour a little base oil into a saucer and add 2–3 drops of the essential oil.

There are many good books and courses available on massage. Massage can be a relaxing, tension and stress-relieving process; it can also be stimulating, toning and re-energizing, or it can be a mixture of both. It is a skill that we feel all of us can have and it is a method of communication. Giving someone permission to touch your body requires trust and a willingness to be receptive and vulnerable. When you are working on a person's body you are giving to them of yourself and are communicating that you care. Learn to express yourself through massage for therapeutic reasons as well as for enjoyment.

There are several other ways essential oils can be used, for example:

BASE CREAM
Use in a similar way as a base oil, although a lower percentage of essential oil should be added – not more than 1 per cent. It may be easier to use when a very oily base is not required.

OIL BURNER OR DIFFUSER
Oils can be a very effective way to help clear the atmosphere. They mask unpleasant smells, can be used to fumigate a room from contagious diseases or create a change in the atmosphere. Put 2–3 drops of essential oil into a water-filled receptacle above a candle and the room will be slowly fragranced. Be careful that the water does not dry out, leaving the oil to burn. Olibanum (frankincense) is particularly good, and sandalwood, cedarwood and rosewood are all excellent to help atmosphere change. Use antiseptic oils for fumigation: *Eucalyptus citriodora* is particularly good when combined with lavender or lemon. Try out different combinations: mixing a citrus oil with a sweeter or woody oil will give a more rounded, fuller scent, for example mandarin with ylang-ylang or sandalwood.

INHALATIONS
Add 3–4 drops of oil to a bowl of steaming water and cover the head and bowl with a towel to inhale the oils. This is particularly useful for respiratory complaints and congestion. It can also be good for skin problems. One suggestion for spotty, clogged pores is to pour boiling water onto 30g (1oz) of chamomile and elderflower herb mix before adding the oil of your choice, such as lavender or rose.

BATHS
One of the easiest ways to use oils is by adding them to a hot bath. In order to disperse the essential oil molecules, so that they cannot irritate delicate mucous

membranes, they must be prediluted before adding to the bathwater. Add 5–10 drops of the essential oil or blend to 10ml of base oil, milk or dispersing oil base, and then add to the bathwater when run. Adding the oil of your choice just before you get in will give you the benefit of the aroma. Allow yourself at least 15 mins in the bath to derive full benefit. It is especially good to help relieve tension. If you are feeling too detached or overwhelmed or find yourself ignoring outside needs or not coping with affection – all signs of stress – a bath with oils such as geranium and lavender can be of great benefit. It can also be good when a really cleansing bath is required. Combine with a bagful of herbs and a few drops of Bach walnut or crabapple flower remedies when you wish to rid yourself of outside influences and regain contact with yourself. Adding a blend of oils to a bath can help eliminate toxins and help sluggish conditions – rosemary is especially good for this.

COMPRESSES

Oils can be used in compresses in similar ways to that described in the general information on herbs on pages 184–92 but extra care must be taken as they are so concentrated.

CAUTION: Always remember that essential oils are highly concentrated and never apply them directly to the skin. Some should only be used after some experience and knowledge of both the oils and the person you are treating. Anyone with sensitive skin should do a patch test before using a new oil extensively. In general, treat all oils with caution, but in particular the spice oils: black pepper, cinnamon and clove can irritate the skin. Citrus oils must be used with care, and the following oils should be avoided during pregnancy: basil, camphor, hyssop, nutmeg, oreganum, pennyroyal, sage, and wintergreen.

Do not use essential oils on babies and be very careful with children – never use more than 1 per cent dilution. Do not continue using an oil over a prolonged period of time: once a day for 3 weeks is the maximum unless directed otherwise by a qualified practitioner.

Never take the oils internally, unless a medically qualified aromatherapist has directed you to do so.

Homoeopathic Remedies

Unlike herbalism, homoeopathy has not been established as a system of healing for much longer than 200 years. The 'law of similars' though, on which the principles of homoeopathy are based, was a concept understood amongst ancient civilizations. What creates imbalance is also that which can create balance. It has been well known amongst herbalists that a herb given in small amounts will cure symptoms that it will create in larger doses. For example, valerian in small doses relieves tension; larger amounts can cause headaches. Datura is an excellent remedy for lung complaints, but in larger quantities it is a poison. Belladonna, a major homoeopathic remedy, will cure violent, sudden complaints – headaches, sweating, fever, convulsions, etc. – whereas in its plant form it will cause these symptoms. Apis mel is another remedy, made from the sting of a bee, which is a homoeopathic cure for painful red swellings.

In recent medical history, we have come to separate the person from their symptoms; treatments have been directed towards specific ailments, and these can be detrimental to the whole body. Medical practitioners have often failed to understand what a cure is. Dr S. Hahnemann (1755–1843), who devised the system of homoeopathy as we know it, defined cure as 'a recovery undisturbed by after-suffering'. With homoeopathy, the aim is to restore balance to the person.

There are a great many homoeopathic remedies. The skill of the homoeopath is to match the most appropriate remedy 'picture' to that of the person. This is done by accurate observation of the individual. All the tiny details are noted and are seen as clues to choosing the right remedy. It is important to look at the whole person, and her habits on mental and emotional levels as well as the physical.

CHOOSING A HOMOEOPATHIC REMEDY

In this *Materia Medica* section, the homoeopathic monographs give a rough outline of the main problems that are covered by the remedy. Before selecting one that has been mentioned in the section on systems, make a note of all the changes that have taken place while you or the person you are treating has been ill. Carefully observe the symptoms. Your friend has a bad cold; is there an accompanying headache? Aching limbs? A flushed face? Does she feel very cold or hot? Is she feeling congested? Check whether she feels better or worse lying down, sitting up, etc. Also, learn to observe changes in mood and thought patterns – everything you notice will lead to making the right decision.

PLEASE NOTE: when you read through a monograph, remember that it does not matter if you do not have all the symptoms covered by a particular remedy. What does matter is that all the symptoms felt by you, or the person you are treating, are included in the homoeopathic remedy picture. Unlike herbs, it is best not to combine homoeopathic remedies.

CHOOSING A POTENCY

Homoeopathy is a very subtle form of healing. A remedy is made from a substance from one of the three kingdoms – animal, vegetable or mineral. It is reduced to such an extent that it does not contain sufficient matter to act directly on the tissues. An amount of the original substance is taken, mixed with alcohol and made into a tincture (mother tincture). If one tenth of this is taken out and added to nine-tenths of alcohol, it is shaken (succussed), and this results in a 1X remedy. A 6X potency has therefore been diluted and succussed six times. A C potency is based on a different method of division. One part in 100 is taken out each time and added to another 99 parts. This is done 200 times to produce a 200th (200C) potency. The more times the remedy is diluted the higher the potency. It is paradoxical to our materialistic way of thinking that the more reduced the original substance becomes, the more profound the action of the remedy. Do not let these processes put you off using homoeopathic remedies: it is safe to use the lower potencies and these can be given on a repeated basis.

DOSAGE

When the symptoms are very acute a 6X potency can be given hourly or even more frequently. But for longer term, chronic conditions give one dosage in the morning and one at night. A 30C potency can be given for more dramatic, acute symptoms, where the whole body is involved and a more profound reaction is needed. Give one or two doses.

For example, arnica 6 can be given repeatedly for bruising, aches and pains. When the injury involves some shock to the body use arnica 30. This can be repeated once or twice, preferably eight hours apart, but it is advisable not to use any 30 potency over a prolonged period of time. Arnica 200 would be much more effective if the person were in a severe state of shock after an accident, and one dose should be sufficient. It is important to remember to *stop* taking the remedy when the symptoms start improving. If the symptoms return, repeat the remedy. Keep an eye on the symptom picture; if it changes, change the remedy. If there is no change in the condition after about six doses, look for a better alternative or get advice. Do not give a high potency of one remedy and then follow it up with a lower potency of the same remedy, however if a remedy works but the beneficial effects disappear, try a higher potency.

Homoeopathic remedies do work; they are used very effectively by vets on animals and recently a few controlled tests have been done to prove their effectiveness. We cannot really explain *how* they work other than by suggesting that they encourage the natural forces of the body to restore a healthy balance by stimulating the person's vitality and directing energy where it is needed. It is a truly holistic form of healing. The fact that the more refined (i.e. diluted) the remedy the more profound the effect suggests it may be possible, in the future, to stimulate the body's healing processes without any remedy at all. This takes us into the area of spiritual healing which is in fact the basis from which shamans and witch doctors operate in non-materialistic societies. It is an ability that has been largely lost, but perhaps it will be acknowledged more in the future.

Until then it is worth remembering that homoeopathic remedies have no side-effects, they are cheap to produce and do not deplete natural resources. This makes them ideal for countries such as India, where homoeopathy is widely practised and recognized.

A final comment on homoeopathic medicines: they are sensitive and need to be treated with care – store them in a cool, dark place away from strong smells. It is advisable to avoid taking coffee, peppermint, menthol, camphor or eucalyptus while using a homoeopathic treatment. They may antidote it, and it would be a shame to risk this happening.

Flower Remedies

Flower remedies are a wonderfully accessible way of helping emotional and mental states. Often imbalances in these areas will give rise to problems on the physical level.

Flower remedies were first used by Dr Edward Bach (1886–1936). He discovered that remedies could be made from flowers, where the vitality of the plant was received by the water placed close by, and this would help feelings of fear, anxiety and irritation. His medical researches led him to the understanding that much of our ill health has its origin in our emotional and mental state rather than in the physical body.

Each of the 'remedy-states' that Dr Bach described has a positive and negative aspect and he saw the negative conditions as the true cause of illness and disease. The flowers embody the positive state; their natural vibrations help us to enjoy life and return to health.

Since Bach remedies have been used to such effect, there has been a proliferation of other remedies made by many different people from all over the world in many different habitats. Some of the more widely used ranges include the Californian essences, the Bush Flower remedies, Bailey remedies, etc.

Bach Flower Remedies

Thank you to Julian Barnard for the following information.

DIAGNOSIS AND DOSAGE
Select from the list any remedies that feel appropriate. It is best to limit the number to no more than five or six.

To make a medicine strength mixture: take 2 drops from each chosen stock remedy and put into a small bottle of water, about 30ml, adding brandy if desired, as a preservative. If Five Flower Remedy is chosen, then 4 drops of stock are used. Dosage is then 4 drops, 4 times daily. Alternatively, for short-term problems, put 2 drops of each stock remedy into a glass of water and sip at intervals until relief is obtained.

Benefit is derived from small regular doses rather than by the volume of remedy that is taken. An inappropriate remedy will not hurt or cause adverse reaction. There is no need for fear of overdose or error – feel confident and trust yourself. Remedies may be taken direct from the stock bottle, but this has no greater benefit than the diluted remedy.

FIVE FLOWER REMEDY
Dr Bach chose five of the 38 remedies as a first aid combination, naming them the *Rescue Remedy*. This may be used in any kind of emergency, trauma or in circumstances when we need immediate help, before and after moments of difficulty, for accidents and upsets of every kind.

This first aid combination is always helpful bringing calm, restoring peace and emotional balance. It will help both the people affected and those who assist or watch. It is also good for plants and animals, with the addition of other single remedies as appropriate. *Dosage:* Mix the Five Flower Remedy to medicine strength using 4 drops in a small bottle (30ml) of brandy and water, then take 4 drops as often as required. Alternatively put 4 drops into a glass of water and sip frequently.

THE REMEDIES
The remedies were grouped by Dr Bach under seven headings. In these brief descriptions the negative state is given first with some positive aspects at the end *in italics*. The full description for each remedy state, as given by Dr Bach, can be found in *Twelve Healers* (C.W. Daniel, 1933).

FOR FEAR:

Aspen	Vague, unknown, haunting fears, trembling apprehension and premonitions; *trusting the unknown.*
Cherry Plum	Fear of losing control, doing dreaded things, desperation; *mental calm and sanity.*
Mimulus	Fear of specific, known things – animals, heights, pain, etc., nervous, shy people; *bravery.*
Red Chestnut	Worry for others, anticipating misfortune, projecting anxiety; *trusting to life.*
Rock Rose	Panic, terror, hysteria, horror, dread; *the courage to face an emergency.*

FOR UNCERTAINTY:

Cerato	Distrust of self and intuition, easily led and misguided; *confidently seek individuality.*
Gentian	Discouragement, doubt, melancholy; *take heart and have faith.*
Gorse	No hope, accept chronic illness or difficulty, pointless to try; *the sunshine of renewed hope.*
Hornbeam	Weary and can't cope, temporary fatigue; *strengthens and supports.*
Scleranthus	Cannot resolve two choices, indecision, alternating; *balance and determination.*
Wild Oat	Lack of direction, unfulfilled, drifting; *becoming definite and purposeful.*

INSUFFICIENT INTEREST IN PRESENT CIRCUMSTANCES:

Chestnut Bud   Failing to learn from life, repeating mistakes, lack of observation; *learning from experience.*

Clematis   Dreamers, drowsy, absent-minded; *brings down to earth.*

Honeysuckle   Living in memories; *involved in present.*

Mustard   Gloom and despair suddenly cloud us, for no apparent reason; *clarity.*

Olive   Exhausted, no more strength, need physical and mental renewal; *rested and supported.*

White Chestnut   Unresolved, circling thoughts, mental turmoil; *a calm, clear mind.*

Wild Rose   Lack of interest, resignation, no love or point in life; *spirit of joy and adventure.*

FOR LONELINESS:

Heather   Longing for company, talkative, overconcern with self; *tranquillity and kinship with all life.*

Impatiens   Irritated by constraints, quick, tense, impatient; *gentle and forgiving.*

Water Violet   Withdrawn, aloof, proud, self-reliant, quiet grief; *peaceful and calm, wise in service.*

OVERSENSITIVE TO IDEAS AND INFLUENCES:

Agrimony   Anxiety and worry hidden by a carefree mask, apparently jovial but in agony; *steadfast peace.*

Centaury   Kind, quiet, gentle, anxious to serve, weak, dominated; *an active and positive worker.*

Holly   Jealousy, envy, revenge, anger, suspicion; *the conquest of all will be through love.*

Walnut   Protection from outside influences, for change and the stages of development; *the link breaker.*

DESPONDENCY AND DESPAIR:

Crab Apple   Feeling unclean, self-disgust, small things out of proportion; *the cleansing remedy.*

Elm   Capable people, with responsibility, who falter, temporarily overwhelmed; *the strength to perform duty.*

Larch	Expect failure, lack confidence and will to succeed; *self-confident, try anything.*
Oak	Persevering, despite difficulties, strong, patient, never giving in; *admitting to limitation.*
Pine	Self-critical, self-reproach, assuming blame, apologetic; *relieves a sense of guilt.*
Star of Bethlehem	For consolation and comfort in grief, distress, after a fright, a shock or accident.
Sweet Chestnut	Unendurable anguish, desolation and despair; *a light shining in the darkness.*
Willow	Dissatisfied, bitter, resentful, life is unfair, unjust; *uncomplaining, acceptance.*

OVERCARE FOR WELFARE OF OTHERS:

Beech	Intolerant, critical, fussy; *seeing more good in the world.*
Chicory	Demanding, self-pity, self-love, possessive, hurt and tearful; *love and care that gives freely to others.*
Five Flower Remedy	The combination of cherry plum, clematis, impatiens, star of Bethlehem and rock rose. For use in any emergency.
Rockwater	Self-denial, stricture, rigidity, purist; *broad outlook, understanding.*
Vervain	Insistent, willful, fervent, enthusiastic, stressed; *quiet and tranquillity.*
Vine	Dominating, tyrant, bully, demands obedience; *loving leader and teacher, setting all at liberty.*

FLOWER REMEDY CREAM

This is made from the five flowers in Dr Bach's Rescue Remedy combination with the addition of crab apple for cleansing. The cream may be used freely for any external problem or injury: for bruising, irritation, bites and stings, for dry skin, spots, strains, etc. Like the remedies, it helps the physical condition by helping the subtle energies of the body.

Flower Remedy Cream is made with great care from the purest natural substances using no animal products. It may be used safely and with confidence.

Health improves as our emotional state becomes more positive. 'Any disease,' said Dr Bach, 'however serious, however long standing, will be cured by restoring the patient to happiness, and the desire to carry on with his life work.'

Flower remedies work 'not by attacking disease but by flooding our bodies with the beautiful vibrations of our Higher Nature'. They help to remake the contact with our true self which has become hidden by our reaction to life's difficulties.

While these remedies will not interfere with other treatments, they do not replace professional medical advice if that is appropriate. They are harmless, natural and made in the best possible conditions with love, care and attention. They can be taken in any circumstances by anyone needing help.

⚜ Flower Remedy Combinations

Neal's Yard Remedies has worked with Julian Barnard to produce a range of combination remedies using Bach remedies. They are as follows and can be used for general conditions. It is always best to individualize the combination of remedies to suit each emotional and mental state, but these will be effective for general assistance.

Flower essences have been used successfully worldwide since the 1930s and are reported to influence the emotions positively and thus promote wellbeing. Simple and safe to use, they provide a valued addition to everyday family care, including our pets.

LETTING GO
Holly, Willow, Vine, Beech, Chicory, Water Violet
This blend generates acceptance and understanding when anger and bitterness seem uppermost in the mind and it is difficult to feel life is fair. Could also bring essential insight into the self and therefore the power to change.

Indicated for: *Resentment, intolerance, co-dependence, neediness, unhappiness, relationship problems, attention-seeking, blaming, indifference, uncaring, distancing, controlling, won't change etc.*

FOCUS
Larch, Elm, White Chestnut, Hornbeam, Gentian, Clematis
This blend helps to clear the head, increase confidence in the self and bring a positive attitude to learning and academic work, despite possible setbacks. If working under the pressure of deadlines, this blend can focus the mind and may be taken as often as required.

Indicated for: *Exam formula, interviews, cramming, mental tiredness, overwhelmed, fear of failure, revision, distracted, fuzzy-headed, mental chatter, uninspired etc.*

COURAGE
Honeysuckle, Cherry Plum, Mimulus, Red Chestnut, Rock Rose, Aspen, Agrimony
This blend encourages calm control and courage when fears and apprehensions have taken over. It gently dispels fearfulness and inner turmoil so feelings of security and safety can take root.

Indicated for: *Panic, fright, shyness, trembling, fear for others or the world, specific fears, irrational fears, fear of hurting the self or others, mental torment etc.*

CONFIDENCE AND POWER
Larch, Centaury, Rock Rose, Gentian, Elm, Pine
This blend brings assertiveness and inner strength when life's challenges have sapped motivation and self-esteem. It becomes easier to develop a stronger sense of individuality and to function with greater integrity and conviction.

Indicated for: *Poor sense of self, belittling, apologetic, lack of confidence, powerlessness, inferiority, submissive, self-effacement, discouraged, valueless, self-sacrificing etc.*

OPTIMISM
Gorse, Gentian, Mustard, Sweet Chestnut, Cherry Plum, Heather
This blend brings a renewal of optimism and faith when life feels impossible. It brings about a gentle rebirth as it uplifts the self out of intense darkness and into the light.

Indicated for: *Moody adolescents, gloom, despondence, discouraged, hopelessness, pessimistic, despairing, dark night of the soul, loneliness etc.*

S.O.S.
Clematis, Impatiens, Rock Rose, Star of Bethlehem, Cherry Plum
Dr Bach's rescue combination promotes feelings of calm and serenity and is indicated during life's most extreme challenges or situations. Also bringing essential balance and control, frequent use is suggested during such times, as the effect is thought to be cumulative.

Indicated for: *Emergencies, bereavement, interviews, life dramas, emotional situations, travel, public speaking, exam nerves, dizziness, anguish etc.*

DIRECTION
Scleranthus, Wild Oat, Cerato, Walnut, Mimulus, Wild Rose
This blend offers valuable support during times of personal transformation when direction may be lost and it can become difficult to make decisions. It

promotes essential inner clarity, alongside an increased understanding of the self and the ways we inhibit our positive progress in life.

Indicated for: *Lack of commitment, mid-life crisis, career changes, vulnerable, house moves, doubt, indecision, vacillation, apathy, fear of the future, lack of responsibility etc.*

REVITALIZE
Olive, Elm, Oak, Crabapple, Hornbeam, Walnut
This essence is revitalizing when the responsibilities of life have taken their toll and there may be extreme fatigue. It helps a depleted system recuperate, by making available essential support and vitality. Take as often as required if feeling low.

Indicated for: *Debilitated, burn-out, overworked, carers, strained, female cycles, drained, no get up and go, overwhelmed, low, fragile, weak, out of sorts, congested etc.*

UNWIND
Vervain, Impatiens, Agrimony, Rock Water, Walnut, Aspen, White Chestnut
The pressure to continually function at our best is an accepted part of a modern hectic lifestyle. However, it demands a lot emotionally. This blend brings welcome relief when it becomes increasingly difficult to relax, switch off and recharge with a refreshing night's sleep.

Indicated for: *Uptight, overwrought, striving, driving, over intense, impatience, perfectionism, worry, restless nights, bad dreams, wakeful etc.*

INSTRUCTIONS FOR USE
Add 4 drops to small glass/bottle of water. Sip from glass/bottle at 4-hourly intervals throughout the day. Take more frequently if indicated. Make up new glass/bottle daily. Alternatively take 4 drops under the tongue direct from the dosage bottle every 4 hours.

Australian Bush Flower Remedies

Thank you to Ian White who has given us permission to include the following information.

Australia has the world's oldest and highest number of flowering plants which have both beauty and strength. Also Australia is relatively unpolluted and metaphysically has a very wise, old energy.

At this time there is a tremendous new vitality in this country. This, combined with the inherent power of the land, is why the Australian Bush Flower Essences are unique. Practitioners and prescribers worldwide are now incorporating the Australian Essences to form an integral part of their therapy.

The Bush Remedies not only help to give clarity to one's life but also the courage, strength and commitment to follow and pursue one's goals and dreams. They help to develop a higher level of intuition, self-esteem, spirituality, creativity and fun. The more the Essences are used, the more one is likely to experience greater awareness and happiness in one's life. Then everyone benefits – the individual, society and the planet. The effect of these Essences is similar to that of meditation in that they enable the person to access the wisdom of their Higher Self. This releases negative beliefs held in the subconscious mind and allows the positive virtues of the Higher Self – love, joy, faith, courage etc. – to flood their being. When this happens the negative beliefs and thoughts are dissolved and balance is restored.

ADMINISTERING THE REMEDIES
The majority of the remedies should be used for a maximum of two weeks at a time. If at the end of that period it appears that the remedy has not totally resolved the problem, take a week's break, then repeat or use a different Essence to address the issue, if necessary.

DOSAGE
Seven drops from dosage bottle taken morning and night on rising and retiring. Take for 10–14 days unless otherwise specified. This dosage is most effective and easy to remember.

REPERTORY OF MENTAL AND EMOTIONAL STATES

Abandoned, feels	Tall yellow top
Absent-minded	Red lily
Abuse – *see* Sexual Trauma	
Accident-prone	Jacaranda; Mountain devil; Red lily
Acknowledgment, unable to receive	Philotheca
Adopted child	Tall yellow top

Agoraphobia	Flannel flower
Aimless	Silver princess
Alienated	Tall yellow top
Aloof	Yellow cowslip orchid
Anger	Dagger hakea; Mountain devil
Anticipation	Dog rose
About public speaking:	Bush fuschia
Apathy	Kapok bush; Silver princess
Apologetic	Sturt's desert rose
Apprehension	Dog rose
Aura, damaged	Fringed violet
Authority, issues around	Red helmet orchid
Autism	Red lily
Awkwardness, social	Kangaroo paw

Belonging, no sense of	Tall yellow top
Bitterness	Dagger hakea; Mountain devil
Blaming others	Dagger hakea; Mountain devil; Southern cross; Yellow cowslip orchid
Bonding issues	
Doesn't feel at home anywhere:	Tall yellow top
To promote between mother and child:	Bottlebrush
To promote between father and child:	Red helmet orchid
To promote between couples or partners:	Wedding bush
To promote between groups:	Slender rice flower
Bored easily	Peach-flowered tea tree

Centred, to promote feeling of being	Crowea; Jacaranda
Chakras, blocked	
Heart chakra:	Bluebell; Tall yellow top
Base chakra:	Bush iris
Changeable	Jacaranda
Clumsiness	Jacaranda; Kangaroo paw
Commitment, lacking	Kapok bush; Peach-flowered tea tree; Wedding bush
Communication, to improve	
Between couples or family members:	Bush gardenia

Public speaking:	Bush fuschia
With the higher, intuitive self:	Paw paw; Turkey bush
Concentration, poor	Red lily; Bush fuschia
Confidence – *see* Self-confidence	
Courage, lacking, during time of crisis	Waratah
Creativity, blocked	Turkey bush
Critical	Yellow cowslip orchid
Criticism, oversensitive to	Red grevillea

Daydreaming	Red lily; Sundew
Death, patients close to	Bush iris
Defiant	Red helmet orchid
Despair	Waratah
Detail	
Excessive attention to, nitpicking:	Yellow cowslip orchid
Lack of attention to:	Red lily; Sundew
Direction, lacking	Silver princess
Disconnected	Red lily; Sundew
Discouraged easily	Kapok bush; Old man banksia
Distracted easily	Jacaranda; Red lily; Sundew
Dithering	Jacaranda
Domineering	Isopogon
Dullness of mind	Bush fuschia
Dutiful	Sturt's desert rose
Dyslexia	Bush fuschia

Emotional pain, especially buried	Sturt's desert pea
Emotions closed off	Bluebell; Tall yellow top; Yellow cowslip orchid
Energy, lacking	Banksia robur; Macrocarpa; Old man banksia
Enthusiasm, lacking	Old man banksia; Silver princess
Lacks ability to follow through:	Peach-flowered tea tree
Etheric body	
To align etheric and astral bodies with physical:	Crowea; Fringed violet

Fanaticism	Hibbertia; Yellow cowslip orchid
Fantasizing	Red lily; Sundew
Fears, general	Dog rose; Grey spider flower
Commitment:	Wedding bush
Death:	Bush iris; Dog rose
Extreme fears and phobias:	Grey spider flower
Fire, flames, hot objects:	Mulla mulla
Illness:	Dog rose; Peach-flowered tea tree
Intimacy:	Wisteria
Poverty:	Bluebell; Sunshine wattle
Psychic attack:	Fringed violet; Grey spider flower
Rejection:	Illawara flame tree
Touch or physical contact:	Flannel flower; Fringed violet; Wisteria
Female energy, to balance	She-oak; Wisteria
Focus, lack of	Jacaranda; Red lily; Silver princess; Sundew
Forgiveness, to promote	Dagger hakea; Mountain devil
Frustration	Banksia robur; Old man banksia; Red grevillea; Wild potato bush
Generosity, excessive	Philotheca
Lacking:	Bluebell
Greed	Bluebell
Grief	Sturt's desert pea
Guilt	Sturt's desert rose
Hatred	Mountain devil
Heaviness	Little flannel flower; Old man banksia; Waratah
From exhaustion:	Macrocarpa
From emotional pain:	Sturt's desert pea
From guilt:	Sturt's desert rose
From bodily limitations:	Wild potato bush

Hopelessness	Sunshine wattle; Waratah
Hurried	Black-eyed Susan
Hypochondriac	Peach-flowered tea tree

Impatience; always on the go	Black-eyed Susan
Indecision	Jacaranda; Paw paw; Red lily; Sundew
Know what they need to do but not how to do it:	Red grevillea
Inept	Kangaroo paw
Infertility, from emotional causes	She-oak; Turkey bush
Inhibition	Little flannel flower; Turkey bush
Inner child, to help release	Little flannel flower
Insensitive	Flannel flower; Kangaroo paw
Intellectual	Hibbertia; Isopogon; Tall yellow top; Yellow cowslip orchid
Intuition, to develop	Paw paw; Turkey bush
To promote integration of right and left brain:	Bush fuschia
Isolation	Tall yellow top

Jealousy	Mountain devil; Slender rice flower

Learning difficulties	Bush fuschia
Life's purpose, to help determine	Silver princess
Loneliness	Tall yellow top
Love	
Lacking in love for self and others:	Mountain devil
To increase self-love and self-acceptance:	Five corners

Male energy, to balance	Flannel flower; Wisteria
Manipulative	Isopogon; Mountain devil
Martyr	Southern cross
Materialistic	Bush iris
Meditation, to enhance	Bush iris

Memory, poor	Isopogon
Mood swings	Peach-flowered tea tree

Narrow-minded	Slender rice flower
Nationalistic	Slender rice flower
Nightmares	Dog rose; Grey spider flower
Fires or being burnt:	Mulla mulla

Obsessive thoughts	Boronia
Out-of-sorts feeling	Crowea
Overwhelmed	
By major life changes:	Bottlebrush; Red grevillea
By responsibility:	Illawara flame tree
By sudden fear or panic:	Grey spider flower
With decision-making:	Paw paw
By new information or ideas:	Paw paw

Panic	Grey spider flower
Past life experiences	
Traumas involving fire or being burnt:	Mulla mulla
Pessimistic	Sunshine wattle
Pining	Boronia
Planetary concern, to develop	Red helmet orchid
Pride	Slender rice flower
Psychic protection	Fringed violet; Grey spider flower

Racist	Slender rice flower
Rape – *see* Sexual Trauma	
Read, inability or disinterest	Bush fuschia
Rebellious	Red helmet orchid
Rejection, feelings of	Illawara flame tree; Tall yellow top
Relationships	
Breaking down, between family members:	Bush gardenia
Broken, after:	Boronia; Dagger hakea; Mountain devil; Sturt's desert pea; Waratah

Commitment lacking in couples: Wedding bush
Discomfort around social relationships: Kangaroo paw
Loss of passion and interest between
couples: Bush gardenia
    Sibling rivalry: Mountain devil
    With father or authority figures: Red helmet orchid
Resentment   Dagger hakea; Mountain devil;
        Southern cross

    Hidden, towards those who were once
    very close: Dagger hakea
Resignation   Kapok bush; Southern cross;
        Waratah

Resistance
    To change, new ideas or people: Bauhinia
    During transitions: Bottlebrush
Responsibility, fear of   Illawara flame tree
    Over-responsible: Old man banksia
Restricted, feels   Wild potato bush
Revengeful   Mountain devil
Rigidity
    With resistance to change: Bauhinia
    With dogmatism and self-denial: Hibbertia
    With seriousness: Little flannel flower
Routine, stuck in   Bottlebrush; Red grevillea

Sadness   Sturt's desert pea
Scattered   Jacaranda
Self-absorbed   Kangaroo paw
Self-blame   Sturt's desert rose
Self-confidence, lacking   Dog rose; Five corners;
        Illawara flame tree; Turkey
        bush

    When speaking in public: Bush fuschia
Self-discipline and control, excessive   Hibbertia
    Lacking: Wedding bush
Self-disgust   Billy goat plum
Self-esteem, poor   Five corners; Philotheca; Sturt's
        desert rose; Tall yellow top

Self-image, poor   Five corners
Self-pity   Southern cross
Selfish   Red helmet orchid
Sensitivity
    Lacking: Kangaroo paw; Red helmet
                                       orchid
    In males: Flannel flower
    Excessive psychic sensitivity: Fringed violet
    Oversensitive to criticism: Red grevillea
Separation, sense of   Tall yellow top
Seriousness   Little flannel flower
Sex
    Inability to enjoy: Billy goat plum; Wisteria
    Revulsion: Billy goat plum
    Excessive desire: Bush iris
Sexual trauma/abuse, after   Billy goat plum; Flannel
                                       flower; Fringed violet;
                                       Sturt's desert rose; Wisteria

Shock, trauma, bad news etc., to aid
    recovery from: Fringed violet; Waratah
    From burns or fires: Mulla mulla
Slowness   Old man banksia
Spaciness   Red lily; Sundew
Spirit guides, to develop awareness of in
    children   Little flannel flower; Sundew
Spirituality
    To enhance spiritual awareness: Bush iris; Little flannel flower
    To balance spiritual and earthly planes: Red lily
Split feeling   Red lily; Sundew
Spontaneity, lacking   Little flannel flower; Turkey
                                       bush

Stress
    Busy people, always on the go: Black-eyed Susan; Jacaranda
    Exhaustion from: Macrocarpa; Old man banksia
Stuck feeling   Red grevillea; Wild potato
                                       bush
    Creativity blocked: Turkey bush
    In the past: Sunshine wattle

Stuttering	Bush fuschia
Subconscious mind, to open up	Isopogon
Subtle bodies, to align	Crowea
Suicidal thoughts and feelings	Waratah
Superiority, feelings of	Hibbertia; Yellow cowslip orchid
Survival skills, to bring forth	Waratah
Suspicious	Mountain devil

Terror	Grey spider flower
Timidity	Dog rose; Five corners; Philotheca
Transitions, to assist during	Bottlebrush; Red grevillea
Trapped feeling	Red grevillea

Unclean feeling	Billy goat plum
Ungrounded	Red lily; Sundew

Vagueness	Red lily; Sundew
Victim, feelings of	Southern cross; Sunshine wattle
To illness:	Spinifex
Visualization, to enhance	Bush iris

Weariness	Macrocarpa; Old man banksia
In those usually dynamic:	Banksia robur
Worry	Crowea

RECOMMENDED DOSAGE

Seven drops from dosage bottle mornings and night, on rising and retiring. Take for 10–14 days unless otherwise specified. This dosage is the most effective, is easy to remember and builds up a rhythmic healing frequency.

FLOWER ESSENCE DESCRIPTIONS

ALPINE MINT BUSH   *Prostanthera cuneata*
Positive: Revitalization, joy, renewal
Negative: Mental and emotional exhaustion, lack of joy, weight of responsibility

ANGELSWORD   *Lobelia gibberoa*
Positive: Attaining spiritual truth/protection, access to gifts from past
   lifetimes, repairs whole energy field
Negative: Spiritual confusion, interference with true spiritual connection,
   spiritual gullibility, looking for answers outside of self, spiritually
   'possessed'

BANKSIA ROBUR   Swamp Banksia
Positive: Enjoyment of and interest in life
Negative: Loss of drive and enthusiasm

BAUHINIA   *Lysiphyllum cunninghamii*
Positive: Acceptance and open mindedness, embracing new concepts/ideas
Negative: Resistance to change, rigidity, annoyance

BILLY GOAT PLUM   *Planchonia careya*
Positive: Sexual pleasure, enjoyment; acceptance of one's physical body
Negative: Sexual revulsion, loathing or disgust of an aspect of oneself

BLACK-EYED SUSAN   *Tetratheca ericifolia*
Positive: Slowing down, ability to turn inward and be still, inner peace
Negative: Rushing, always on the go, impatience, always striving

BLUEBELL   *Wahlenbergia* sp.
Positive: Opens the heart, joy, sharing
Negative: Cut off from feelings, fear of lack or greed

BOAB   *Adansonia gregorii*
Positive: Releases past negative actions within families – abuse, prejudice.
   Releases negative thought patterns, releases deep-held emotion
Negative: Taking on negative family thought patterns, repetition of past
   negative experiences

BORONIA   *Boronia ledifolia*
Positive: Serenity, clarity of mind and thought
Negative: Obsessive thoughts, pining for recently ended relationships

BOTTLEBRUSH   *Callistemon linearis*
Positive: Bonding between mother and child, serenity, letting go
Negative: For going through and overwhelmed by major life changes

BUSH FUCHSIA   *Epacris longiflora*
Positive: Allows one to integrate information, develops intuition
Negative: Inability to balance the logical and rational with the intuitive and
   creative, switched off, ignoring gut feelings.

BUSH GARDENIA   *Gardenia megasperma*
Positive: Renews interest in others, improves communication, passion
Negative: Taking for granted, unaware of others, self-centredness

BUSH IRIS   *Patersonia longifolia*
Positive: Spiritual insights, understanding beyond the material/physical
Negative: Fear of death, materialism, atheism, excessiveness

CHRISTMAS BELL   *Blandfordia nobilis*
Positive: To help manifest one's desired outcome
Negative: When experiencing a sense of lack

CROWEA   *Crowea saligna*
Positive: Balances and centres the individual
Negative: Worrying, out of balance, feeling 'not quite right'

DAGGER HAKEA   *Hakea teretifolia*
Positive: Forgiveness, open expression of feelings
Negative: Resentment, bitterness towards close family, friends, lovers

DOG ROSE   *Bauera rubroides*
Positive: Confidence, courage, belief in self
Negative: Fearful, shy, insecure, apprehensive of others, niggling fears

DOG ROSE OF THE WILD FORCES   *Bauera sessiliflora*
Positive: Emotional balance, calmness, sanity in times of turmoil
Negative: Fear of loss of control, physical pain with no apparent cause

FLANNEL FLOWER   *Actinotus helianthi*
Positive: Gentleness, sensitivity in touching, joy, trust, sensuality
Negative: Dislike of being touched, lack of sensitivity – especially in males

FRESH WATER MANGROVE   *Barringtonia acutangula*
Positive: Ability to fully experience, open-hearted, open-minded
Negative: generational mental prejudice, prejudice without experience, closed
    mind and heart

FRINGED VIOLET   *Thysanotus tuberosus*
Positive: Removes effects of past or present distress, psychic protection
Negative: Distress, damage to aura, drained by others/situations

FIVE CORNERS   *Styphelia laeta*
Positive: Love and acceptance of self, celebration of own beauty
Negative: Low self-esteem, dislike of self, held-in personality

GREEN SPIDER ORCHID   *Caladenia dilatata*
Positive: Attunement, ability to guard information, release of terrors and
    phobias
Negative: Nightmares, needing acceptance, phobias

GREY SPIDER FLOWER   *Grevillea buxifolia*
Positive: Faith and courage
Negative: Terror, panic

GYMEA LILY   *Doryanthes excelsa*
Positive: Humility, awareness and appreciation of others
Negative: Pride, dominating personality, status seekers

HIBBERTIA   *Hibbertia pedunculata*
Positive: Acceptance of self and own innate knowledge
Negative: Fanaticism – self-improvement/discipline/knowledge

ILLAWARRA FLAME TREE   *Brachychiton acerifolius*
Positive: Self-approval, self-reliance, confidence, inner strength
Negative: Sense of rejection, being left out, fear of responsibility

ISOPOGEN   *Isopogon anethifolius*
Positive: Able to learn from past experiences, remember the past
Negative: Unable to learn from past experience, controlling personality

JACARANDA   *Mimosifolia* sp.
Positive: Decisiveness, clear-mindedness, quick thinking
Negative: Scattered, changeable, dithering, aimless, rushing

KANGAROO PAW   *Anigozanthos manglesii*
Positive: Relaxed, sensitivity, *savoire faire*, enjoyment of people
Negative: Socially immature, clumsy, gauche, insensitive to others' needs

KAPOK BUSH   *Cochlospermum fraseri*
Positive: Persistence, willingness to 'give it a go', application
Negative: Easily discouraged, resignation, apathy

LITTLE FLANNEL FLOWER   *Actinotus minor*
Positive: Playfulness, joy, ability to have fun
Negative: Denial of the 'child' in the personality, seriousness

MACROCARPA   *Eucalyptus macrocarpa*
Positive: Renews enthusiasm. Strong affinity to the adrenal glands, bringing
    about energy, strength, vitality
Negative: Personally drained. Tired, exhausted, burnt-out, low immunity

MINT BUSH   *Prostanthera striatflora*
Positive: Calmness, ability to move on, readiness for initiation
Negative: Spiritual trial and tribulation, despair, overwhelm, perturbation and
    confusion

MONGA WARATAH   *Telopea mongaenis*
Positive: Strengthens one's will; self-empowerment
Negative: Neediness, disempowerment; addictive personality

MOUNTAIN DEVIL   *Lambertia formosa*
Positive: Unconditional love, forgiveness, happiness
Negative: Hatred, anger, jealousy, holding of grudges, suspicious

MULLA MULLA   *Ptilotus atripicifolius*
Positive: Reduces the negative effects of fire and the sun's rays
Negative: Distress/trauma associated with exposure to fire, heat and sun

OLD MAN BANKSIA   *Banksia serrata*
Positive: Ability to cope with whatever life brings. Energy, enthusiasm,
    enjoyment of and interest in life
Negative: Disheartened, weary. Plethoric, low in energy, sluggishness, low
    thyroid activity

PAW PAW   *Carica papaya*
Positive: Focus and clarity
Negative: Overwhelmed, burdened by decisions

PEACH-FLOWERED TEA TREE   *Leptospermum squarrosum*
Positive: Balance, responsibility for own health
Negative: Mood swings, lack of commitment

PHILOTHECA   *Philotheca salsolifolia*
Positive: Ability to accept praise, acknowledgment and love
Negative: Excessive generosity, inability to accept acknowledgment

PINK MULLA MULLA   *Ptilotus exaltatus*
Positive: Overcoming obstacles, opening up, forgiveness
Negative: Deep hurt, guarded/isolated, feeling blocked

RED GREVILLEA   *Grevillea speciosa*
Positive: Strength to leave unpleasant situations, boldness
Negative: Feeling stuck, affected by criticism, reliant on others

RED HELMET ORCHID   *Corybas dilatatus*
Positive: Helps father/child bonding, sensitivity, respect
Negative: Rebelliousness, selfish, problems with authority

RED LILY   *Nelumbo nucifera*
Positive: Grounded, focused, living in the present
Negative: Vagueness, indecisiveness, daydreaming

RED SUVA FRANGIPANI   *Suneiria rubra*
Positive: Feeling nurtured, equanimity, calmness
Negative: Turmoil, emotional upheaval, sadness

ROUGH BLUEBELL   *Trichodesma zeylanicum*
Positive: Unconditional love, openness, compassion sensitivity
Negative: Openly malicious, total lack of concern for others' feelings,
    manipulative, hurtful

SHE-OAK   *Casuarina glauca*
Positive: Overcomes imbalances in females. Fertility, conception, hormonal
    balance
Negative: Distress associated with infertility. Infertility, female hormone
    imbalance, PMS

SILVER PRINCESS   *Eucalyptus caesia*
Positive: Life purpose and direction, motivation
Negative: Aimless, despondent, lacking life direction

SLENDER RICE FLOWER   *Pimelea linifolia*
Positive: Co-operation, humility, appreciation of beauty in others
Negative: Racism, narrow mindedness, comparison with others

SOUTHERN CROSS   *Xanthosia rotundifolia*
Positive: Personal power, positive attitude, responsibility for self
Negative: Victim mentality, poverty consciousness

SPINIFEX TRIODIA   sp.
Positive: Empowers through emotional understanding to heal the physical,
    works well topically on cuts and lesions
Negative: Sense of being a victim to illness. Herpes, chlamydia, fine cuts

STURT'S DESERT PEA   *Clianthus formosus*
Positive: Diffuses sad memories, allows one to let go, motivates
Negative: Deep hurt, sadness, emotional pain

STURT'S DESERT ROSE   *Gossypium sturtianum*
Positive: Allows one to follow own inner convictions and morality
Negative: Guilt, low self-esteem, easily led

SUNDEW   *Drosera spathulata*
Positive: Grounded, focused, similar to Red Lily – specifically for those under
    28 years of age
Negative: Disconnected, split, lack of focus

SUNSHINE WATTLE   *Acacia terminalis*
Positive: Optimism, acceptance of the beauty and joy in the present
Negative: Struggle, stuck in the past, expectation of a grim future

SYDNEY ROSE   *Delphinium consolida*
Positive: Feeling safe and at peace; heartfelt communication
Negative: Feeling separate; deserted; unloved or morbid

TALL MULLA MULLA   *Ptilotus helipteroides*
Positive: Feeling secure with people, social interaction
Negative: Feeling scared, lack of interaction, feeling unsafe

TALL YELLOW TOP   *Senecio magnificus*
Positive: Sense of belonging
Negative: Alienation, lonely, isolated

TURKEY BUSH   *Calytrix exstipulata*
Positive: Inspired creativity, renews artistic confidence
Negative: Creative block, disbelief in own creative ability

WARATAH   *Telopea speciosissima*
Positive: Courage, tenacity, faith, adaptability, survival skills
Negative: Black despair, hopelessness, inability to respond to crisis

WEDDING BUSH   *Ricinocarpos pinifolius*
Positive: Commitment in relationships, dedication to life purpose
Negative: Difficulty with commitment in relationships

WILD POTATO   *Solanum quadriloculatum*
Positive: Freedom to move on in life
Negative: Sense of being weighed down and encumbered

WISTERIA   *Wisteria sinensis*
Positive: Fulfilling sexual relationship
Negative: Women who feel uncomfortable and uptight about their sexuality.
   Fear arising from sexual abuse

YELLOW COWSLIP ORCHID   *Caladenia flava*
Positive: Humanitarian concern, impartiality, balances pituitary
Negative: Critical, judgemental, bureaucratic

COMPANION ESSENCES
AUTUMN LEAVES
Positive: Letting go; in one's last days before passing over; increases awareness
   and communication with loved ones in the spiritual world
Negative: Difficulties in the transition of passing over from the physical plane
   to the spiritual world

GREEN ESSENCE
Positive: Harmonize the vibration of any yeast mould or parasite to one's own
   vibration; purifying
Negative: Emotional distress associated with intestinal and skin disorders

LICHEN
Positive: Eases one's transition into the light; assists separation between the
   physical and etheric body; releases earth-bound energies
Negative: Not knowing to look for and move into the Light when passing
   over; earth bound in the astral plane

19

Materia Medica

Aconite   *Aconitum napellus*

This is the remedy to give at the beginning of an illness. Use for people that are generally healthy and robust and who fall ill suddenly. Aconite can be the first remedy to give after a shock or fright. It may also be appropriate for those who have never been well since a profound incident affected them. Give at any time where there is a rapid onset of symptoms. Aconite is a remedy that must be given quickly, before other symptoms set in, and it works fast. In this way it is very useful to give to children.

Mental and emotional indications: Symptoms must be accompanied by fear and oversensitivity. The person may be nervous and excitable and suffer from great anxiety. There may be fears, often irrational, about being mugged, drowning, earthquakes, war, flying, operations, etc. Patients may be prone to panic attacks and feel they are going to die. But they may also have had a terrifying incident in their past, for example they may have been victims of rape. This is a remedy for women in labour who fear they will never get through the experience and will die in childbirth.

Physical: Complaints are marked by feverishness. Pains are sudden and sharp, sticking or tearing. The person is sensitive to cold, dry, windy weather. This remedy is excellent given at the onset of a cold. Give for respiratory complaints and earache, the onset of chills, sore throats and where there is a burning thirst for water.

Cough: Where the cough comes on after a chill. Cough is dry, croupy, painful, worse in evening or after drinking or breathing in. Relieved by lying on the back.

Eyes: Use for conjunctivitis, especially after exposure to cold winds, for photophobia and for loss of sight after shock.

Head: Feels heavy and hot, with possibly a bursting headache and burning sensation like a hot tight band around the head. Give for the after-effects of the sun and fevers with extreme headaches. Senses are acute; great sensitivity to noise, light, smells. The face looks anxious and will alternate between being red and pale.

Heart: Remedy for high blood pressure and hard full pulse. Use at the beginning of heart-attack symptoms.

Stomach: Give when gastritis has been brought on by drinking cold water after being overheated. Thirsty. Pains in abdomen which extend to the chest on waking.

Children: Indicated when the child wakes up in terror, screaming. Use to bring down temperatures, where there is restlessness and throwing off of bedclothes. Hot and cold in waves. Good for cramps.

Modalities: Symptoms get worse from fright, shock, chills, cold, dry wind in the evening, night-time, at midnight. They are accompanied by fear, nightmares that wake you up. They improve by being in the open air, from rest, warmth and sweating.

Agnus Castus   *Vitex agnus castus*

Synonyms: Chaste tree, chasteberry, monk's pepper

Parts used: Fruit collected in autumn

Habitat: Native to Mediterranean and western Asia

Main constituents: Alkaloids, bitters, flavonoids, volatile oils

Actions: Hormone regulator, lactogogue, progesterogenic

Main uses: Traditionally a symbol of chastity and held to be capable of warding off evil, agnus castus was also thought to reduce sexual desire and libido, hence was chewed by monks. Research has confirmed that it acts as a hormonal regulator. It is used in the treatment of irregular menstrual cycles, symptoms of pre-menstrual syndrome such as bloating, swollen and tender breasts, irritability, headaches, mood swings and associated problems and acne. It is also believed to increase fertility in women and the flow of milk in breast-feeding. It is often indicated as an alternative to HRT for menopausal women and for withdrawal symptoms for those giving up the pill. It has a calming, relaxing effect on the reproductive system.

Toxicity: None.

Contraindications: Should not be taken with progesterone drugs. May counteract the effectiveness of birth control pills. Avoid during pregnancy, unless used to prevent miscarriage due to progesterone insufficiency in the first trimester.

Dosage: 300mg 2 tablets 3 times daily. Tincture: 1:1 in 25 per cent alcohol, 10–20 drops every morning. Can increase for irregular periods.

⚘ Agrimony *Agrimonia eupatoria*

Synonyms: Cocklebur
   Parts used: Aerial parts, harvested in summer
   Habitat: Native to Europe, likes wet and waste grounds
   Main constituents: Coumarins, flavonoids, tannins
   Actions: Astringent, bitter tonic, cholagogue, diuretic, haemostatic, hepatic, vulnerary
   Main uses: This is a gentle liver tonic and digestive herb. Used for acid indigestion, sluggish liver functioning. Helps with assimilation of nutrients. Good for convalescence, general weakness and diarrhoea. Helps tone the bladder and can be used for incontinence. Good for bleeding, including nosebleeds. Apply externally for sores and cuts.
   Toxicity: None.
   Contraindications: None.
   Dosage: Take 1 teaspoon of herb to 1 cup of boiling water 3 times daily. Tincture 1:5 in 45 per cent alcohol. Take 1–4ml daily.

⚘ Alfalfa *Medicago sativa*

Synonyms: Lucerne
   Parts used: Aerial parts and sprouting seeds, harvested in summer
   Habitat: Native to Europe, Asia, North Africa, grown as a crop, green manure and on waste land
   Main constituents: Alkaloids, coumarins, essential enzymes, isoflavones, rich in vitamins and minerals
   Actions: Anti-anaemia, anticholesterol, anticoagulant, antihaemorrhagic
   Main uses: A wonderfully good source of vitamins and minerals, therefore excellent for debility and convalescence. Use for bones, teeth, weight loss. Helps rebuild damaged tissues and repair arthritic conditions. Can be beneficial for symptoms of menopause and PMS.

Contraindications: Avoid use in autoimmune diseases.

Dosage: Eat the sprouts in salads. Tincture: 1:1 in 45 per cent alcohol, 5–15 drops in water daily.

Allium Cepa   *Allium cepa*

This homoeopathic remedy has no marked mental indications. It is used to treat excess secretions of the mucous membranes in the nose, eyes, larynx, etc. It is good where there is burning in the nose, throat and mouth.

Colds: This remedy treats symptoms which include mucus streaming from the nose and eyes, with frequent sneezing and profuse acrid, burning discharge from the nose, that excoriates lips and nose. Profuse, bland lachrymation (this is the opposite in euphrasia). The person feels hot and thirsty. Symptoms get worse indoors, in the evenings and in a warm room. The symptoms improve in the open air.

Cough: This is incessant, hacking, tickling which is worse in cold air. There is a desire to suppress the cough because it is so troublesome.

Hayfever: Allium cepa can be used to treat hayfever if the symptoms already mentioned fit. They get worse from warmth.

Laryngitis: The larynx tickles, the throat feels hoarse and raw and the pain extends to the ears. There is a sensation of a lump in the throat. Coughing seems to tear the larynx (you need to hold the throat when coughing).

Modalities: Symptoms get worse in a warm room and from wet feet. They improve from cool, open air, motion and from bathing.

Aloe Vera   *Aloe barbadensis*

Synonyms: Lily of the desert, plant of immortality (both translated from African languages)

Parts used: Gel which is found inside the spiky cactus-type leaves

Habitat: Native to South and East Africa, also widely grown in South America and world wide as a crop

Main constituents: Anthraquinones, minerals, tannins, vitamins

Actions: Antibiotic, astringent, bitter, coagulant, demulcent, vulnerary

Main uses: Alloeh means 'bitter' in Arabic. Aloe vera is a remedy known throughout the world. It is great for most skin conditions – sore, weeping or dry. Use for burns, sunburn, eczema, wound healing. Use in a mouthwash for dental problems. Internally, take for digestive cleansing and stimulating the digestion, constipation, ulcers, parasites. As a food supplement, aloe vera aids digestion as well as the functioning of the kidneys, liver and gall bladder.

Contraindications: Avoid internal use during pregnancy and in cases of intestinal obstruction, ulcerative colitis and acute inflamed intestines.

Dosage: For external use, it is best to break off a fresh leaf and apply the gel directly onto the skin (aloe is an easy plant to grow in most dry and warm conditions; keep it in sandy well-drained soil, preferably in the shade). Internally, use the juice 5ml 3 times daily. Buy juice that is organic if possible, packed fresh with the minimum of preservatives.

Alumina   *Alumina*

This homoeopathic remedy will be indicated by an overall dryness, debility and lack of reaction. There will be sluggishness and exhaustion. It is a good remedy for old people and long-term chronic complaints, e.g. constipation. The appearance may be thin, withered, wrinkled and old-looking.

Mental and emotional indications: Marked by confusion, irritability, obstinacy and absent-mindedness, with poor concentration and memory. There will be dullness, a feeling of sluggishness and aversion to work. Alumina can help more serious states of mental confusion when everything seems unreal and there is a marked fear of insanity or suicide, even to the point where the person cannot look at a knife without fearing the desire to kill themselves or others. Time seems to pass slowly and although appearing to be in a state of haste, things are actually done slowly. There may be disturbance in co-ordination or mistakes in speech. The alumina type will feel guilty, as though having committed a crime.

Physical: Marked by a dryness of all mucous membranes, except in the genitals.

Abdomen: Constipation is marked by a lack of desire, as though the rectum is paralysed, and there is a need to strain even though the stools are soft or lumpy and covered with mucus. There may be a craving for indigestible things such as chalk, charcoal or soil. There is a need to sit down all the time due to weakness in the legs.

Skin: Complaints are dry, rough, burning, itchy and accompanied by a desire to scratch until blood is drawn (similar to sulphur).

Women's complaints: Periods which are early, pale, short and scanty will leave the woman feeling physically and mentally exhausted. Leucorrhoea during the daytime can be very profuse and burning, and is better after washing with cold water. The vulva may be sore and itchy.

Modalities: Symptoms get worse in winter, warm rooms, when eating potatoes and while talking. They get better in damp air and with cold washing.

It is always best to avoid using aluminium pans, especially when cooking eggs, or for fruit or making tea. Although people use less aluminium at home, it is still widely used in restaurants, hospitals, etc. If you feel you are having to eat a lot of food cooked in aluminium, it may be worth considering taking the occasional dose of this remedy to allay any of the above symptoms. It is also used in anti-perspirants so choose a deodorant which is not an anti-perspirant, or check to see if it contains aluminium.

Angelica Root   *Angelica archangelica*

Parts used: Root, rhizome, lifted in autumn
   Habitat: Europe
   Main constituents: Bitters, malic acid, tannins, volatile oil
   Actions: Antibacterial, antifungal, bitter, carminative, diaphoretic, diuretic, expectorant, smooth muscle relaxant, tonic
   Main uses: Use for cold damp conditions, infections of the respiratory system. Good for coughs, colds, bronchitis, asthma and TB. Tones the nervous system. Good for nervous debility and depression. As a bitter it increases the appetite; in smaller doses it decreases the gastric acidity and can help with ulcers.
   Contraindications: Pregnancy.
   Dosage: Decoction of root, 25g to 1litre water. Take 15ml 3 times daily. Tincture: 1:5 in 45 per cent alcohol. Take 2–5ml 3 times daily.

Aniseed   *Pimpinella anisum*

Parts used: Seeds, collected after flowering
   Habitat: Worldwide
   Main constituents: Volatile oil
   Actions: Antiparasitic, antispasmodic, carminative, expectorant, oestrogenic

Main uses: Good for all coughs, whooping cough and dry infections of the respiratory system. Relieves gut tension and digestive problems where there is wind or colic. Soothing to the nervous system and helps racing heart and palpitations. In South American tradition, aniseed is used for PMT and is thought to eliminate sad thoughts. Helps milk production in nursing mothers. Give for teething problems.

Contraindications: Allergy to anise and anethol.

Dosage: A few seeds in water infusion.

ANISEED OIL

This oil is not often used due to the toxic accumulative effects of the oil. It may be used with caution in very small quantities in a massage blend for scabies and other infestations.

Ant Crude   *Antimonium crudum*

The keynote of this homoeopathic remedy is overindulgence. It is primarily a gastric remedy and is good for children and for old people.

Mental and emotional indications: Ant crude will suit a person who is greedy, gluttonous and fat, with a dislike of life. They feel weary of living but are sentimental and love moonlight, twilight or soft lighting. The child is fretful and cries when touched or looked at; they are angry when they get attention and get weepy from touch, coughing or during sleep. An indication of ant crude is becoming sulky, snappy and resentful if disturbed. There is varying delirium during a fever and a vicious temper when they feel sick and want to be left alone. They blame other people for their troubles, although very often problems are caused through their own indulgences.

Physical: There is a bitter taste in the mouth, also vomiting and belching. A key symptom for this remedy is a thickly-coated white tongue. There can be a violent thirst accompanying diarrhoea. They may have detached gums that bleed, toothache, cracks in the corner of the mouth and nostrils, redness of the eyelids, split or deformed nails, corns and rheumatoid arthritis. Ant crude is a good remedy for pimples, vesicles, pustules and scaly, pustular eruptions that are itchy and burning and become worse at night. It is useful for chickenpox and measles as long as they are accompanied by the general and emotional symptoms of this remedy. Other symptoms indicated: callouses, brittle hair and hair loss.

Modalities: Worse with cold bathing, damp, water, heat of summer and over-eating. Better in the open air, with rest and moist warmth.

Ant Tart   *Antimonium tartaricum*

This is a good homoeopathic remedy for acute heart cases where there's heart failure, or for extreme cases of pneumonia and bronchitis where the skin has become blue, pale and sweaty.

Mental and emotional indications: Ant tart is a remedy for a worn-out, exhausted body, and any mental symptoms will reflect this; there is apathy, great sleepiness or sleeplessness, drowsiness, a bad temper and irritability, especially when being touched or looked at.

Physical: They feel the cold but dislike stuffiness, thirstlessness.

Abdomen: Symptoms include frequent stools, diarrhoea with mucus, summer diarrhoea. Violent pain in the lumbar-sacral region. The slightest movement causes cold, clammy sweating.

Cough: One of the keynotes of this remedy is coarse rattling in the chest. It is good to give in cases of whooping cough, asthma, pneumonia and bronchitis. The rattling is accompanied by a feeling of oppression and suffocation and it is more comfortable to sit up. There may be intense nausea which is relieved after vomiting. It is a good remedy for old people who have no reactive power. When their chests are full of rattles and wheezes, the lungs have filled up and there is no power to raise phlegm. It is also a good children's remedy for coughs when the child is angry and for nursing babies who let go of the nipple and cry, reaching for breath. The child feels better if he is carried around or is upright.

Head: Ant tart is a 'last gasp' remedy *(see also* carbo veg) where the face is pale, sickly drawn, with sunken eyes and dark rings around them. Lips are pale and shrivelled. Nostrils dilate and flap. There is a death-like face with coldness and cold sweat.

Skin: It is a good remedy for pustular eruptions such as chickenpox, herpes, impetigo and spots that are slow to come out with accompanying chest complaints.

Modalities: Worse in a warm room, with warm clothing and warm weather, from anger and lying down. They improve with expectoration and sitting up.

❋ Apis   *Apis mellifica*

This homoeopathic remedy will suit the type of person that is busy, active and industrious.

Mental and emotional indications: They can be spiteful, rather excitable, jealous and fidgety. They always appear restless and possibly clumsy, awkward and prone to dropping things. Often they are absent-minded and indifferent or apathetic. A remedy to treat ailments after anger, jealousy, grief or fright. The apis-type person is often hard to please or irritable, and is said to demonstrate 'foolish, childish behaviour'. This may come from the person being very changeable and tearful, with no obvious cause, and prone to tantrums or shrieking or screaming suddenly, even when asleep.

Physical: The main physical characteristic for which this remedy is used is oedema or watery swellings. This remedy is made from the sting of a bee, so any symptoms that resemble this – painful, red, hot, swollen, swelling – are indicated. The pains are stinging and pricking, with a dry, burning heat (compare with belladonna). There can be swellings under the eyes and in the hands and feet. Symptoms will be mainly right-sided and there will be thirstlessness. It is also excellent where there is anaphylactic shock (allergic reaction) to the sting.

Women's complaints: Features of apis also include ovarian cysts, stinging pains in the ovaries and burning in the breasts. There may be a tendency to miscarry in the first months of pregnancy. It will be good for oedema in pregnancy and for cystitis where the urine is scanty, perhaps bloody, almost suppressed and accompanied by a frequent desire to urinate. The passing of urine may be helped by pressing on the area of the bladder. It may also be good for urine retention in newborn babies (*see also* aconite).

Modalities: Symptoms get worse from heat, touch and after sleep. They get better from cold, cold air and cold applications.

❋ Arg Nit   *Argentum nitricum*

This is one of the main homoeopathic remedies for fears.

Mental and emotional indications: People needing arg nit may object to any idea or suggestion through fear. This is especially true of children. They fear open and confined spaces or heights and have fear of anticipation. The nervous system is taut. They are highly-strung individuals who are impulsive, hurried and jumpy. They are always early because they are afraid of being late, they are always in a rush and they will be hot and flustered. Also, they are full of suspicions that things are going to happen to them and that people are out to get them: they always check that doors are locked. These fearful people often manage to just avoid dangerous things, like stepping into a deep hole. They will make certain that they sit at the end of a row of people. They will not travel on the underground because they suspect that they will be robbed and they are fearful of taking medicines. They walk and eat fast, and play mental games and build up fantasies about 'What if …?' They are obsessive and talk easily. They get frightened of flying and crossing bridges. Excessive mental exertion causes headaches, and if they are overtired they become trembly and paralysed. This remedy has been useful for multiple sclerosis sufferers; it can also help premature ejaculation due to excitement, and speech impediments. Arg nit is very good to take for anticipatory ordeals such as exams, a driving test or public speaking (the person will very likely get diarrhoea before the event).

Physical indications: An arg nit person will probably be thin, wiry and look prematurely old, having lived on his nerves and emotions. These people worry about their health and desire fresh air, cold food and drinks.

Digestion: Many digestive problems arise through anxiety. Arg nit types crave sweets and sugar, although sugar tends to bring about diarrhoea. They also like salt and strong cheeses. There may be flatulence, bloating and abdominal pain after eating. Complaints are caused or made worse by eating. There may be strong feelings of nausea which will lead to vomiting. In children and babies, it may be the remedy for discharges from the eyes. Symptoms of heart palpitations, vertigo and fainting, also headaches and pains are splinter-like, cutting, tearing and get worse from lying on the right side.

Modalities: Symptoms get worse with emotion, anxiety, from sugar and lying on the right side. They improve from the cool and open air.

Arnica   *Arnica montana*

This homoeopathic remedy must form part of any first aid kit. It is the first remedy to think of in the case of an accident or shock. It is used where there is throbbing, burning and stitching pains, but the underlying or main sensation is one of being bruised. It can be used for physical trauma or accidents, where there is extensive bruising and shock to the system, e.g. car, head or sports injuries, surgical operations, dental extractions and childbirth. It can also be used where there is overexertion. Arnica works by removing any shock caused by physical trauma; the complaints may heal in themselves but a feeling remains of not being quite well. Arnica will heal on all levels, but where complaints are caused by emotional trauma other remedies are probably more appropriate.

In the general symptom picture there is great oversensitivity to pain or discomfort, for example the bed feels too hard, making the person feel restless, and there is a fear of being touched or approached. The face may be red-hot but the body is cool and the extremities cold.

Mental and emotional indications: The arnica-type person may say there is nothing wrong and believe that he is well, especially just after an accident, or when there clearly *is* something wrong. One symptom of arnica is that a person may come out of a state of unconsciousness or delirium to answer a question and then return back to her previous state.

Physical: Include burping where there is a taste of rotten eggs, and also a similar-smelling flatulence.

Women's complaints: It is the first remedy to consider for a threatened miscarriage after an injury or fall, and it is often the only remedy routinely given during and after labour. It can help where there is soreness in the body and uterus during pregnancy (*see also bellis perennis*) and for varicose veins in pregnancy, but there must be the accompanying bruised sensation. Arnica can be used for postpartum haemorrhage and for afterpains, and in some cases of septicaemia; also in mastitis where the nipples are bruised and sore.

Modalities: Symptoms get worse from injury and touch; they get better from lying with the head low.

Dosage: 6C for overexertion, bruising, etc., and repeat as necessary; 30C for more serious injuries, and, for example, in labour and childbirth, take 2 times a day for 3 days; 200C for injuries to the head or before and after operations, etc., take 1 or 2 doses. Externally arnica ointment and tincture can be applied locally for stiffness and bruising etc., but be careful not to use on any open cuts or wounds. Use homoeopathic arnica before a visit to the dentist and repeat the dose after any treatment where bruising has occurred.

Astragalus   *Astragalus membranaceus*

Synonyms: Huang qi, milk vetch
   Parts used: Root
   Actions: Antimicrobial, adaptogen, diuretic, immune stimulant, tonic
   Main uses: An important energy tonic that helps to build up resistance to weakness and disease. It is a tonic to the immune system, heart and blood. It is mainly used as a tonic for younger people (under 40 years) and is a specific remedy for ME. Astragalus is also used for treating cancer patients and AIDS because of its strong immune-enhancing properties. It can be used as a blood tonic to strengthen exhausted and debilitated women, especially after heavy menstrual bleeding. It can help build up resistance after recurrent infections.
   Dosage: Tincture: 1:5 in 45 per cent alcohol. Take 2–3ml 3 times daily. Decoction of 5–10g in 1 cup of water 3 times daily.

Aurum   *Aurum metallicum*

This homoeopathic remedy is good for depression, destruction of tissue, memory weakness, restlessness and headaches. It is made from gold and symbolically it can be said to be good when the light has gone out of a person's life.
   Mental and emotional indications: There is blackness and loss of the love of living, the person feels weary and has a desire to die. Suicide is a real possibility. There is no enjoyment of anything or anyone – work, family, and so on. Aurum types are pessimistic and gloomy; they feel thwarted. They feel unworthy and that they have neglected their responsibilities; they feel that they have failed to do what they should have done. Aurum could be appropriate for people whose business has failed. They sit and brood. They feel much worse at night, becoming worse during the evening, dwelling on their failings. Pains come on during the night-time and drive them to despair. They may improve during the day and stop being broody by becoming angry or even violent. They are very impatient. These states can come on from prolonged physical pain, worry, too much responsibility or loss of property or a business. They can hold everything together intellectually and keep up appearances, but the will goes, and they can shock everyone with their collapse.
   Physical: Aurum is good for heart disease. It is the remedy to use when there is a weight on the chest as if the heart has stopped, if it feels as though the heart is giving a large thump; or there are violent beatings, palpitations, breathless-

ness on exertion and watery swellings of the lower limbs and ankles, also waves of violent heat and flushes as if the blood is bursting out of the veins, with rushes of blood in the head. The liver feels large, hard and inflamed. There are bone pains, which are aching, boring pains going down long bones, especially those in the legs. Joints are affected, the cartilage around the joints swells and becomes painful, especially at night, and prevents sleep or wakes the person up. This leads to depression. Pain will make mild depression severe. There is a fear of death, a destruction of bones in the ears and nose, ulcers in the mouth and throat and on skin which is near to bones. Headaches are really bad with a tearing pressure, throbbing and rushes of blood to the head. Complaints that can be helped by this remedy also include swollen testes and prolapse of the uterus.

Modalities: Symptoms get worse at night, in the cold air, from mental exertion, from resting and in the winter. They improve from warmth, movement and walking and in the summer.

❋ Avens Sativa *Avens sativa*

See Oats.

❋ Balm *Melissa officinialis*

Synonyms: Lemon balm, melissa
  Parts used: Aerial parts, collected while still fresh and before flowering
  Habitat: Southern Europe, Asia, Africa
  Main constituents: Flavonoids, polyphenols, tannins, volatile oils
  Actions: Antidepressant, antihistamine, antiviral, carminative, diaphoretic, nervine, relaxant
  Main uses: This is a gentle herb that also calms and tones the heart where there are palpitations or a nervous disposition. It acts as a tranquillizer on the nervous system and is particularly good for insomnia and panic attacks. Drink as a tea during fevers and for disorders of the digestive system such as indigestion, bloating and nausea. Known to help cold sores both topically and internally. Good for insect bites.
  Contraindications: None. Safe to use for children and adults.
  Dosage: Drink infusion 10g to 1 cup of water 3 times daily. Tincture 1:5 in 45 per cent alcohol, 5ml 3 times daily.

Barberry Bark   *Berberis vulgaris*

Parts used: Root, bark or fruit gathered in autumn
   Habitat: Europe
   Main constituents: Alkaloids, berberine, chelidonic acid, oxyacanthine
   Actions: Antibacterial, astringent, hepatic, stimulates bile secretion
   Main uses: This is a good tonic for the liver, assists bile production and helps gallstones and jaundice. Has a direct action on the spleen. Good to use where there are protozoan infections of the gut, e.g. amoebic dysentery, giardiasis.
   Contraindications: Pregnancy and diarrhoea.
   Dosage: Decoction of 5g to 1 cup of water. Tincture: 1:10 in 25 per cent alcohol, 5ml 3 times daily.

Basil Oil   *Ocimum basilicum*

A well-known culinary herb that is steam-distilled in Europe, North Africa and the USA. The oil usually available is distilled from *Ocimum basilicum* or sweet basil oil.
   Main constituents: Alpha terpineol, phenols, linalool, estragole, methylengeunol and monoterpenes.
   Main uses: It is a wonderful reviving oil and also has a relaxing effect on the nervous system. It is an excellent nerve tonic because it is restorative, uplifting and strengthening. It can relieve brain fag, nervousness, anxiety, depression, tension headaches and nervous insomnia. Basil is a useful oil for the digestive system – it helps indigestion and nervous dyspepsia. It will stimulate the appetite and, being antiseptic, will help intestinal infections. It can also promote sweating, so it can be used to help bring down a fever, and because it is antispasmodic it will assist respiratory conditions such as whooping cough, asthma and bronchitis. Basil oil can also help stimulate menstruation and generally help tone the female reproductive system.
   Safety and applications: Do not use more than 1 per cent dilution. In higher doses the content of estragole is possibly carcinogenic. Avoid use during pregnancy. This oil should not be used for prolonged periods of time, as it can become an irritant. Primarily, basil oil is good for the person who is worn out and debilitated, either from illness or overwork. It can be combined with a wide range of other oils, for example with fennel for the digestion; with rosemary, melissa or bergamot for overwork; with eucalyptus for sinus problems;

and with bergamot, geranium or neroli for anxiety. These are just a few suggestions. It is worth experimenting to find out which combinations you find effective and prefer.

Belladonna   *Atropa belladonna*

One of the major homoeopathic remedies for any first aid kit is belladonna – it is for usually healthy people and children who fall ill. It is a strong, robust remedy when symptoms suddenly appear. It is the first remedy to think of for children's fevers.

Physical: These will be marked by redness, burning heat and brilliant eyes, with dilated pupils; there may be a wild look and expression. Pains are throbbing with a hot head and cold hands and feet. There can be a high fever which is accompanied by a rapid, full pulse; the tongue and throat can be bright red. There is a need for cold drinks. As the fever gets higher it can develop into delirium, with biting, spitting, tearing at bed clothes, trying to escape, laughing and talking. The senses can become very acute.

The violence and suddenness of the onset of any complaint is one of the main identifying aspects of belladonna. It is excellent for turmoil in the brain, as with strange delusions. Pains are violent and throbbing; there is sensitivity to draughts. In women, periods may be early, profuse, with hot, bright red blood, and painful, often accompanied by a throbbing headache. It is one of the main remedies for period pains. There may be mastitis with bright red patches on the breast, accompanied by a fever. Belladonna is the main remedy for bright red skin complaints and for sunstroke.

Modalities: Worse in sun, draughts, touch, motion, noise and light.

Benzoin   *Styrax benzoin family: Styracareae*

This may be used by aromatherapists but it is not strictly an essential oil; it is a sticky, strong, sweet-smelling/tasting resin that must be diluted in alcohol or warmed before it can be packed or used.

Parts used: Solvent extraction of the resin tears made by incising the tree
Main constituents: Benzoic acid, benzoresinol, vanillin
Fragrance: Vanilla-like, sweet-balsamic, heavy

Main uses: This is a warming resin traditionally used for respiratory, skin and circulation problems. It has strong antibacterial actions and is used as an expectorant for coughs. Combine in mixture for sore throats and hoarseness. Also good for cold, mucus conditions where the person is feeling chilled. Use for urinary infections; particularly indicated for cystitis. Can help soothe arthritic conditions when the pain is worse from cold. Benzoin is appropriate for weak appetite, slow, sluggish digestion and poor absorption. Excellent to use in a combination for cold, blocked, clammy skin or where there are lesions and cracking. Has been used in the treatment of ezcema. Use for mouth ulcers and as a mouthwash.

Safety and application: There is no known toxicity, but may be a skin irritant in quantity. Include with oils such as lemon and rose in a base cream for the hands and feet. Combine with frankincense and myrrh as an incense. Use 2–3 drops diluted in a cup of water as a mouthwash. When diluted in an alcohol base, use as an essential oil, 1 per cent dilution.

Berberis   *Berberis vulgaris*

This homoeopathic remedy is most frequently used in the treatment of urinary organs, liver and gall bladder. The pains radiate and are shooting, sticking and burning, and change locality and character. There are gurgling or bubbling sensations, and symptoms seem to fluctuate, e.g. thirsty one minute and no thirst the next. The person looks generally distressed, pale and sickly.

Physical indications: Nephritis, cystitis and soreness in the lumber region and kidneys, where there is a need to step carefully as any pressure or jolting is intolerable. Use berberis for burning, sticking pains in the kidneys; bubbling sensations, pain in the bladder, frequent urination, burning in urethra when not urinating, renal colic; pains are more common on the left side; pains that start in the kidney region or along the course of the urethra and radiate out; and pains that go up to the kidneys and down to the bladder. There can be an urge to urinate and this is accompanied by pain on urination in the groin and thighs. The urine usually contains a sort of mucousy, grey deposit or a sandy, reddish sediment. It is dirty looking but not offensive or bloody. Berberis is an excellent remedy for kidney stones and gallstone colic, and for sticking pains that get worse from pressure.

Modalities: Symptoms get worse with motion.

❋ Bergamot Oil   *Citrus bergamia*

This is a pleasant, light green oil that provides the well-known fragrance and flavour in Earl Grey tea.

Family: Rutaceae

Parts used: Oil expressed from unripe fresh citrus fruit of the bergamot

Main constituents: Aldehydes, coumarins, lactones, linalyl acetate, sesquiterpenes

Fragrance: Tea-like, fresh, citrus

Main uses: This is a great oil to use for emotional and mental problems, as it is uplifting and restores the spirits. Use in the winter during the short hours of sunlight. Bergamot has an antispasmodic action and can be used for digestive complaints, colic, flatulence and indigestion. Its antiseptic qualities make it suitable for urinary infections and cystitis. Use for skin problems, herpes, acne, psoriasis, bites, scabies, lice. Use in a compress to draw out thorns and boils.

Safety and application: The bergaptene component in bergamot is photosensitizing, so always try to obtain an oil where the bergapten has been removed. For wounds, it is a wonderful oil to use in combination with lavender. For digestion, combine with chamomile. For cystitis, use with eucalyptus or juniper. Use maximum 2 per cent in a base oil or cream.

❋ Beth Root   *Trillium erectum*

Parts used: Rhizome and root

Habitat: Native to North America

Main constituents: Fixed oil, steroidal saponins, tannins

Actions: Alterative, antihaemorrhagic, antiseptic astringent, emmenagogue, uterine stimulant

Main uses: Known by the Native Americans to help with childbirth, to lessen bleeding, heavy periods and heavy bleeding during menopause, beth root contains precursors of the female sex hormones which not only make it a good uterine tonic but will also act like oxytocin, the hormone released during labour. This helps the uterus to contract and stimulates the flow of breast milk. Good as a general tonic for women, it can also be used for bleeding in other parts of the body, e.g. lungs, kidneys, bladder, skin. Use in a wash for cuts and piles.

Contraindications: Do not use in pregnancy until onset of labour.

Dosage: Decoction 10g in 1 litre of water. Take ½ cup 3 times daily.

❋ Black Cohosh   *Actaea racemosa*

Synonyms: Black snakeroot
   Parts used: Root and rhizome
   Habitat: Native to North America, also now in Europe
   Main constituents: Isoferulic acid, isoflavones, resin, salicylic acid, tannins, triterpene glycosides
   Actions: Analgesic, anti-inflammatory, antispasmodic, emmenogogue, nervine, sedative
   Main uses: Traditionally used for gynaecological complaints and to relieve pain in childbirth. Due to its oestrogenic constituents it is particularly used where there are hormonal imbalances, as in period pains and menopausal problems, especially hot flushes. Helps PMT, pains and bloating. During childbirth will give strength to weakened contractions and will stimulate the uterus to contract. Will help the womb to involute after birth and soften after-birth pains. Use for skin complaints that are cyclical. Use for its sedating properties to relax the heart and circulatory system, also to reduce the swelling and pains of rheumatism. Also known to help tinnitus, back pain, aching muscles, stress-related asthma, stress-related indigestion and colitis.
   Contraindications: Do not give during pregnancy (until onset of labour), or when breastfeeding.
   Dosage: Decoction of 5g in ½ litre of water. Take ½ cup daily. Tincture: 1:10 in 60 per cent alcohol. Take 10–30 drops in water as needed or daily.

❋ Black Pepper Oil   *Piper nigrum*

One of the oldest and most important spices, black pepper has been valued for centuries. The oil is obtained by steam distillation and is traditionally produced in India, Africa and other tropical areas of the world.
   Family: Piperaceae
   Parts used: Seeds
   Fragrance: Fresh, spicy, warm
   Main constituents: Ketones, monoterpenes, sesquiterpenes
   Main uses: As a stimulating oil, black pepper alleviates sluggish conditions of the digestive system. Use in a massage oil for constipation and indigestion. It will also be useful for mucus, colds and respiratory problems, but this oil is best used in a massage blend for stimulating and warming stiffness and aching

joints and muscles. It relieves rheumatism, sprains and any wasting condition of the muscles.

Safety and application: This oil is not toxic, yet it may be an irritant if used on sensitive skin and in excess. Do not use in greater dilution than 1 per cent. It blends well with lemon, marjoram or sandalwood.

❀ Blackcurrant   *Ribes nigrum*

Synonyms: Cassis
   Parts used: Berries or leaves
   Habitat: Europe, Asia
   Main constituents: Flavonoids, proanthocyanidins. The seeds contain essential fatty acids, prodelphinidins, tannins; volatile oil is in the leaves only; the fruit have a high vitamin C content.
   Actions: Antirheumatic, astringent, diuretic, febrifuge
   Main uses: Strengthening effect on the blood vessels. Use to cool the early stages of fevers. Cleansing herb for urinary congestion. Aids elimination of urine and uric acids. Use for rheumatic complaints and gout.
   Contraindications: None.
   Dosage: Infuse 25g to ½ litre of water. Drink as a tea. Use the fruit as purée, syrup or fresh.

❀ Bladderwrack   *Fucus vesiculosus*

Synonyms: Kelp
   Parts used: Thalus (whole plant)
   Habitat: North European and North American coastal areas
   Main constituents: Minerals including iodine, mucilage, polyphenols, polysaccharides
   Actions: Antihypothyroid, anti-obesic, antirheumatic, endocrine gland stimulant, stimulates circulation of lymph, tonic
   Main uses: Has a regulating effect on the thyroid. Use for thyroxin deficiency, sluggish metabolism, obesity and constipation. Indicated for lymphatic swellings and rheumatism, arthritis and gout. Nourishing and soothing for the skin, particularly when dry and flaking. Use as a hair rinse and in the bath or footbath.
   Contraindications: Not recommended in hyperthyroidism.

Dosage: Infusion of ½ teaspoon of powder to 1 cup of boiling water. Tincture: 1:5 in 25 per cent alcohol. Take 5ml 3 times daily. You can also use bladderwrack in cooking or take it as capsules.

Blue Cohosh   *Caulophyllum thalictroides*

Synonyms: Squaw root, papoose root
  Parts used: Roots and rhizome
  Habitat: Native to North America, grows in damp north-facing wooded areas
  Main constituents: Alkaloids, resin, steroidal saponins
  Actions: Anti-inflammatory, antispasmodic, emmenagogue
  Main uses: This is a traditional women's herb used by the Native Americans. It is an excellent uterine tonic. Taken in the last few weeks of pregnancy it will help prepare the uterus for labour, making the delivery shorter and easier. During labour, use to stimulate weak or irregular contractions. It can be used for delayed, painful periods and for inflammation of the vagina. Indicated for rheumatic pains during the menopause.
  Contraindications: Do not use during pregnancy until the last few weeks, when it should be used under the supervision of a herbal practitioner.
  Dosage: ½ teaspoon decocted in cup of water. Drink 3 times daily or as needed. Tincture: 1:10 in 70 per cent alcohol, 1–2ml 3 times daily.

Borage   *Borago officinalis*

Synonyms: Star flower
  Parts used: Aerial parts
  Habitat: Grows in southern Europe, now cultivated for its seed production
  Main constituents: Seeds contain gamma linolenic acid, mucilage, pyrrolizidine alkaloids, tannins
  Actions: Adrenal gland restorer, antidepressant, demulcent, galactogogue
  Main uses: This is a cheerful plant with a tradition of lifting the spirits. Good for stress, depression, tiredness. It helps to sweat out fevers and restore wellness, strengthens the adrenal glands and is good for those who have been ill for a long time or who have come off steroids. Soothes the respiratory system. The oil is said to be good for the skin.

Contraindications: The plant must be used with caution, as it is potentially toxic to the liver. Do not take for more than 3–4 weeks at a time. The seed oil does not contain the alkaloids and is not under question.

Dosage: 1 teaspoonful herb to 1 cup of water 3 times daily. Tincture: 1:10 in 45 per cent alcohol. Take 1–5ml in water 3 times daily.

Borax   *Borax veneta*

A homoeopathic remedy that is mainly used for thrush and mouth ulcers.

Mental and emotional indications: The main features of this homoeopathic remedy are anxiety, especially around downward motion, and fear of going downhill, downstairs, being put down or in babies, being swung. There is an oversensitivity to noise and a tendency to become excessively startled and frightened of sudden or unusual sounds, such as coughs, sneezes and fireworks. It has been an effective remedy when given to very nervous animals. It is good for babies who cry out in their sleep as if they are frightened of a dream, or those who cling to the side of a cot because they are afraid of falling. Babies who fit this remedy picture often cry or scream before passing a stool, urinating or whilst nursing. They are fidgety, the skin is often unhealthy and the hair gets matted at the back of the head. They may have ingrowing eyelashes.

Physical: Include injuries that suppurate and are slow to heal. The nose can be red and shiny and the nostrils may get inflamed and crusty. There may be ulceration and thrush of the mucous membranes and mouth ulcers that may bleed while eating or when touched. The person feels worse from eating sour or salty food. In babies, thrush in the mouth is hot and tender and will make it difficult to suck. There can be soreness in the vagina, accompanied by itching, and hot smarting pains; the vulva may be itchy. Leucorrhoea appears like uncooked eggwhite and is excoriating. There can be erosion of the cervix. Periods can be too early, profuse or accompanied by colic, which can be griping and nauseous. If the symptom picture fits, borax may help conception, which is often prevented by the acrid leucorrhoea.

Modalities: Symptoms get worse from downward motion, sudden noise, damp and cold; they get better from pressure.

⚛ Bryonia   *Bryonia alba*

This is one of the main homoeopathic remedies used for problems of the respiratory system, headaches, pains and constipation.

Mental and emotional indications: Bryonia is indicated by intolerance of disturbance. Suffering from extreme irritability and anger, the person will want to be left alone with no interference. She is anxious about the future and has no sense of security. She is confused and can become delirious. She may also be quietly morose, with great fear of poverty and uncertainty. The confusion will become worse when she is talked to or moved, even when sitting up or walking.

Physical: Symptoms will start slowly, unlike with aconite or belladonna. The person will want rest, quiet and no attention. Complaints are generally right-sided and may start as the weather changes, or after getting cold. Pains are usually intense – stitching or bursting. These seem better when lying on the painful side and with pressure. This is a remedy for respiratory complaints, coughs, bronchitis, pneumonia. Where the pains are acute, sticking and get worse by breathing deeply, there may be accompanying pains in the joints, which can be swollen, hot and red. The face may look dark red and bloated, with dry lips. Bryonia is indicated by suppressed discharges, excessive dryness of the mucous membranes of the whole body, dry stools, parched lips and dry, hard and racking cough, with very little expectoration and dark and scanty urine. The person will want to drink large quantities but infrequently.

Digestive system: Constipation with large, hard, crumbling and dry stools, as if burnt. There may be 'summer diarrhoea', which comes on from being chilled after overheating, stools are like dirty water.

Head: Dizziness, fainting on rising, headache that is bursting. The pain feels bursting when the person stoops or coughs. She can wake with a headache that gets worse during the day – often this is a pain behind the eyes.

Women's complaints: Periods may be replaced by frequent nosebleeds. Periods may be early and profuse or suppressed altogether and there may be a headache before the period starts. There may be sticking pains in the ovaries. Breasts may be swollen and sore during periods; bryonia is a remedy for mastitis where there are sticking pains in the breasts.

Modalities: Worse from motion, sitting up, stooping, coughing, exertion, deep breathing, getting hot, touch and anxiety; better from pressure, lying on a painful part, coolness and open air.

❋ Burdock   *Arctium lappa*

Parts used: Leaf, root, seeds

Habitat: Native to Europe, Asia and America

Main constituents: Leaf: inulin, mucilage, tannins, terpinoids; root: acetylenic compounds, amino acids, inulin, mucilage, phenolic acids, pytosterols, tannins, volatile oils

Actions: Leaf: depurative, diuretic, mild laxative; root: alterative, antibacterial, antibiotic, antirheumatic, diaphoretic, diuretic, mild laxative

Main uses: Burdock has traditionally been used as a blood purifier and to treat gout, fevers and kidney stones. Now it is more often used as a detoxifying agent for conditions caused by a build-up of toxins, such as acne, spots, eczema, psoriasis, arthritis, gout, urinary stones, gravel and fevers. Use externally for sores and infections. The leaf is also used for poor digestion, stomach problems and anorexia.

Dosage: Decoction of root, 2–6g 3 times daily. Tincture: 1:5 in 25 per cent alcohol (leaf or root), 1–2ml 3 times daily.

❋ Caladium   *Caladium seguinum*

This homoeopathic remedy is good for mosquito and insect bites that burn and itch intensely. There can be nervous excitability and great sensitivity to noise; intense itching of the genitals, with burning; and dryness in areas which are usually moist. There may be a red, dry stripe down the centre of the tongue which gets wider towards the tip. The person is usually thirstless and wants to lie down and not move. This remedy may help modify the craving for tobacco.

Modalities: Symptoms get worse from movement, sudden noises, tobacco and sexual excess; they improve with cold air, short sleeps and sweating.

❋ Calc Carb   *Calcarea carbonica*

This is a remedy to help give support and stability, particularly through times of transition. It can also be an excellent homoeopathic remedy for children. Whether teething or for childhood ailments. The typical calc carb person will be fair, tend to be overweight and clammy.

Mental and emotional indications: Calc carb is a remedy for chilly people. Children are worse from heat and push away bed covers, but as they get older they get chillier and may wear socks in bed until the feet get too hot and they take them off. Diarrhoea is pale and may alternate with constipation. They feel better when they are constipated. They are thorough and methodical people, they like to do things in their own time. Maybe sensitive and peevish. Tendency to get depressed. Mental agility tends to slow down as they get older, thoughts churn around and they take longer to understand and will pause before answering. They may get anxious about the future and their health, the more tired they become, the greater the anxiety. They become worried about how others see them. Although they don't like to admit they have a fear of death, it dominates their lives.

Physical: Symptoms will be marked by chilliness and dampness.

Circulatory system: It is also good for all kinds of arthritic conditions which get better in dry heat and worse in the cold and damp. The sluggishness in the circulation leads to chilblains, varicose veins and then leg ulcers.

Head: A tendency for headaches which come on after exertion but get better from lying on the left side. There may be vertigo on descending stairs and severe vertigo on suddenly turning the head. They get headaches if they do not eat, eruptions and cracks behind the ears. There is a continual feeling of emptiness which gets better from eating.

Respiratory system: Calc carb may be a good remedy to use for those who catch colds easily or suffer from chronic catarrh where the mucus goes down the back of the throat.

Women's complaints: Breasts may get swollen and painful before a period, with accompanying constipation. Periods are often early, painful and heavy. It is a good remedy to consider for uterine fibroids. There is often a strong sexual impulse.

Children: Children who need this remedy may have a desire to eat indigestible things, such as coal and chalk; as a baby, they smell sour, vomit milk and have a poor appetite. They often appear to have large heads where the fontanelle is slow to close. They can be slow to teethe and many have pot bellies, frequently have colds and tend to whine and grumble. They may suffer from nightmares that wake them. Symptoms can arise after vaccinations.

Modalities: Worse: exertion (both physical and mental), cold air, bathing, cooling, dentition, pressure of clothes. Better: dry weather, after breakfast.

✳ Calc Fluor   *Calcarea fluorica*

Calc fluor is one of the 12 homoeopathic remedies known as tissue salts, so called as they are present in the tissues of the body. It is used to improve elasticity in the skin, veins or glands.

Physical: This remedy is used for swollen glands or for swellings that have become hard, e.g. swollen tonsils or hard nodes in the breast. It is one of the best remedies to help distended varicose veins, inflamed skin and stretch marks in pregnancy. It can really help if it is used on a regular basis. It is also good for piles during pregnancy. Calc fluor can be used to accompany a diet or fast to help with the elasticity of the skin when excess weight is lost too quickly.

Teeth: Used for enamel deficiency; take with calc phos, give twice daily for a fortnight to children with forming teeth. Give this twice a year.

Modalities: Worse: starting to move, cold, damp. Better: moving.

✳ Calc Phos   *Calcarea phosphorica*

Calc phos is one of the 12 homoeopathic remedies known as tissue salts, so called as they are present in the tissues of the body. Calcium phosphate is an essential part of good nutrition and proper growth. It is found in blood, saliva, gastric juices, bones, connective tissue and teeth. Calc phos will help to give solidity to bones, promoting cell growth, assisting digestion and assimilation. It acts as a tonic for debility and during convalescence.

Physical: Use calc phos for all bone diseases, osteoporosis or brittle bones. Calc phos would be a good supporting remedy with symphytum for the non-union of fractures. It will help speed up the healing process. It is very good for slow-growing, slow-teething children, or for those with rickets. Give for growing pains in children and adolescents. Other symptoms may include a stiff neck which comes on after being in a draught; rheumatism caused by cold weather. Cramps, spasms, numbness; cold hands and feet, moaning during sleep.

Mental and emotional indications: These are influenced by overall mental weakness – an inability to sustain any mental effort, impaired memory, confusion, tiredness from over-talking or mental work. The calc phos type feels discontented and complains. There may be a nervous restlessness, with sighing and a desire to get away or travel, a feeling of wanting to be on the move and an irritability which gets worse when tired.

Digestive system: Calc phos can be used for digestive problems where there is heartburn, flatulence and colic. There can be a large appetite, particularly for salted or strong-tasting foods. The abdomen can be flabby with hot, watery, offensive, spluttering stools. Diarrhoea gets worse in the summer and with fruit or when it accompanies teething.

Head: Use for schoolchildren who have headaches brought on by over-study or anaemia. They are nervous, restless and the head feels cold to touch. It is made worse by cold air and draughts and improves with bathing.

Respiratory system: There is a tendency to catch colds easily and often from becoming chilled. Coughs will have yellow expectoration.

Teeth: Calc phos is an excellent remedy to give for teething which is painful, difficult or slow. Also for teeth which are soft and decay easily and gums which are pale, painful and inflamed.

Throat: Indications include a sore, aching throat, swollen glands, radiating pain on swallowing and chronic enlargement of tonsils. It is a good remedy for bronchitis where there is inflammation of the middle ear, the glands are swollen and the ear aches.

Women's complaints: Calc phos is particularly appropriate for rapidly grow-ing young people with anaemia, or for those suffering from heavy periods. It is good for women who have lost a lot of body fluids, for girls with discharges. Use for periods occurring during breastfeeding. Periods that are painful where the pains get worse as a result of a change of weather and improve when the flow starts. Excessive bleeding. For tiredness during pregnancy where breasts may be sore. Calc phos is excellent for anaemia caused by heavy periods, or for weakness after prolonged breastfeeding. Use for prolapse after weakness.

Modalities: Worse: weather changes, draughts, colds, teething, mental exer-tion and adolescence. Better: warm, dry weather, lying down.

Calc Sulph   *Calcarea sulphurica*

Calcium sulphate is one of the 12 homoeopathic remedies known as tissue salts, so called as they are present in the tissues of the body. This mineral acts on the connective tissue. It is a cleanser, it heals wounds, purifies the blood and is good for conditions that arise from toxicity.

Physical: Calc sulph helps with elimination of toxins. It is good to use for cleaning out what is left from coughs and colds. Use where catarrh is persistent and to help clear skin problems. It will help conditions that suppurate and have thick, yellow, lumpy or blood-streaked pus. Calc sulph is very good for adolescent acne or for pimples, particularly on the face and shoulders. It is good for painless abscesses around the anus. Use to treat old oozing ulcers where the pus is thin and watery, or for purulent discharges that will not heal. Use calc sulph for burning, itching soles of the feet, or when there is oversensitivity of the nerves and the person is feeling on edge.

Modalities: Worse: draughts, touch, cold, water, heat of a room. Better: open air, eating, heat when applied locally.

Cantharis   *Cantharis vesicatoria*

This homoeopathic remedy is especially appropriate for conditions affecting the urinary and sexual organs. It is one of the most specific remedies for cystitis.

Mental and emotional indications: Irritability and anger get worse with pain. Use of foul language. There may be a general oversensitivity, anxiousness and restlessness. Liable to contradict, attempts to do things but cannot accomplish them.

Physical: Normally pale individuals but become flushed during bouts of pain. Pains are cutting, biting, smarting, burning and they accompany all ailments. They cause great mental excitement. There is oversensitivity in all parts of the body. There is burning in the body, both internal and external.

Head: Feels heavy, inflamed eyes that are burning, flushed face. Throat burns making swallowing difficult and very painful. Reluctant to drink through fear of increased pain.

Skin: Use for raw, painful burns and scalds, before or just after blisters form.

Urinary: The urinary and generative organs feel very sensitive. The kidney area is sensitive to the slightest touch. Urine is burning, scalding, with constant desire to urinate. This becomes intolerable as the cutting, burning pains get worse before and after urination. They are accompanied by spasms and a sore, raw sensation. Urine can be bloody and burns like fire. Urine passes in drops. Cantharis is the most frequently indicated remedy for cystitis; it is also good for nephritis and renal colic.

Modalities: Worse: urinating, sound of water, cold. Better: warmth, rest, massage.

Carbo Veg   *Carbo vegetabilis*

This is a life-saver remedy. It can be used after a haemorrhage where there are cold sweats, cold feet, cold breath, a thready, weak pulse, a need for cold air and a blueness in the face. It can be used for a newborn in this state – in this case use a single 200C potency. Carbo veg can be used after an exhausting illness and it is good for children who have never totally recovered from measles, whooping cough or a loss of body fluids. It is a remedy for people who are greatly debilitated, weak, in a state of collapse and are without vitality, e.g., someone who has nearly drowned.

Mental and emotional indications: The person will feel pale, chilly, exhausted and needing air. There is a weakness of memory, a slow grasp of things, confusion, irritability, anxiousness or indifference.

Physical: Give when someone faints and needs air. Use for asthma attacks or persistent nosebleeds

Digestive system: This is one of the major remedies for flatulence, bloated rumblings, indigestion, a distended stomach, which is worse from lying down but improved by burping, and there is excessive gas in the stomach and intestines.

Modalities: Worse: eating rich, fatty foods, pressure of clothes around waist, walking. Better: belching, farting, lying down, from air.

Cardamon Oil   *Elettaria cardamomum*

The seeds and pods have been used for centuries as a digestive ingredient for food. The fragrant oil is distilled from the seeds and produced mainly in India and the USA.

Family: Zingiberaceae

Parts used: Crushed seeds and pods

Fragrance: Spicy, warm, slightly lemony

Main constituents: Cineole, esters, oxides, monoterpenes, terpineol

Main uses: This is a warming oil that works well for digestive complaints, particularly when they are due to being in a nervous or tense state. It is an anti-spasmodic oil and can be used in a massage blend for griping indigestion, heartburn, colic and flatulence. It has a calming yet toning effect and will bring relief to headaches, lift depression and help to calm fears of sexual relation-ships. Traditionally the seeds have been used as a breath freshener. A few can be chewed after a meal or a couple of drops can be dissolved in alcohol and made into a mouth rinse. Use also as an incense mixed with myrrh and frankincense.

Safety and application: This is a safe oil to use in dilution of 2 per cent in massage blends. Cardamon blends well with frankincense, geranium, lemon, mandarin and palmarosa.

❊ Catnip   *Nepeta cataria*

Synonyms: Catmint, cat's wort
   Parts used: Aerial parts
   Habitat: Europe
   Main constituents: Bitter principle, iridoids, tannins, volatile oil
   Actions: Antidiarrhoeal, antiflatulent, diaphoretic, digestive, emmenagogue, febrifuge, sedative
   Main uses: Helps with colds and 'flu associated with fever and digestive upsets with flatulence. Good for colic cramps. Good for children. Recent research suggests that it is an effective mosquito repellent.
   Contraindications: Not to be used during pregnancy.
   Dosage: 1 teaspoon herb to 1 cup of water. Drink as needed. Tincture: 1:5 in 25 per cent alcohol. Use as insect spray with added citronella oil.

❊ Caulophyllum   *Caulophyllum thalictroides*

This is a great homeopathic remedy for women. It will be indicated where there is weakness and debilitation either during pregnancy and labour or due to the symptoms of PMT.

Mental and emotional indications: Extreme exhaustion, irritability, mood swings, fearfulness, feeling unable to carry on. Restlessness.

Physical: This remedy helps improve the uterine tone. Give where there is a danger of miscarriage during the first few weeks of pregnancy. Give during labour when the contractions are irregular and ineffective or disappear due to exhaustion. Indicated for very painful contractions, pain like pricking needles in the cervix, late dilation of the cervix. Useful for prolonged and painful after-pains and profuse lochia. Indicated for periods where there are erratic, cramping, labour-like pains which start in the small of the back and are accompanied by nausea. Can also be used for rheumatism where the toes, fingers and joints are affected. The pains are severe, cramping and move around.

Modalities: Worse in the evening, better for warmth.

✳ Causticum   *Causticum*

This is one of the main homoeopathic remedies for grief as well as being excellent for coughs and burns.

Mental and emotional indications: This person will have a defeatist outlook, as she has been worn down by emotional disappointments and now copes with life by suppressing her emotions. Such people can be pessimistic, apprehensive, weepy and despair of any chance of recovery. They are afraid that something will happen, of the dark and twilight; distrustful and absent-minded. They are sympathetic and easily upset by other people's suffering and get very concerned and worried about their own family and loved ones. They have a very low sexual drive. Ailments come on from grief, loss of sleep and anger. They are chilly people, with tears near to the surface; they may have a sallow, sickly look. It is a remedy for carers, especially those who have nursed another through a terminal illness.

Physical: Causticum can really help where there is weakness on a physical level as well as mental. It can be very good for multiple sclerosis, neuralgia, rheumatoid conditions and one-sided paralysis. There can be burning sensations and vertigo, with a tendency to fall forwards or sideways which gets worse from lying down, stooping or during a period. There can be a sensation of space between the brain and the skull, and also paralysis of single areas, such as the face, voice, eyelids, throat or limbs. Causticum is a remedy for conditions that occur after cold winds, e.g. Bell's Palsy. It can be given for rheumatism which gets worse in cold dry weather and better in damp conditions.

Abdomen: There can be paralysis in the rectum and constipation with no urge to pass a stool even when soft. There may be burning, stinging piles which get worse when touched or washed. Causticum is a remedy that is often given for cystitis. It is appropriate when symptoms are brought on by a cold or chill. There is only a small amount of urine passed, sometimes after a long wait. There's involuntary urination on sneezing, laughing, coughing or sudden movement.

Eyes: Water in the open air, vision can become dim through paralysis in the optic nerve, there can be drooping eyelids, cataracts or tiny warts on the upper lids.

Respiratory system: There may be a loss of voice or a burning hoarseness in the morning, with rawness in the throat. There is an inability to raise phlegm, as it slips back. The expectoration can taste greasy. The chest is full of mucus. Involuntary urination when coughing. A hollow tickling cough brought on by cold air, improved by drinking cold water.

Skin: It is a remedy for warts that bleed easily. It is excellent to give for second- or third-degree burns, for burning pains and to help relieve continuing discomfort even after initial healing.

Stomach: The person likes stimulants, e.g. coffee, tea, spicy food, etc., and can sit down to a meal feeling hungry but then the actual smell of food is upsetting. She can feel ravenous but then a little food makes her feel full. There's a desire for salt.

Modalities: Worse: cold, dry air, wind, evening, twilight and darkness, extremes of temperature, changes of weather, between 2 and 4 a.m. Better: damp, rainy, moist conditions, cold drinks, washing, the warmth of bed and gentle motion.

✳ Cayenne   *Capsicum frutescens*

Synonyms: Chillies, red pepper
  Parts used: Fruit
  Habitat: Tropical areas of America, India, Africa
  Main constituents: Alkaloids, capsaicinoids, fatty oil
  Actions: Analgesic, antiseptic, antispasmodic, carminative, stimulant; externally as counterirritant, rubefacient
  Main uses: This is a very warming herb. It will help conditions where there is cold and low vitality, e.g. promoting circulation in the elderly or those with hypothermia. It stimulates the circulation and is excellent to make into a salve to rub onto cold feet and hands. Use also for arthritis or where there are cold neuralgic pains. Good to use where there is cold, 'flu and general weakness. Will help relieve wind and colic and other gastric conditions where there is weakness and debility.
  Contraindications: Do not use on broken or very sensitive skin, or near the eyes. Internally, excessive dosage can cause gastrointestinal irritation in sensitive individuals.
  Dosage: Tincture 1:3 in 60 per cent alcohol. Make into a salve to apply locally or use the macerated oil for local massage.

Cedarwood Oil   *Cedrus atlantica*

Cedar, native to the Atlas Mountains in Morocco and Algeria, has been highly valued for centuries as a building material that repels insects.

Family: Pinaceae

Parts used: The oil is steam distilled from the wood chips and branches of the tree.

Main constituents: Alcohols, ketones, sesquiterpenes

Fragrance: Woody, slightly sweet

Main uses: This oil has a strengthening power best used to both soothe and tone the nervous system. Great for people with chronic nervous complaints. As an astringent oil, use for chronic diarrhoea, chronic catarrh and coughs, chronic cystitis. Good for arthritis, rheumatism and to help move toxicity. Use as an antiseptic for oily skin, hair, acne, dandruff. Stimulates hair growth. Use for alopecia. Use for fungal infections and as a parasiticide for lice and scabies. Cedarwood oil blends well with frankincense and rosemary.

Safety and application: Non-toxic, non-sensitizing, non-irritating. Use always in a base oil, dilution of 2 per cent.

Celery   *Apium graveolens*

Parts used: Seeds, stalks

Habitat: Native to Europe

Main constituents: Apiol, coumarins, fixed oil, minerals, volatile oil

Actions: Antigout, anti-inflammatory, antirheumatic, antispasmodic, carminative, diuretic, lowers blood pressure, urinary antiseptic

Main uses: Commonly used as a vegetable, this plant cleanses the urinary system and reduces acidity in the body. Use for cystitis, bladder problems and inflammation of the urinary tract. Helps detoxify the body and improve the circulation. Particularly good for rheumatism and stiffness. Use for asthma and bronchitis. The seeds are more potent than the vegetable and are often used to treat arthritis and gout.

Contraindications: Do not take the seeds in pregnancy. Individuals with kidney disorders should use it with caution.

Dosage: Celery stems can be eaten raw in salads or juiced to make a cleansing drink. Decoction of seeds: ½ teaspoon to 1 cup of water taken 3 times daily. Tincture 1:5 in 90 per cent alcohol. Take 2–5ml 3 times daily.

❋ Chamomile (German)   *Matricaria recutita*

Parts used: Flowerheads

Habitat: Europe and all temperate climates

Main constituents: Bitter principle, flavonoids, tannic acid, volatile oil (containing azulene)

Actions: Analgesic, anti-inflammatory, antiseptic, antispasmodic, bitter, carminative, sedative, vulnerary

Main uses: This is a great herb with a whole range of uses. It is not surprising that chamomile tea has become one of the most popular herbal teas in the stressful, polluted environment that we live in. As a herb to aid digestion, chamomile will be soothing and calming for gastric ulcers, spasms, indigestion and nausea. Take for nervous, excitable conditions, tension, insomnia, restlessness, migraines and other headaches. For the respiratory system, use for inflammation and sore throats. Use for PMT, candidiasis. Use as a douche for vaginal bruising and inflammation. Externally, this is a herb that can be used in a wash for treating inflamed, sore, irritated skin conditions, burns and wounds. It helps to soothe allergic reactions, both internally and externally. Use in an eyewash for conjunctivitis and for sore, puffy, sticky eyes, and use in a rinse for gum infections. Give to children for teething, fretful states.

Contraindications: None. Safe for infants.

Dosage: Infuse 1 teaspoon to 1 cup of water. Leave to stand for 5 mins. Tincture 1:5 in 45 per cent alcohol.

❋ Chamomile Oil   *Matricaria chamomilla*

One of the favourite oils to use, distilled in increasing quantities in Britain, this oil is a distinctive blue due to the high content of azulene in it.

Fragrance: Intense, sweet, bitter

Main constituents: Alpha-bisabol oxide, sesquiterpenes (chamazulene)

Main uses: As the healing properties of azulene are now attracting the interest of scientists, chamomile is at last receiving medical recognition, even though it has been used for centuries. Chamomile oil has calming, sedating properties which make it ideal for nervous, excitable conditions. Use for headaches, insomnia, stress and irratibility. Use with St John's Wort for sciatica or neuralgia. Use for painful and inflamed joints, tense, aching muscles. Use for digestive problems in a massage oil to treat colic, indigestion and diarrhoea.

As an antispasmodic, chamomile will help with menstrual cramps. Include in a soothing massage oil for menopausal symptoms. A great skin healer and soother, good for all skin conditions. Use in an oil blend with bergamot, lavender and rose or in a cream base for wounds and dry skin conditions.

Toxicity and application: Non-toxic, use 1–2 per cent in dilution. Use in oil, cream bases and in the bath.

⚹ Chamomilla   *Matricaria chamomilla*

This is a valuable soothing homoeopathic remedy and particularly helpful for teething children.

Mental and emotional indications: The person who fits this remedy will have a short temper, be irritable, dissatisfied, quarrelsome, excitable, nervous or obstinate. She may dislike being spoken to or even looked at. She will be oversensitive to pain and will feel that it seems unbearable. Chamomilla treats ailments arising from anger, excitement or abuse of stimulants. Women in labour may need this remedy if their pain is unbearable and they blame their partner! Children needing chamomilla will seem impossible. Their pain will be bad, but they will be difficult to convince that you are doing all you can to help. They will want to be carried, but may also reject whatever they have just asked for.

Physical: All symptoms will be worse in the heat and the person may feel hot and sweaty, and will be restless, particularly when sleeping or at night between 9 p.m. and midnight. The child that is teething will have one cheek that is red and hot while the other remains pale and cool. Diarrhoea may accompany teething pains. It will be green and watery and smell sulphurous. The baby may arch his back or draw his legs up in pain.

Head: Chamomilla is often good for earache if the pain is acute, the face is flushed and the patient is irritable. Also use for toothache which is worse from heat, hot food and drinks.

Women's complaints: Chamomilla is excellent to give in labour when pains are excessive and spasmodic. It is very good for the transition stage and at any time when the woman becomes abusive. Give 200C as necessary during this time. It is also good for after-pains. Use for inflamed, tender nipples which make breastfeeding painful.

Modalities: Worse: Teething, stimulants, draughts, heat, 9 p.m.–midnight. Better: Sweating, cold applictions, being carried, mild, wet weather.

Chickweed *Stellaria media*

Parts used: Aerial parts
   Habitat: Northern Europe
   Main constituents: Coumarins, flavonoids, glucosides, saponins, vitamins
   Actions: Alterative, cooling, demulcent, emollient, reduces itching
   Main uses: This is a cleansing herb which is good for the respiratory system, skin and joints. Use for lung problems where there is yellow, hot phlegm, a loose cough or a very hard, dry cough. Good for dry, itching, cracked skin conditions, eczema, psoriasis, boils, abscesses and painful spots. Use internally as well as externally in a wash; use herbs in the bath or a cream. Helpful for rheumatism where joints are hot and painful, chickweed also calms the heart, especially palpitations which arise as a result of tiredness.
   Contraindications: None.
   Dosage: Infuse 2 teaspoons to 1 cup of water, drink 3 times daily or use as wash. Tincture 1:5 in 45 per cent alcohol, 5ml 3 times daily.

China *Cinchona officinalis*

This is a good homoeopathic remedy for any weakness and debilitation arising through loss of fluids, blood, sweat, etc. It is used in dealing with the effects of long-term heavy discharges or recurrent fevers such as malaria or after a long bout of 'flu.
   Mental and emotional indications: Marked by touchiness, a tendency to overreact, nervousness, excitability. The china picture includes people who feel and think intensely, they may be oversensitive to noise and colour. They tend to be discerning and find communication difficult. They may try to avoid talking, as they can be hurtful or sarcastic. They tend to be opinionated, quietly aggressive and self-sufficient. They may have strong feelings and consider themselves ill-used, even though they tend to be loyal. They may have a fear of dogs.
   Physical: China is a good remedy for exhaustion, especially nervous exhaustion. Use for nerve-based pains, neuralgia and sciatica. Useful after a haemorrhage to help replenish the blood more quickly.
   Digestion: Often a history of wasting and weight loss from long illness and poor digestion. Gallstones and gallstone colic. Bloating and fermentation which does not improve with farting. Desire to loosen clothing. Appetite after

starting to eat or a sense of fullness after the first mouthful. Everything tastes bitter. Tongue is flabby and yellow-coated. Stools may be undigested and watery, but painless.

Cina   *Artemisia maritima*

Useful children's homoeopathic remedy and effective in the treatment of worms.

Mental and emotional indications: Marked by the child's apparent indifference to or dislike of being cuddled. Complaining and cross. Such children are sensitive, inclined to hit out and disinclined to play. They cannot bear being looked at or approached, although they may want to be carried. They want things but then reject them when they get them.

Physical: The face is pale and sickly with bluish-white around the mouth, dark rings around the eyes and dilated pupils. They pick the nose until it bleeds. The nose will itch and the child will rub its nose constantly. Remedy for threadworms. Ravenous hunger soon after a meal, constant craving for sweets and bread. The child may develop a distended, hard abdomen and have twisting pains which are better with pressure, or there may be cutting, pinching pains from the worms, with an itchy anus. When a child has worms, it is good to give the remedy in 200C. Give one dose at night-time and one the following morning, then no more. *(See pages 198–9 on homoeopathic dosage.)*

Skin: Restless sleep, night terrors or crying out. The child may grind its teeth during sleep.

Modalities: Worse: being touched, night-time. Better: lying on stomach.

Clary Sage Oil   *Salvia sclarea*

Family: Lamiaceae (Labiatae)

Main constituents: Alcohols, esters, linalylacetate, linalool oxides, sesquiterpenes

Fragrance: Tenacious, bitter-sweet, herbacious

Main uses: This oil gently stimulates and strengthens one's vitality as well as having a soothing effect on the nervous system. It is sedating, anti-convulsive and regenerating. It is useful during convalescence, and in all forms of mental and physical debility, where the person has become weakened and depressed. It can be used in a blend for the treatment of post-natal depression or when

recuperating from a breakdown. Clary sage strengthens the kidneys and digestive system, and is particularly good for the female reproductive system. It
strengthens a weak uterus and is good for absent, scant or painful periods.
It will also be helpful for asthma and cramps, and it lowers the blood pressure.

Safety and application: Non-toxic, non irritant, it can cause dizziness. Do
not combine with alcohol. Clary sage may often be used instead of sage as it is
safer; it combines well with basil, geranium, jasmine, lavender, etc. Use 2–3
drops in a saucerful of base-massage oil.

Cleavers   *Galium aparine*

Synonyms: Clivers, goosegrass
  Parts used: Aerial parts
  Habitat: Northern Europe
  Main constituents: Anthraquinones, flavonoids, glycoside asperuloside,
iridoids, polyphonic acids
  Actions: Adaptogen, alterative, anti-inflammatory, astringent, diuretic
  Main uses: Helps the lymph to flow and helps drain the lymph nodes. Use
to treat conditions of the urinary system, painful infections, cystitis and
bedwetting. May relieve mastitis. This is one of the main herbs for sluggish,
dull skin. Use also for dry skin conditions. Can be used as a spring tonic to
help cleanse the body and beautify the skin.
  Contraindications: None.
  Dosage: Infuse 1 teaspoonful to 1 cup of water. Take 3 times daily. Tincture
1:5 in 25 per cent alcohol. Take 5ml 3 times daily.

Clove Oil   *Syzygium aromaticum* or *eugenia caryophyllata*

A spice oil used in perfumery, the food industry and in dentistry. Distilled in
the West Indies and India.
  Family: Myrtaceae
  Fragrance: Hot, spicy, woody
  Main constituents: Oxides, phenols, sesquiterpenes, terpenes
  Main uses: As a powerful antiseptic and analgesic, clove oil is excellent to
use for toothache. Apply a drop on a cotton bud and place on the infected

tooth. Add to alcohol or tincture to use as a mouthwash. As a stimulating warming oil combine in blends to help with problems due to slow circulation. Will help dullness or confusion. Clove oil can be blended with other oils and used as an insect repellent. Use with chamomilla or eucalyptus against moths.

Safety and application: Clove oil is an irritant. Do not use in any blend concentration above 0.5 per cent of total. Do not use during pregnancy or breastfeeding.

Coccus Cacti   *Coccus cacti*

A good homoeopathic remedy to use where the bronchial tubes are full of mucus.

Physical: There may be rawness of the air passages, or a sensation of a crumb or lump behind the larynx which causes coughing, and there is a desire to swallow constantly.

Coughs: This remedy can be given for whooping cough. A child can be seized by violent fits of coughing ending in vomiting, or where clear, ropey mucus hangs in strings from the mouth. Attacks of coughing will come on at night-time with tickling in the larynx. This remedy can be considered for an early-morning cough which starts off being dry and barking, and then brings up stringy mucus. Expectoration can be stringy, yellow or reddish. It is viscous and sour-tasting.

Modalities: Worse: from heat and warm rooms, lying down, waking up, irritation of the throat, the slightest exertion, brushing teeth. Better: cold, washing in cold water, cold drinks and walking.

Coffea   *Coffea canda*

Coffea is a homoeopathic remedy for insomnia that is caused by over-stimulation. It may be the remedy for a hyperactive child.

Mental and emotional indications: If you are familiar with the effects of a strong cup of coffee, recognizing the symptoms of coffea should not be too difficult. There is a sense of exhilaration and excitement, the mind is restless, full of ideas and plans, the memory is alive. All the senses are heightened, symptoms can be brought on by the shock of good or exciting news.

Physical: Difficult to get off to sleep. Insomnia from sudden emotion. The coffea type is wide awake and the body is overactive. They may feel hot and agitated which can bring on headache. Use for toothache if pain improves with cold water.

Modalities: Worse: cold air, noise, overstimulation. Better: rest, cold water.

Colocynthis   *Citrullus colocynthis*

The main action of this homoeopathic remedy is on the abdominal area. It is excellent when ailments come on after anger, frustration, grief, humiliation or embarrassment.

Mental and emotional indications: Marked by restlessness and nervousness, crying out from intense pain but there is a strong dislike of being questioned.

Physical: Abdominal pain which causes the person to double up. It is often indicated for babies with colic when they pull their legs up and the pains seem cutting and griping. An adult will clutch the area of pain or apply hard pressure to bring relief. It is good for colic which comes on after anger and is accompanied by vomiting or diarrhoea. Colocynthis is a good remedy for period pains where there are severe cramping pains in the uterus and the menstrual flow is either early or suppressed. It is relieved by warmth. Pains may be accompanied by dizziness when the head is turned to the left. Colocynthis can be used for sciatica where there are cramping pains in the hip.

Modalities: Worse: emotional states especially anger, movement and at night. Better: hard pressure, doubling up, heat and rest.

Coltsfoot   *Tussilago farfara*

Parts used: Aerial parts

Habitat: Europe

Main constituents: Flavonoids, mucilage, pyrrolizidine alkaloids, vitamin C, zinc

Actions: Anticatarrhal, anti-inflammatory, antispasmodic, expectorant

Main uses: A traditional and great remedy for coughs, nervous coughs, smoker's cough, dry cough of the elderly. Use as a tonic to strengthen the lungs. Helps reduce or prevent mucus forming. Helps with unproductive coughs, asthma and whooping cough.

Contraindications: Due to pyrrolizidine alkaloids, use with care. Not to be used where there are any indications of liver problems. Take for no more than

2–3 weeks at a time. Avoid in pregnancy and whilst breastfeeding.

Dosage: It is best to boil the leaves as a decoction and reduce the risk to the liver. Use 25g to 500ml water. Use only as an expectorant. Combine with thyme and elecampane to make syrup.

⚜ Comfrey   *Symphytum officinalis*

Synonyms: Knitbone
Parts used: Leaves and roots
Habitat: Europe
Main constituents: Allantoin, mucilage, phenolic acids, pyrrolizidine alkaloids, steroidal saponins, tannins
Actions: Demulcent, expectorant, speeds up cell division, vulnerary
Main uses: Has been used for many years as a herb for healing all wounds. In digestive tract, use for healing any ulceration – bleeding from the stomach, lungs, bladder, bowels. Use as an expectorant for dry coughs. For the bones, use to speed up the healing of fractures, sprains and ligament damage. Use externally either as a poultice, tincture or macerated oil. Comfrey promotes or regulates the overgrowth of skin tissue, is effective for psoriasis and skin ulcers and helps clear bruises and heal scar tissue. Helps relieve the inflammation caused by gout and rheumatic joints. Promotes rapid healing.
Contraindications: Due to the pyrrolizidine alkaloids, mainly present in the root, do not use the root internally.
Dosage: Infusion of leaves: 1 teaspoon per cup of water 3 times daily for maximum of 6 weeks. Tincture (leaf): 1:5 in 45 per cent alcohol, take average 2–6ml 3 times daily for maximum of 6 weeks. Poultice: Liquidize fresh herb for application as desired. Macerated oil: Infuse dried or fresh in olive oil. Combine either oil or tincture into cream base, minimum 10 per cent.

⚜ Cornsilk   *Zea mays*

Parts used: The silky threads (styles and stigma) surrounding the corn on the cob
Habitat: Native to South America, cultivated worldwide
Main constituents: Allantoin, flavonoids, potassium, saponins, vitamins C and K, zinc

Actions: Antihypertensive, anti-inflammatory, cholagogue, demulcent, diuretic, reduces blood sugar

Main uses: Used most significantly as a diuretic. With its silicea and potassium content, it can be used for most urinary problems. Soothing to the urinary tract, it relaxes and relieves pain, irritation and constant desire to urinate. Use for cystitis, kidney stones, bedwetting, hypertension, liver cirrhosis, bleeding of the gums and nosebleeds.

Contraindications: None.

Dosage: Infusion: 1–2 teaspoons in cup of water. Take 3 times daily or as required. Tincture: 1:5 in 25 per cent alcohol. Take 5–15ml 3 times daily.

Couchgrass   *Elymus repens*

Synonyms: Twitch, *chien dents* (Fr.), *triticum repens*
   Parts used: Rhizome
   Habitat: Throughout Europe as an invasive weed
   Main constituents: Mucilage, tricitin, vitamin A
   Actions: Anti-inflammatory, demulcent, diuretic, laxative
   Main uses: Soothing for the urinary tract infections, cystitis, urethritis. Helps tone the bladder and is good to combine with marshmallow when the urine is dark and gritty. Use couchgrass as an eliminating and detox tea to improve the skin.
   Contraindications: None.
   Dosage: Decoction: 3 teaspoons in 1 cup of water 3 times daily. Tincture: 1:5 in 25 per cent alcohol, 5ml 3 times daily

Crampbark   *Viburnum opulus*

Synonyms: Guelder rose
   Parts used: Dried bark and root bark
   Habitat: Europe, America
   Main constituents: Coumarins, hydroquinones, resin, tannins, valerianic acid, viburnins
   Actions: Antispasmodic, astringent, nervine, sedative
   Main uses: Use for muscular cramps, spasms, uterine pains, flooding periods, nervous tension. Its main use is for period pains.

Contraindications: Not advised in pregnancy without professional advice.

Dosage: Decoction: 1 teaspoon in cup of water, 3 times daily or as needed. Tincture: 1:5 in 70 per cent alcohol. Take 5ml in water 3 times daily.

Cranberry   *Vaccinium oxycoccos*

Parts used: Fruit

Habitat: North America, North Asia

Main constituents: Flavonoids, tannins, vitamin C

Actions: Antiseptic, astringent

Main uses: A great tonic for the urinary system and in the treatment of cystitis and infections of the urinary tract. Good source of vitamin C.

Contraindications: Use under supervision for kidney infection.

Dosage: Drink fresh juice, 1 glass per day, for mild urinary infections.

Cypress Oil   *Cupressus sempervirens*

A light oil reminiscent of the trees and areas around the Mediterranean.

Family: Cupressaceae

Parts used: Twigs and leaves

Main constituents: Monoterpenes, alcohols: a-terpineol, esters, sesquiterpenes, oxides

Fragrance: Light, woody, resinous, fresh

Main uses: One of the key oils for circulation, being astringent and refreshing, it will be useful for varicose veins, broken capillaries and haemorrhoids. It can be combined to treat circulatory disorders, especially chilblains. Use for excessive discharges, hot burning diarrhoea, frequent urination, nosebleeds. Has a toning effect on the uterine muscles and pelvic area, use for heavy, prolonged periods and symptoms of the menopause. Particularly useful combined in creams for wrinkled, oily, loose skin. It checks perspiration and can be used for footbaths. It has a strong antispasmodic effect and can be used in the treatment of coughs, asthma and whooping cough.

Safety and application: Non-toxic oil. Use in combination with ginger, lavender and rosemary for varicose veins. Be sure to massage only at the bottom of the vein, furthest from the heart. Use maximum 2 per cent in massage oil or cream, 10 drops in footbath.

❀ Daisy   *Bellis perennis*

This homoeopathic remedy is a kindred one to arnica, hypericum and calendula. It is chiefly used for the effects of accidents, sprains and bruises. It is good to use where muscles have become sore and bruised after heavy work.

Physical: Use daisy for injuries to the back or slipped discs, after major surgical operations, injuries or blows to the breasts and where tumours develop from injuries. It can be especially effective for elderly people and for those who have difficulty getting well.

The indication for this remedy is tiredness; the patient wants to lie down. The joints and muscles feel sore. There are pains down the thighs and the wrists feel contracted, as if held by elastic bands. This remedy is good to use during pregnancy where there is difficulty in walking and the uterus can feel sore and squeezed. Waking up early can be an indication of daisy, but it is also known that giving this remedy in the evening can cause waking at 3 a.m. It is therefore a good idea to give it during the day.

Modalities: Worse: touch, cold bathing, cold drinks, becoming chilled after being hot, hot baths, a warm bed and surgical operations. Better: continued motion, cold applications.

❀ Damiana   *Turnera diffusa*

Synonyms: Damiana aphrodisiaca
    Parts used: Leaves and stems
    Habitat: South America
    Main constituents: Arbutin, bitter substance, damianin, fixed oil, flavonoids, gum, resin, tannins, volatile oil
    Actions: Antidepressant, aphrodisiac, diuretic, thymoleptic, tonic
    Main uses: Used as a general tonic, good for low spirits, weakness, exhaustion. Strengthening for the genito-urinary system. Used to improve libido (aphrodisiac) in men and relieve depression.
    Contraindications: None.
    Dosage: Infusion 3 times daily, 1 teaspoon to cup of boiling water. Tincture: 1:3 in 60 per cent alcohol, 2–4ml 3 times daily.

✸ Dandelion   *Taraxacum officinalis*

Parts used: Leaves and roots

Habitat: Native to northern Europe

Main constituents: Minerals, especially potassium, sesquiterpene lactone, vitamins. In the leaf also carotenoids, coumarins. Root: phenolic acids, taraxacoside.

Actions: Antirheumatic, bitter tonic, diuretic, laxative, increases flow of bile, regulates the flow of pancreatic secretions, stimulates the production of breast milk

Main uses: An important diuretic used to rid the body of toxins and waste matter. Supports the actions of the liver and gall bladder. Use for diabetes, hepatitis. Helps stimulate the digestive processes. Use for indigestion, lack of appetite, anorexia, digestive headaches, constipation. Stimulates the metabolism and helps improve the condition of the skin. Use for acne, eczema, psoriasis. Will help relieve swellings of rheumatism, gout and arthritis. Good for heart problems where there is oedema and high blood pressure.

Contraindications: Do not use where there is gall bladder blockage.

Dosage: Use young leaves in salads and roast the dried roots as a substitute for coffee. Infuse 2 teaspoons dried leaves in boiling water 3 times daily or as required. Tincture: 1:5 in 25 per cent alcohol, 2 teaspoons 3 times daily.

✸ Dill   *Anethum graveolens*

Parts used: Seeds

Habitat: Europe

Main constituents: Coumarins, flavonoids, volatile oil

Actions: Antispasmodic, carminative

Main uses: Particularly good as an infusion for breastfeeding mothers. Will help to relieve colic and wind in the baby. Will also help increase the flow of milk.

Dosage: Infuse 1 teaspoon of crushed seeds in 1 cup boiling water. Can give 2–3 teaspoons of strained infusion to the baby.

Drosera   *Drosera rotundifolia*

This is a good homoeopathic remedy for whooping cough or dry violent or rapid coughs.

Physical: Several coughs may follow, one from another, which end up with a whooping noise as the person runs out of breath and tries to inhale. The person may rest for a few minutes and then the cough will start up again. It can be deep, barking, choking and incessant. It can end up with gagging, choking and vomiting. Food will be vomited. The child holds the stomach as it hurts so much from coughing. There may be a red, congested face from the effort of coughing. The person feels exhausted. Tickling in the throat can promote the cough. Although the cough may not be very noticeable during the day, as soon as the head touches the pillow at bedtime it can become constant, with gagging and vomiting.

Modalites: Worse: midnight, lying down, warmth of bed, singing, drinking and laughing.

Echinacea   *Echinacea angustifolia, E. purpurea, E. pallida*

Parts used: Mainly roots, leaves also

Habitat: North America, now grown in Europe

Main constituents: Alkamides, flavonoids, polysaccharides

Actions: Anti-inflammatory, antimicrobial, antiseptic, detoxifying, immune stimulant, tonic, vulnerary

Main uses: This is an important herb which is a natural antibiotic and immune system stimulant. Bacteria entering the body produce hyaluronidase to dissolve the cell walls. Echinacea inhibits this enzyme to help prevent bacterial access to healthy cells. Its polysaccharides have a neutralizing effect and stop the bacteria from spreading, leaving white blood corpuscles to combat the local infection. It is possible to use echinacea as a prophylactic, especially for colds and 'flu during an outbreak. It increases the activity of the immune system by activating the coding of T-cells. Antibacterial and antifungal, it is used to work against all infections, particularly those of the respiratory and urinary systems. Use for skin and fungal conditions, thrush, ringworm, athlete's foot, acne, spots, burns and bites, also allergies, tonsillitis and dental infections. Also used for viral infections such as colds and 'flu.

Contraindications: AIDS, leukaemia.

Dosage: Decoct root and leaves, 1 teaspoon in 1 cup of boiling water 3 times daily. Tincture: 1:5 in 45 per cent alcohol. Take 2–5ml 3 times daily.

Elder *Sambucus nigra*

Parts used: Flowers, leaves and berries

Habitat: Europe

Main constituents: Flavonoids, phenolic acids, tannins, volatile oil. Berries: anthocyanins, vitamins A and C

Actions: Anticatarrhal, anti-inflammatory, diaphoretic, expectorant (when taken hot), laxative

Main uses: A lovely herb to use. Infuse the flowers for colds and 'flu, especially when combined with peppermint and yarrow. In the summer, drinks of elderflower and lemon are cooling and delicious. The berries make an excellent syrup for coughs, sore throats and colds. The flowers tone the mucous membranes and can be used for all infections of the respiratory and urinary tract. Use for ear infections, sinusitis, tonsillitis, allergies, catarrh and hayfever. It will increase sweating and will help speed the process of fevers, such as whooping cough, measles and chickenpox. On the skin, elderflowers are a well-known emollient, being soothing, calming and anti-inflammatory. Help capillaries. Use to soothe the eyes. The berries are more nutritious and have greater expectorant qualities. Anthocyanins, purple pigments found in elderberries, possess significant free-radical scavenging activity and can enhance the immune function because they can boost the production of cytokines, proteins that act like messengers in the immune system and help regulate immune response, thus helping to defend the body against disease. Research has found that elderberry extract significantly shortens the recovery time from physical exertion and significantly reduces the effects of stress.

Dosage: Infuse 2 teaspoons of dried flowers in 1 cup of boiling water and drink 3 times daily or as required. Taken hot it is stimulating; cool, it is soothing. Tincture: 1:5 in 45 per cent alcohol, 2–5ml 3 times daily. Follow traditional recipes for wine-making. Combine tincture or flower water into creams by substituting the water part. Use for hand and face creams.

✳ Elecampane   *Inula helenium*

Parts used: Roots and rhizomes
  Habitat: Asia and Europe
  Main constituents: Inulin, phytosterols, sesquiterpenes lactones
  Actions: Alterative, antiseptic, antispasmodic, diaphoretic, expectorant
  Main uses: An excellent herb for lung complaints, it helps promote mucus and sweating during fevers. Use for chronic lung complaints where there is weakness and lack of appetite. Traditionally used for TB, asthma and whooping cough. A refreshing herb, it can be given to children as a tonic. As a bitter, it contains helenin, which helps expel worms.
  Contraindications: Not recommended in pregnancy or when breastfeeding.
  Dosage: Boil ½ teaspoon in 250ml water and drink twice daily. Tincture: 1:5 in 25 per cent alcohol, 1–4ml 3 times daily.

✳ Eucalyptus Oil   *Eucalyptus globulus; other varieties: E. citriodora, E. radiata*

The eucalyptus tree family is native to Australia. It has been used medicinally for thousands of years as an antibacterial, healing herb and oil.
  Family: Myrtaceae
  Parts used: Leaves and twigs
  Main constituents: Alcohols, 1.8 cineole, esters, ketones, oxides, sesquiterpenes, terpenes
  Fragrance: Strong, medicinal, camphorous
  Main uses: One of the key areas of action of the eucalyptus family of oils is the effect that they have on the immune system, being warming, drying oils with excellent antiseptic and stimulating properties. Having antispasmodic and expectorant actions, eucalyptus is frequently used to heal respiratory conditions where there is much unexpelled mucus. Use for asthma, bronchitis and catarrh. Good for colds, 'flu, coughs, sinusitis and throat infections. Use effectively in steam inhalations.
  Eucalyptus globulus has a toning effect on the nervous system. Use to treat neuralgia, sciatica, headaches and general weakness, also for contagious diseases – chicken pox, measles. It will help protect against infection. Use for rheumatism where symptoms are worse from cold, damp conditions. Use where there is stiffness and loss of mobility. Good for cystitis when it is brought on by a

chill, also for vaginal discharges and infections. Eucalyptus is a very drying oil and is good to use with fennel oil for digestive infections.

Eucalyptus citriodora is a lemony-fragranced eucalyptus. This is used to greater advantage over the other two where there is more heat in the system. It has a more cooling action. Use more for fungal infections and where the discharge is yellow, also for herpes, insect bites, as an insect repellent and for skin complaints.

Eucalyptus radiata is a peppermint-smelling variety which can be used in a similar way to the *globulus*. It has a stimulating and energizing effect, making it more effective to use for infections and fevers. It has a greater strengthening action on the nervous system and, being less fiery than *globulus*, it will be more appropriate for treating more sensitive catarrhal conditions.

Safety and application: These oils are non-toxic and non-irritant if applied externally, but are very toxic if taken internally. Use with caution. For massage, use maximum 1 per cent in diluted blends. Use any of the eucalyptus varieties to disinfect the room, using an atomizer, diffuser or burner.

Eupatorium   *Eupatorium perfoliatum*

This is one of the major homoeopathic remedies for colds, 'flu and fevers, where there is a bruised feeling all over the body, as if the bones are broken. The person moans with pain and with violent aching.

Head: Symptoms include sore, throbbing pain which feels worse with sweating and is better for vomiting.

Eyes: Sore, aching, yellow eyeballs with a headache.

Nose: There is nasal catarrh with sneezing and aches around the face.

Mouth: Yellow tongue, bitter taste and cracks on the corner of the mouth.

Respiratory symptoms: Hoarseness which is worse in the morning, a cough with soreness of the chest and a desire to hold the chest.

Main indications: Use this remedy when there is thirst or nausea and a violent, aching chill which begins in the small of the back. Bitter vomiting after a chill or during heat. Burning heat. Sweat is scanty. There is an insatiable thirst, before and during a chill and fever although drinking water will make the symptoms feel worse.

Modalities: Worse: in the cold air, during periods, with motion, from coughing, the sight or smell of food and lying on the affected part. Better: with vomiting bile, from conversation, with sweating (except with a headache) and lying on the face.

❋ Euphrasia　*Euphrasia officinalis*

Euphrasia is the main homoeopathic remedy for allergies and hay fever that affect the eyes.

Physical: Euphrasia is good for tired eyes, where they feel as though there is something in them or there is in fact something there. There is a redness of the eyeball, with a marked sensitivity to light and profuse watering from eyes and nose. The secretion from the eyes is acrid, itchy and burning. The eyes may water constantly, the margins of the lids can be red, swollen and burning. This can be accompanied by a dimness of vision and a sense of contraction in the eyelids, or twitching.

Take for conjunctivitis and for the first stage of measles. Also, for hayfever where there is a lot of sneezing and tears. Use for colds where the eyes are very watery and the nose is streaming. Euphrasia is also excellent for sticky eyes where there is a thick, yellow, acrid discharge. Use for cases of whooping cough when there are excessive tears accompanying the cough during the daytime. The headache is bursting, there is catarrh and discharge from the eyes and nose.

Modalities: Worse: bright light, indoors, p.m., warmth. Better: dark rooms.

❋ Eyebright　*Euphrasia officinalis*

Parts used: Aerial parts

Habitat: Wild areas of northern Europe

Main constituents: Flavonoids, iridoid glycosides, tannins

Actions: Antihistamine, anti-inflammatory, astringent

Main uses: Used internally or externally. It can work as a tea to strengthen the eye muscles and generally on the eyes and the respiratory tract. Good for catarrhal conditions and as an antiseptic for infections of the ear, sinusitis, hayfever and colds. Externally, use as an eyewash for conjunctivitis, red eye, itching eyes, styes.

Dosage: Infuse 1 teaspoon in 1 cup of boiling water. Take 3 times daily. Use also when cool in an eyebath. Tincture: 1:5 in 45 per cent alcohol, 1–4ml 3 times daily.

⚘ False Unicorn   *Chamaelirium luteum*

Synonyms: Helonias
    Parts used: Roots and rhizome
    Habitat: Native to North America
    Main constituents: Glycosides, steroidal saponins (precursors of oestrogen)
    Actions: Balancing ovarian and uterine tonic, diuretic, emetic, emmenagogue
    Main uses: Combined with agnus castus, this herb will be good for all weaknesses of the uterus. It has a regulatory effect on all uterine functions. Good for prolapses, discharges. Being an oestrogen-balancing herb, it may be used for infertility and menopausal symptoms. Use for tired women with backache and depression. It can equally be beneficial to men in the treatment of impotence.
    Contraindications: Not to be used in pregnancy.
    Dosage: Decoct 1 teaspoon in 1 cup for 5–10mins. Take 3 times daily. Tincture: 1:5 in 45 per cent alcohol. Take 2–5ml 3 times daily.

⚘ Fennel   *Foeniculum vulgare*

Parts used: Roots, leaves, seeds
    Habitat: Southern Europe
    Main constituents: Coumarins, flavonoids, volatile oil
    Actions: Anti-inflammatory, antispasmodic, aromatic, carminative, diuretic, stimulant, warming
    Main uses: Helps to expel wind from the gut and can be used as a mild laxative. Use with crampbark and liquorice for constipation. For intestinal spasms or as a digestive tea, combine equal parts aniseed, chamomile, fennel and orange peel. Use a similar mix to relieve swollen feet and ankles. Use in syrup for coughs or as infusion for teething problems. Can be combined with uva ursi for treating cystitis. Use in dental preparations for taste and to relieve swellings. Use in eyewash for sore or inflamed eyes. Fennel will help to increase flow of breast milk and is said to help with reducing weight.
    Contraindications: Oestrogenic properties may stimulate periods. Do not use in excess.
    Dosage: Infuse 1 teaspoon fresh or dried leaves/root in 1 cup of boiling water. Take 3 times daily. Can also crush ½ teaspoon seeds into 1 cup of boiling water.

✴ Fennel (Sweet) Oil   *Foeniculum dulce*

The taste and fragrance of fennel have been used for thousands of years. The plant was considered to be able to ward off evil.

Family: Umbelliferae

Parts used: Seeds

Main constituents: Alcohols, ketones, monoterpenes, oxides, phenols

Fragrance: Sweet, spicy, aniseed-like, fresh

Main uses: Refer to Fennel *(see previous page)* for the uses are the same. The oil is more concentrated, but may be safely used in massage blends. This is a great oil to use with lavender and marjoram for muscular aches and pains. For the stomach, combine with chamomile and aniseed to relieve bloating and spasms. For the reproductive system, fennel can be blended with geranium and rose to relieve cramps and menopausal symptoms and to stimulate the milk flow in breastfeeding mothers. As fennel is an unblocking oil, use in a detoxifying blend for the skin.

Safety and application: Possible sensitization. Do not use more than 1.5 per cent in massage blends.

✴ Fenugreek   *Trigonella foenum-graecum*

Parts used: Seeds

Habitat: Around the Mediterranean, North Africa

Main constituents: Alkaloids, flavonoids, minerals, saponins, vitamins, volatile oil

Actions: Anti-inflammatory, demulcent, lowers fever, nutritious, soothing

Main uses: Soothing for gastric ulcers and gastritis, colic, dysentery, diarrhoea. Helps put on weight. Increases milk in breastfeeding mothers. Use where the mucous membranes are affected, for mouth ulcers, coughs and urinary complaints.

Contraindications: Do not take in therapeutic doses during pregnancy.

Dosage: Chew seeds and use as digestive after meals. Infuse 1–2 teaspoons crushed seeds in boiling water. Use as required.

❋ Ferrum Phos   *White phosphate of iron*

This is one of the range of 12 homoeopathic tissue salts found in the blood. It carries oxygen to all parts of the body. It is a very useful remedy for the first stage of an illness, before any discharge starts. It is good for anaemia, inflammation and fever.

Mental and emotional indications: These people are talkative, excited and oversensitive, with alternating moods. There is weakness of memory, forgetfulness and anxiety about the future, sadness, listlessness and depression.

Physical: The person feels much better after a sleep. Use ferrum phos for fevers where the face is flushed and the skin is hot and dry, where there is a quick, full pulse, thirst, pain and redness. It is also good for haemorrhages from any part of the body when the blood is bright red. Ferrum phos indications include right-sided shoulder pains, a bruised soreness of the chest, shoulders and surrounding muscles. It is better to give this remedy in the morning.

Digestion: Vomiting of bright red blood or undigested food, stomach aches. Use for haemorrhoids that are inflamed and bleeding bright red blood.

Ears: Good for the first stage of an ear infection, inflamed ears, radiating pains and pulsating, chronic catarrh of the middle ear.

Eyes: Inflamed, red, burning sensation as if there is dust under the eyelid.

Head: This is the remedy when the head feels dull and top heavy, with pains which feel as if a nail is being driven in on one side or hammering pains that are worse on the right side and feel better with nosebleeds and cold pressure. Ferrum phos is good for children's headaches when they also have red eyes and a red face.

Nose: Take ferrum phos for the first stage of all colds. Good for those who catch colds easily and have nosebleeds, especially for children when the blood is bright red. Congestion of the mucous membranes.

Respiratory system: Good for the first stage of all inflammatory respiratory conditions: bronchitis, painful tickly cough, hard, dry cough with soreness in the lungs, croup, loss of voice with hoarseness.

Throat: Sore, dry, red, inflamed with much pain; an ulcerated throat.

Women' complaints: Take for profuse periods that are painful with bright red blood, anaemia (combine with calc phos for this), periods every three weeks, heavy pains, dry vagina, stress incontinence.

Modalites: Worse: night, especially between 4 and 6 a.m., suppressed sweat, touch, movement. Better: cold applications, lying down, sleep.

❋ Feverfew   *Tanacetum parthenium*

Parts used: Leaves

Habitat: Europe and now worldwide

Main constituents: Sesquiterpene lactones, volatile oil

Actions: Antimigraine, antirheumatism, antispasmodic, bitter, sedative, reduces fevers

Main uses: Research in the 1980s showed that this herb was able to significantly help migraine sufferers. More generally, those with migraines that are relieved by warmth will find this herb helpful. Use as a preventative. Helps with dizziness, tinnitus, painful and late periods, menstrual depression. Use for osteoarthritis and rheumatic, painful swellings. Use for reducing fevers in headachy colds and 'flu.

Contraindications: Fresh leaves may cause mouth ulcers and sore tongue in some people. Do not use during pregnancy.

Dosage: Tincture: 1:5 in 45 per cent alcohol. Make the tincture straight after collection. Take 1ml as required or 3 times daily. As a preventative for migraines, eat 2–3 fresh leaves between bread daily or take as capsules.

❋ Frankincense Oil   *Boswellia sacra*

Frankincense oil is still collected in traditional ways in the Middle East and East Africa. Drops of resin form along incisions made in the trees and are collected and traded before being distilled into oil. The resin has been used for centuries as incense specifically to change atmospheres and for meditation. Also known as olibanum.

Family: Burseraceae

Parts used: Tears of resin

Main constituents: Alcohols, esters, monoterpenes

Fragrance: Softly medicinal, sweet and spicy, light and lifting

Main uses: This is a toning, uplifting oil. It is rejuvenating emotionally, good for depression and concentration. It has an antispasmodic and calming effect on the nervous system. It is also astringent and anti-inflammatory which contributes to its reputation as being great for respiratory, circulatory and skin problems. It is cooling and calming for the lungs and respiratory system. Use for catarrhal conditions, asthma, bronchitis and other chest infections. It helps to calm the circulation and has a stimulating effect on the immune system. For the skin, frankincense will treat ageing skin, wrinkles and scar tissue. Use for wounds and ulcers.

Safety and application: Non-toxic and non-sensitizing, this oil combines well with lemon, neroli and sandalwood for skin treatments. Combine with cypress and vetiver for circulation. Traditionally frankincense was mixed with myrrh as an incense, each having a balancing effect on the other. Use in blends of 2–3 per cent dilution.

Garlic   *Allium sativum*

Parts used: Cloves of the bulb
  Habitat: Native to Asia
  Main constituents: Minerals, vitamins, volatile oil
  Actions: Antibiotic, anti-infection, antiparasitic, antispasmodic, antiviral, cholagogue, detoxifying, diaphoretic, expectorant
  Main uses: Used for thousands of years and recommended for many ailments through the ages, garlic will combat respiratory infections and loosen phlegm. Use for coughs, asthma, colds, catarrh, discharges and ear infections. Tones the gut, good for sluggish digestion, especially in the elderly. Use for expelling worms. Will lower cholesterol and regulate high or low high blood pressure. Use to lower blood sugar level. Good for allergies, Candida and fungal infections. Use to help improve the condition of the skin. Garlic is generally an excellent cleanser and detoxifier.
  Dosage: Eat as much fresh garlic as you can! Eat 2 cloves with bread 2 or 3 times daily for infections.

Gelsemium   *Gelsemium sempervirens*

The keynote of this homoeopathic remedy is weakness. Everything is depressed, there is physical weakness, a lack of vitality and the mind appears disconnected, unable to think or fix attention. It is the first remedy to think of for 'flu.
  Mental and emotional indications: There is weakness in reaction to stimuli, the person is inclined to be hysterical, confused, dazed, apathetic, slow to answer and brooding. It is an anticipatory remedy which is good for stage fright, exams, interviews, when the legs tremble and feel like jelly, or when the knees go weak in labour. It can be used for fear that has a particular past association and creates trembling. The person is pathetic in his weakness. He is

easily influenced, e.g. by the weather or passive sympathy. He gets tired very easily. Worry, drugs, 'flu and colds can bring on extreme weakness, fear of heights and air travel.

Physical: Pains in the legs. The central nervous system is affected. The person will tremble, and experience spasms and use the wrong words. Irregular heart beats, palpitations and feelings that the heart will stop if she keeps still.

'Flu: Gelsemium is the number one 'flu remedy, for hot, flushed face and a heavy feeling. The onset is slow and accompanied by severe aching pains. Stiffness in the cervical region of the neck, aching in all the muscles, shivers run up and down the spine. A remedy for those who have never fully recovered from a bout of 'flu.

Head: The eyelids feel heavy, vision becomes blurred, headaches feel better after urinating and are associated with catarrh, 'flu, periods or emotional upsets. They are mostly at the back of the head but then they move forward to over the eyes. The tongue feels thirsty and dirty.

Modalities: Worse: emotional stress, shock, dread, ordeals, humidity, cold, damp, sun. Better: alcohol, shaking, sweating, urinating.

Geranium Oil   *Pelargonium graveolens*

Native to South Africa, the fragrant and abundant geranium plant has many varieties and as many different types of oil. Traditionally distilled in Egypt, *graveolens* is the main cultivated variety.

Family: Geraniaceae

Parts used: Partly dried green leaves

Main constituents: Alcohols, aliphatic aldehydes, esters, ketones, sesquiterpenes

Fragrance: Sweet, heavy, floral, rose-like, slightly minty

Main uses: This oil has a cooling, moistening, regulating effect, with tonifying properties on the nervous system. It is particularly good for restlessness and anxiety. Blend with bergamot, melissa or rose for calming and cooling the heart. Useful for palpitations, neuralgia and panic attacks. Very useful for those that wake in the night feeling hot and clammy. Particularly good for regulating symptoms of the menopause and PMT. Tonic action on the liver and kidneys, helps to cleanse the body, good for cystitis and urinary infections and gallstones. Use to treat addictions. Its balancing effect on the skin makes it good for either oily or dry skin conditions. Use in a lotion or compress for inflamed skin. Combine with lavender and rose (also balancing for the hormones), also citrus oils and sandalwood.

Safety and application: Do not exceed 1–2 per cent in dilution. May be a skin irritant. Do a test before giving a full massage.

✳ Ginger   *Zingiber officinale*

Parts used: Fresh or dry rhizomes

Habitat: Grows in all tropical areas, but native to Asia

Main constituents: Gingerols, mucilage, phenolic compounds, volatile oil

Actions: Anti-emetic, anti-inflammatory, antiseptic, carminative, diaphoretic, expectorant, stimulating

Main uses: Promotes sweating during fevers and cools the body down, helps with nausea during pregnancy, radiotherapy and travel, eases colic and irritable bowel. It promotes the appetite, especially in the elderly, and helps with intestinal problems. Being an antiseptic, it will help with gut problems due to bad food. Ginger is a great warming herb for the circulation, warms the hands and feet, is good for mental fatigue and low blood pressure problems. Stimulating and warming to women who feel the cold, have suppressed periods and lack libido.

Contraindications: The dry root is contraindicated in pregnancy in large therapeutic doses (fine as a spice or fresh ginger root); also hypertension, hypokalaemia.

Dosage: Best to combine with food or in drinks. Combine 2–3 fresh slices in boiling water with lemon and honey at the onset of colds and 'flu. Tincture: 1:5. Average dose 1.5–3ml twice daily.

✳ Ginger Oil   *Zingiber officinale*

A wonderfully warming oil, invaluable in the flavouring and perfumery industries.

Family: Zingiberaceae

Parts used: The oil is steam distilled from the dried rhizomes.

Main constituents: Alcohols, aliphatic aldehydes, esters, ketones, monoterpenes, sesquiterpenes

Fragrance: Spicy, pungent, hot, sweet, familiar

Main uses: A strongly stimulating oil, ginger can be used for all cold and weak conditions. Use to strengthen the nervous system and to increase confidence or where there is exhaustion and weakness or neuralgia and cramps. Blend with black pepper and cypress to stimulate the circulation for conditions such as angina, varicose veins and chilblains, or where the extremities are cold. For the digestive system, ginger is warming, aids assimilation and can bring relief to constipation, diarrhoea, heartburn, wind, colic, nausea, hangovers, travel sickness and sickness in pregnancy. One of the main actions of ginger is on the respiratory system. It is moistening for the lungs and excellent for all colds and cold conditions. It strengthens the adrenal cortex and encourages the immune system and sweating. Use for fevers and infectious diseases. Ginger is one of the best oils to use for stiffness in the muscles and joints, particularly where the conditions are worse from damp and cold. Use for arthritis, numbness, the aches and pains of muscle fatigue. Use in warming up before sports.

Safety and application: Non-toxic, non-irritant, non-sensitizing. Use in blends up to 2 per cent dilution, in hot baths or footbaths up to 4–6 per cent. Blend in base oil before adding 2 tablespoonfuls to the water.

Ginkgo   *Ginkgo biloba*

Synonyms: Maidenhair tree
    Parts used: Leaves, harvested in autumn, and seeds
    Habitat: Native to China, grown in Europe
    Main constituents: Flavonoids, ginkgolide B (a platelet-activating factor), tannins
    Actions: Anti-inflammatory, circulation stimulant, energizing
    Main uses: Traditionally the seeds are used for their anti-inflammatory action on the respiratory system in treating diseases such as asthma. Ginkgo leaves, on the other hand, have become one of the top-selling herbs for their action in stimulating the circulation, especially to the head. Ginkgo increases the blood flow, and research has proved that its use brings a marked improvement in Alzheimer's disease, memory loss, mental fatigue, tiredness leading to depression and headaches. Also use for cold hands and feet, thrombosis and varicose veins.

    Contraindications: Not to be taken with anti-platelet drugs/anticoagulant drugs.

    Dosage: Decoction of half a cup of leaves 3 times daily. Tincture: 1:5 in 45 per cent alcohol, average dose 2–4ml 3 times daily or capsules as recommended.

Ginseng   *Panex ginseng*

Habitat: Native to China, now cultivated, as the wild plants are rare

Main constituents: Glycosides, gum, resin, saponins, starch

Actions: Adrenal hormone stimulant, antistress, antiviral, aphrodisiac, tonic, adaptogen

Main uses: This is the oldest known herb used in China (records show for 4,000 years). It helps to raise immunity and gives resistance to diseases. It is a heart tonic and raises vitality. Thought to be a man's herb, particularly in old age, it is both sedative and stimulant, promoting energy, strength and endurance. Retards build-up of lactic acid, fights fatigue, aids sleep, increases resistance to cold or heat and helps the body to adapt to changed environments. Aids concentration.

Contraindications: Not to be used in pregnancy, during the menopause, for children; not to be taken where there is acute infection, acute asthma or hypertension. Not to be combined with caffeine or taken if on anticoagulant drugs. Do not use for prolonged periods.

Dosage: Decoction of ½ teaspoon of powdered root in boiling water, as required. Tablets: Dose as recommended. Can be included in a soup, add 1g when needed. Tincture: 1:5 in 45 per cent alcohol, average dose 3–5ml twice daily.

Glonoine   *Nitroglycerine*

The keynote of this homoeopathic remedy is quick, violent and bursting pain. It acts on the circulation and is good to give for violent pulsations and a sense of the blood rushing upwards. It is an effective remedy for sunstroke.

Head: Feels enormous, as if the skull is too small for the brain. There are waves of bursting, throbbing, pounding, pulsating pain, as if blood were rushing to the head. The terrible pain gets worse in the sun and improves with vomiting. The pain will tend to increase and decrease as the sun moves higher and lower in the sky. The person holds his or her head, the throbbing pain synchronizes with the pulse, the head throbs with every movement, the veins of the temple are swollen. There is complete intolerance of heat near the head. This remedy can be given for headaches which occur before or after the period or take the place of the period. There may be violent palpitations and throbbing in the ears. It is a remedy to give for nosebleeds that are the result of the heat of the sun. The face may look flushed and hot, or bluish, with the jaws clenched. There may be nausea and vomiting, menopausal hot flushes.

Modalities: Worse: heat, movement, jarring and suppressed periods. Better: open air, lifting the head, cold applications.

Golden Rod   *Solidago virgaurea*

Parts used: Aerial parts
   Habitat: Native to Europe and Asia
   Main constituents: Phenolic glucosides, rutin, saponins
   Actions: Anti-inflammatory, antiseptic, diaphoretic, diuretic
   Main uses: A valuable herb for urinary complaints. Use for infections of the bladder and kidneys, cystitis, nephritis, also candidiasis, thrush, mouth ulcers, sore throat. Use as a douche or gargle. Good for gastric problems, diarrhoea, weak digestion.
   Contraindications: None.
   Dosage: ½ teaspoon in boiling water twice daily. Tincture: 1:5 in 45 per cent alcohol, average dose 1–4ml twice daily.

Goldenseal   *Hydrastis canadensis*

Parts used: Roots and rhizome
   Habitat: Native to North America, now an endangered species, so only the cultivated variety should be used
   Main constituents: Alkaloids (berberine, canadine, hydrastine), resin
   Actions: Alterative, anti-inflammatory, antiseptic, bitter, detoxifying, tonic for the liver, uterine stimulant
   Main uses: This herb acts on all mucous membranes. Use for eye, ear, nose and throat infections. Use for catarrhal conditions, bronchitis, sinusitis or where there is inflammation. For the digestion and intestines, use for heartburn, ulcers, colitis and liver damage. It stimulates the digestion and liver. Good for constipation, jaundice, hepatitis and toning of the gut. Goldenseal can be used for vaginal infections and thick yellow burning discharges. It acts as a uterine tonic by increasing circulation to the uterus, can be given for heavy periods and can be used to encourage labour, but should not be taken during pregnancy. Its antiseptic action makes it suitable

to use as a wash for skin infections and damage. It will have a drying effect on psoriasis.

Contraindications: Do not use when pregnant, breastfeeding or where there is high blood pressure.

Dosage: Tincture: 1:10 in 60 per cent alcohol, average dose 2–4ml in a glass of water. Make an ointment with the tincture or a salve by stirring in 2g powder to 25g beeswax mix. Decoction: Simmer 1g root in ½ litre water for 10 minutes and drink ½ cup 3 times daily.

Gotu Kola   *Centelia asiatica*

Parts used: Aerial parts

Habitat: Native to India, can grow in Europe if protected from frost

Main constituents: Alkaloids, flavonoids, saponins, volatile oil

Actions: Adaptogen, alterative, analgesic, antibiotic, detoxifying, sedative, tonic

Main uses: A herb long used in Ayurvedic medicine. Use as a tonic for the nervous system, for stress, depression and tiredness. Helpful with Parkinson's disease, will aid the memory and help concentration. Tones the digestive tract. Traditionally given to children for diarrhoea. Perhaps best known for its effectiveness with skin disorders. Said to be rejuvenating, good for acne, eczema and healing wounds without scarring. Has excellent antioxidant properties. More recently gotu kola has been used for treating arthritic and rheumatic conditions.

Contraindications: Do not use indefinitely. Recommended duration maximum 6 weeks. Do not use in pregnancy or where there is epilepsy.

Dosage: ½ teaspoon to 1 cup of boiling water 3 times daily. Tincture: 1:5 in 25 per cent alcohol, 2ml 3 times daily.

Grapefruit Oil   *Citrus paradisi*

It is best to buy an organic oil where possible, due to the cocktail of chemicals applied during the standard growing and processing of grapefruit.

Family: Rutaceae

Parts used: Oil is expressed from the fruit.

Main constituents: Alcohols, aldehydes, monoterpenes

Fragrance: Sharp, fresh, citrus

Main uses: This is a detoxifying, uplifting and refreshing oil with a cooling action on the liver. Use for depression. Helps with hangovers. Can help with obesity, by reducing the appetite, and with the digestion of fats. Combine with sea salt to add to the bath to help detoxify and the elimination processes. Grapefruit has an astringent action and will help tone and cleanse the skin and improve skin problems such as acne and oily skin.

Safety and application: Non-toxic, non-sensitizing, non-irritant, a great oil to use in blending, especially for its lifting quality in perfumery. Works well with geranium, jasmine and rose. Use in dilutions of 2 per cent added to skin creams or in massage oils.

Graphites   *Plumbago carbon*

This homoeopathic remedy is useful in the treatment of eczema and impetigo.

Mental and emotional indications: Marked by sadness and despondency. There is an overall fearful foreboding that something terrible will happen. The person is constantly miserable and very easily discouraged and dejected. She lacks vitality and is timid, shy and cautious, with a constant desire to grieve. Her sadness may increase when she listens to music.

Physical: Marked by a chilliness (great sensitivity to draughts). Graphites types are often overweight, have delayed periods and unhealthy skin and nails.

Abdomen: Indigestion, bloated feeling, wind, mouth tastes like rotten eggs. Excessive hunger, pains in the stomach which improve from eating; desire for cold food and an aversion to salt, sweet food or fish. Vomit, sweat and stools all smell sour. Constipation with large stools joined together by mucus, creating fissures in the anus. Numbness in the extremities.

Head: Numb and heavy, as if cobwebs are over the face, and the skin of the forehead is drawn into folds.

Skin: The skin is dry and parchment-like. Every injury suppurates. Eruptions are found between the toes and fingers, on the scalp and behind the ears, on the nipples, labia, in and around the anus. Eruptions contain a sticky, honey-like fluid that exudes from cracks and fissures which are extremely sensitive. Eczema is found on the scalp, face, eyelids and in the folds of the skin. The moist eruptions are covered with scales or crusts. They appear particularly during menstruation.

Women's complaints: Periods are late, scanty and accompanied by feelings of weakness and fainting, painful. Leucorrhoea is burning and profuse.

Modalities: Worse: cold, light, during and after periods, from suppressions, night, hot drinks, music. Better: walking in the open air, hot drinks (especially milk), touch.

Hawthorn   *Crataegus monogyna*

Parts used: Leaves, flowers, berries
   Habitat: Europe and the UK
   Main constituents: Amines, flavonoids, phenolic acids, tannins
   Actions: Antispasmodic, heart restorative, nervine, sedative
   Main uses: This is primarily a heart remedy. It increases the blood flow through the heart and strengthens the heart muscle. Used to treat angina and palpitations, it is a heart restorative, regulating the heart rate by improving the blood flow without increasing the heart rate or blood pressure. It is both hypotensive and hypertensive, and will help to restore the balance from either extreme. Hawthorn can also be used to improve brain function, with improved circulation to the head.
   Contraindications: None.
   Dosage: Infusion: 2 teaspoons per cup of boiling water 3 times daily. With the fruit, decoct 1 teaspoon berries to each cup. Tincture: 1:5 in 45 per cent alcohol. Take 1–2ml 3 times daily. Hawthorn flowers can be made into white wine and the berries into red wine. A glass per day is an excellent heart tonic.

Heartsease   *Viola tricolor*

Parts used: Aerial parts
   Habitat: Native to Europe, gathered in the summer
   Main constituents: Flavonoids, gums, mucilage, saponins
   Actions: Alterative, anti-inflammatory, diuretic, expectorant
   Main uses: Mainly used for its action on the mucous membranes. Combine in a cough syrup or mixture for whooping cough and bronchitis. As a diuretic, combine in mixtures for rheumatism and cystitis. Use as a wash or as a purifying tea for skin disorders, acne, weeping eczema, or allergic reactions.
   Contraindications: None.
   Dosage: Infuse 25g per ½ litre boiling water. Take 1 cup 3 times daily. Tincture 1:5 in 45 per cent alcohol, 3ml 3 times daily.

❋ Hepar Sulph   *Calcium sulphide*

This important homoeopathic remedy is identified by extreme sensitivity and touchiness. It is an important remedy for pus-filled infections.

Mental and emotional indications: The hepar sulph type is dissatisfied and argumentative, prone to fits of anger, easily irritated. She takes offence easily and tends to talk quickly. She is unreasonably anxious and fearful of her own health. The pain makes her feel irritable.

Physical: Use for people who are chilly, who catch colds easily and wear coats in hot weather. Hepar sulph is one of the main remedies for suppuration. Discharges are profuse, yellow and smell offensive. The person will sweat a lot but this does not bring any relief. She is reluctant to uncover herself through fear of getting cold. The sweat, too, is very sour-smelling. Dry coughs will rattle. Inflamed glands and suppurating skin abscesses are other important symptoms. The inflamed area cannot bear any touch. Hepar sulph is an excellent remedy for swellings that have become very painful and splinter-like. It will help to open up and drain an abscess. It is excellent for ulcers, tooth abscesses and boils, and any injury that heals slowly and is red, painful and forms pus.

Colds and catarrh: Symptoms include pain at the base of the nose, sneezing in a cold wind and a running nose. Coughs rattle in the chest with loose mucus, which is difficult to get up and is then thick and yellow. The cough will be barking or choking and get tighter in the cold air. The child will cry before coughing. The cough will get worse in the wind or cold air and when any part of the body is uncovered.

Ears: Hepar sulph can be very good for earache when there are splinter-like pains, when the eardrum is perforated or for mastoid disease.

Throat: Symptoms include swollen tonsils and glands of the neck. The throat seems as though it is being pierced by a fishbone or a splinter, and the pain extends to the ears when yawning or swallowing.

Women's complaints: This remedy covers profuse leucorrhoea, which smells sour or of old cheese, and abscesses on the labia which can be very painful. Someone in need of hepar sulph will like sour things, such as vinegar. Refer to the section on homoeopathic dosage *(pages 198–99)* for the suggested dosage.

Modalities: Worse: cold, wind, air, draughts, being uncovered, touch. Better: heat, warm wraps and hot applications.

✳ Holy Thistle   *Cnicus benedictus*

Synonyms: Cardus benedictus
   Parts used: Dried aerial parts
   Habitat: Waste ground around the Mediterranean and Asia
   Main constituents: Bitter principle, glycoside cnicin, mucilage, tannin, volatile oil
   Actions: Bacteriostatic, carminative, diaphoretic, febrifuge, tonic for the spleen
   Main uses: Used mainly for its gentle action on the liver. Good for digestive problems associated with wind and related to liver problems, gall-bladder disorders, indigestion. Topically, it helps wounds to heal and acts as an antiseptic.
   Contraindications: Can cause vomiting in large doses. Avoid in pregnancy and where complaints are caused by acidity.
   Dosage: Infuse 1.5–3g per cup of boiling water. Take 3 times daily. Tincture: 1:5 in 25 per cent alcohol. Average dose 5ml 3 times daily.

✳ Hops   *Humulus lupulus*

Parts used: Female flower heads
   Habitat: Commercially grown in Europe
   Main constituents: Oestrogens, resin, volatile oil
   Actions: Analgesic, anaphrodisiac, bitter tonic, hypnotic, nervine, sedative
   Main uses: Use for anxiety, excess of sexual energy, headaches, insomnia, nervous restlessness, over-activity in children, stress, tension. More sedating when dried. Good for colitis and for a nervous stomach, where nervous disorders affect the appetite. Hops can help assimilate food and help the body put on weight. Can also be used for gut infections.
   Contraindications: Depression, pregnancy.
   Dosage: The young shoots can be cooked as a vegetable. Infuse one dried flower to each cup of boiling water and take 3 times daily or as required. Tincture: 1:5 in 60 per cent alcohol, average dose 1–2ml. Use hop pillows to aid sleep, if insomnia is due to nervousness.

Horse Chestnut   *Aesculus hippocastanum*

Parts used: Bark, leaves, seeds
  Habitat: Native to Europe and Asia
  Main constituents: Coumarins, oil, polysacharides, saponins, tannins
  Actions: Anticoagulant, anti-inflammatory, astringent, toning, vasodilator
  Main uses: A very useful herb for toning the venous system. Use for varicose veins, leg ulcers, piles. Has the effect of lowering the blood pressure as it causes the excretion of sodium. Lowers blood cholesterol, strengthens cell membranes of the red blood cells, does not affect the iron content.
  Contraindications: Do not use externally on broken skin. Take internally for ulcers, etc. Do not give to children. May not be suitable if taking blood-thinning drugs. Discontinue if there are negative reactions. Do not use if there is kidney disease.
  Dosage: ½ teaspoon of dried seeds infused in 1 cup of boiling water 3 times daily. Tincture: 1:10 in 45 per cent alcohol, 2–5 ml 3 times daily. Combine tincture into salve or cream for external treatment.

Horsetail   *Equisetum arvense*

Parts used: Aerial parts
  Habitat: Native to Europe, Asia, North Africa, America
  Main constituents: Alkaloids, flavanoids, silicic acid, sterols
  Actions: Astringent, haemostatic, styptic
  Main uses: Silicea is helpful for the elasticity of connective tissue. Good to use where the lung tissue is damaged, as in emphysema. Strengthens the tone of the bladder, helps frequent and urgent urination. Good for women who have just given birth and have involuntary urination and for incontinence in the elderly; also for pelvic cramps, heavy bleeding, period pains. Strengthens weak joints. Take for slow-healing fractures, muscle weakness or damage. Use internally to strengthen nails. Use an infusion as a final wash for hair with split ends.
  Contraindications: Pregnancy. Also avoid long-term treatment, due to potential strain on the kidneys or where there is cardiac or renal dysfunction. Take vitamin B to accompany treatment with horsetail.

Dosage: ½ teaspoon to cup of boiling water twice daily. Tincture: 1:5 in 25 per cent alcohol, 1ml twice daily.

Hyssop   *Hyssopus officinalis*

Parts used: Aerial parts
  Habitat: Mediterranean areas
  Main constituents: Flavonoids, mucilage, terpenoids, volatile oil
  Actions: Antispasmodic, diaphoretic, expectorant, tonic
  Main uses: Traditionally hyssop was taken as a general tonic and specifically used for nerves. Now it is used chiefly to treat respiratory infections. Use as a calming herb to allay anxiety; also for coughs, hayfever and bronchial infections where there is much mucus.
  Contraindications: Pregnancy. It is not recommended to use the essential oil without professional supervision.
  Dosage: Infuse 1 teaspoon to 1 cup of boiling water. Take 3 times daily. Tincture: 1:5 in 45 per cent alcohol. Average dose 2–4ml 3 times daily.

Ignatia   *Ignatia amara*

This is one of the best homoeopathic remedies for grief, and for ailments that have come on as a result of grief, for example from bereavement or disappointment in love, where the grief is silent and the mood is changeable and for instability.

Mental and emotional indications: Ignatia is good for ailments that come on after humiliation, sadness or depression. Use for complaints following a fright. The person may be averse to company or consolation and be unable to talk to anyone. They may not be able to stop themselves from crying or they may be unable to cry. They may be hysterical, or sometimes fainting and have times of introspection. Sighing is an important keynote of this remedy, although it is not always obvious. The person who fits this remedy will appear reasonable, often oversensitive and prone to romanticism, also refined, easily offended and finds it difficult to take the slightest criticism. Failings will make them feel angry with themselves. Ignatia is for those who live on their emotions.

Ignatia is usually a remedy for women. These women may fight for a cause and are able to completely devote themselves to that cause, but over a period of time they begin to feel let down and this leads to disappointment. Romanticism often conflicts with the hard realities of life for them. They try not to let others see that they are sensitive.

After shock the mind becomes dazed and is not able to focus clearly. On the emotional level, there may be an inability to speak or cry (can only sigh).

Ignatia is the remedy to give after the news of the death of a loved one. The person will not be able to believe what has happened. She wants to cry but cannot, she feels shocked and cramped on all levels. Ignatia is one of the first remedies to consider for losses such as hysterectomy, rape, miscarriage, or after any major disappointment. The ignatia-type woman tends to fall in love with unobtainable men and this pattern may be repeated. There is a tendency to become infatuated even after meeting casually (e.g. at a bus stop). These women believe that a relationship is ideal. When it ends, the disappointment is very strong and they will vow never to fall in love again. They will want to go a long way away and hide. They go to where the lover may be. They may lose interest in their appearance and femininity. There are suicidal desires but there is no reality to them. If ignatia is given for emotional trauma or delayed shock, it is likely that the person will be able to release the grief. This release may occur even if the remedy is taken several months later where the sense of loss is unexpressed, or manifests on the physical level in headaches, stomach cramps, comfort eating or irregular periods.

Ignatia is a remedy of contradictions. The person may experience roaring in the ears but be better for hearing music, have piles which feel better when walking or a sore throat which gets better with eating food. There may be an empty feeling in the stomach which does not improve with eating, a cough which might get worse from coughing. There may be spasmodic laughter when feeling sad, or sexual desire at the same time as being impotent. When they are chilled they may feel thirsty, but have no thirst during a fever. The mental conditions can change rapidly, swinging from one extreme to another. These contradictions leave the individual feeling mentally and physically exhausted. The main fears that they have are of burglaries and robbers, of being frightened, not sleeping and dying during the night.

Physical: Cramp particularly affects the throat, stomach and solar plexus. There is oppression in the chest, with spasms and trembling. The ignatia type may have a white-coated tongue, a weak trembling voice, spasms and violent yawning. It may be noticeable that there is a tendency to bite the side of the tongue or cheek when speaking. Limbs may jerk during sleep, accompanied by cries and whimpering. There is restriction in the throat which feels as if there is a plug in it. There is a desire for acid, sour, raw, indigestible food. There is either a desire for or an aversion to fruit, smoking and coffee. The abdomen will feel full, the stools may be soft and they are diffcult to pass. The skin can be very sensitive with itching and nettle rash-type eruptions all over the body. This remedy should be compared with staphysagria.

Modalities: Worse: grief, shock, worry, loss, being touched, coffee, tobacco and alcohol. Better: swallowing, eating and lying on the painful side of the body, pressure, solitude.

Ipecac   *Ipecacuanha*

This is a homoeopathic remedy indicated by nausea which is not improved after vomiting. Its other main uses are for coughs and haemorrhage.

Mental and emotional indications: These are marked by anger and indignation, a rather contemptuous, impatient state where ailments come about as a result.

Physical: The face may be pale and with a blueness around the eyes and lips. The nausea and vomiting is accompanied by profuse saliva and a clean tongue. It is a very good remedy to use for morning sickness in pregnancy where there is constant nausea and burping. The stomach can feel as if it is hanging down and there is a desire for food or drink. The person may also have diarrhoea and colic with nausea, cutting pains around the navel, stools coloured grass-green, fermented or slimy and bloody lumps of mucus in the stools.

Respiratory system: Ipecac is also a very effective remedy for coughs which are dry and spasmodic, as in asthma. There can be difficulty in breathing which gets worse with exertion or anxiety. There may also be rattling mucus in the chest, especially when breathing in, but no expectoration. It can be used for whooping cough where there is retching, the child may go rigid and the face may turn red or even blue, and any vomiting may contain mucus. Ipecac can be used for haemorrhaging, where the blood is bright red, gushing and accompanied by nausea (*see also* phosphorus, which is accompanied by more fear), for uterine haemorrhage that occurs during or after labour and when blood is either gushing or in a steady flow. Breathing may be partially suppressed and there are sticking pains from the navel area to the uterus. A woman in need of ipecac may have periods that are typically profuse, bright red and clotted.

Modalities: Worse: warmth, overeating or rich foods and damp. Better: in the open air and with rest.

✳ Jasmine Oil   *Jasminum officinale*

Jasmine is a beautiful, exotic oil with a rich perfume valued over the centuries. It is not strictly an essential oil, but an absolute, as it is produced by use of solvents, generally benzene. It is important to be sure that there are no traces of the solvent in the oil that you buy.

Family: Oleaceae

Parts used: Flowers; the yield is about 0.15 per cent

Main constituents: Alcohols, esters, ketones, phenols

Fragrance: A rich, warm, deeply floral scent

Main uses: This is an oil that will affect the emotions. It is uplifting for depression, restores self-confidence and raises libido. Combine in a massage blend with bergamot, clary sage, neroli or rose to help relieve trauma and grief. Use to relieve menstrual cramps and smooth the passage and symptoms of menopause. Use during labour to keep calm and focused. Will aid childbirth and will be useful to continue use afterwards to encourage milk production. Good as a conditioning oil for dry and sun-damaged skin and to fragrance exotic and warm blends.

Safety and application: Non-toxic. This is a very heady, strong oil and can be used in small quanities, 1 per cent in dilution. Add a few drops to lotions or bath-oil bases, 10–20 drops in 100ml bottle.

✳ Juniper Oil   *Juniperus communis*

Reminiscent of the smells of the Mediterranean, where juniper grows wild on the hillsides from where it is gathered and steam distilled, juniper oil is used in perfumery and as an ingredient of gin. In aromatherapy the twigs, leaves and berries are generally used.

Family: Cupressaceae

Parts used: Twigs and leaves and berries

Main constituents: Alcohols, coumarins, esters, monoterpenes, sesquiterpenes

Fragrance: A light, slightly acrid, woody oil

Main uses: This oil has specific actions on the urinary system. It will stimulate the elimination processes, including the production of urine, and have a detoxifying effect on the blood. Use as a cleanser, combined with cypress for cellulite and oedema. Use for rheumatism, gout and arthritis, backache and stiffness. Use as an antiseptic for respiratory complaints. Will help to decongest bronchial tubes and combat infections. Use to tonify the adrenals and pancreas. As an astringent, use juniper for oily skin. Combine in a lotion or oil base or use in steam facials for acne, blackheads and eczema.

Safety and application: Do not use with inflamed kidneys. Avoid in pregnancy or where there are heavy periods. Use with some caution. Use maximum 1 per cent dilution.

Kali Bich   *Kalicem bichromicum*

This homoeopathic remedy is indicated by catarrhal problems, particularly where the discharges are thick and stringy.

Physical: Marked by pain which can be found in specific, localized spots on the body.

Catarrh: Kali bich is an excellent remedy to give for chronic post-nasal catarrh, for stuffed-up feelings and pressure at the root of the nose. Discharges are thick, stringy, yellow or green and acrid, and they leave the skin surface raw. Other symptoms include a swollen uvula, an ulcerated septum in the nose and a dry throat with abscesses.

Cough: This is deep, croupy, dry and hacking, with a pain that goes through to the back and shoulders. It is difficult to expectorate; mucus is white, tough and stringy.

Headaches: Unable to see but the sight returns as the pain gets worse. They may be localized in one spot, like sinus headaches.

Modalities: Worse: alcohol, 2–4 a.m., in the morning and from the cold and damp. Better: heat, motion and pressure.

Kali Carb   *Kalicem carbonicum*

Mental and emotional indications: People needing this remedy will be feeling weak and exhausted, maybe anaemic. They are often angry individuals who tend towards having fixed or rigid opinions. They don't like to be on their own, are anxious and irritable, sensitive to their environments and fearful about their health.

General Physical: They have a tendency to look puffy and have bags under the eyes. Touchy and chilly, often for older people.

Pains: Stitching pain; pains that get worse from rest or with motion; pains from cold pressure or from lying on the affected side. Pains that affect the pleura, pericardium or joints which are sensitive to pressure and touch. There is a loss of elasticity and power in the ligaments, and around the joints which causes slackness and weakness.

This remedy can be good for weakness in old people, particularly when they have backache, or in women after childbearing. It is also useful for asthma, especially when symptoms get worse in the early morning between 2 and 4 a.m. The asthma will cause the person to sit up and lean forward towards their knees. There is a sensation of no air in the chest; this feels worse when lying down, drinking, from motion or draughts.

Cough: Gets worse at 3 a.m.; asthmatic cough (which must cause bending forward). Cough with sticking pains in the chest or between breaths. Expectoration consists of small, round lumps of blood-streaked mucus or pus. This remedy can be used for pneumonia with sticking pains.

Modalities: Worse: cold winds and cold applications. Better: being warm.

✳ Kali Mur   *Kalicem muriaticum*

This homoeopathic remedy is made from potassium chloride. It forms part of the group of 12 tissue salts so called because they are minerals found in the body. One of the key indicators for this remedy is whiteness; it can be given for all catarrhal conditions where there are thick, white discharges. It is good for all childhood illnesses and to stimulate white blood cell production.

Physical: You can give kali mur for coughs that have thick, white phlegm which is hard to remove, and for loud, noisy 'stomach' coughs or those that are short and spasmodic (e.g. whooping cough). It is excellent for chronic catarrh of the middle ear (glue ear), and when the glands around the ear are swollen. It can be given for deafness that comes on after a cold or when there are noises in the ear. It is the tissue salt for the second stage of colds where the nose is blocked with thick white catarrh. It is also good for inflamed tonsils and when these have grey patches. It is helpful for many conditions with swollen glands.

It can be used for loss of appetite and where rich, fatty foods cause indigestion, or for vomiting of white mucus. It can also be taken when this is a symptom during pregnancy. Another indication of kali mur is light-coloured stools. Skin conditions needing a course of kali mur are those with white, scaly flakes, and any eruptions or patches that have white discharges. It can be given for thick, white, bland leucorrhoea.

Modalities: Worse: fats or rich foods, open air and cold drinks. Better: cold drinks.

Kali Phos   *Kalicem phosphoricum*

This is a homoeopathic remedy made from potassium phosphate. It is a mineral found in nerve tissues and fluids of the body, particulary in the brain and nerve cells. It is one of the 12 tissue salts and is great for the nerves.

Mental and emotional indications: Kali phos acts as a nerve nutrient; it is good for anxiety, nervousness, a weak memory and brain exhaustion, and when these states are made worse from mental exhaustion or hysteria, extreme tiredness and nervous exhaustion. Other indications may be sadness, depression, shyness or being easily startled, either in sleep or when touched. It is indicated when the person seems wound up like a spring and suffers from physical or mental symptoms after excitement, overwork or worry.

Physical symptoms. Abdomen: There may be nervous indigestion and smelly diarrhoea, which can come on after being frightened or with depression and exhaustion. There may be hunger, and a feeling of emptiness even after eating.

Head: Include brain fag, lack of blood going to the head. Headaches are often on the top of the head or one side, arising from overwork; it can be very good for students who study too much. Accompanied by an empty feeling in the stomach. The eyes may be affected, being weak from exhaustion; they may be drooping and hard to keep open.

Pains: Use for backache where the pains are in the spine or for toothache, neuralgia or shingles.

Respiratory system: Kali phos can be very helpful for nervous asthma or hayfever where there is violent sneezing made worse after eating and exertion, such as going up the stairs.

Sleep: It is good for insomnia arising from brain fatigue and worry, and can be given to children who suffer from night terrors.

Women's complaints: Women who need kali phos may have irregular and scanty periods. It is very good to give at frequent intervals during labour, where the contractions have become feeble and ineffectual due to nervous and physical exhaustion. It is often good to give to a person assisting the birth, where the labour is long and exhausting.

Modalities: Worse: the slightest extra mental or physical burden, tiredness, worry. Better: sleep, eating, rest, warmth and gentle movement.

Kali Sulph   *Kalicem sulphuricum*

One of the homoeopathic remedies made from minerals found in the body, known as a tissue salt. The mental picture of this remedy is not particularly significant although there may be sense of a hurriedness and impatience, wanting to lie down but better from a walk.

Physical: Kali sulph is indicated by yellow or green, slimy discharges. It is a remedy for lingering disorders, such as thick catarrh that drags on after a cold. The tongue is yellow and slimy, the person may crave sweets and the anus may be itchy. Kali sulph can be combined with ferrum phos to carry oxygen to different parts of the body. Use for disorders of the scalp and hair, and for hair which is falling out. Nails are brittle with white spots (similar to pulsatilla). The skin flakes, peels or erupts. Lips peel after a cold. Kali sulph is good for the peeling stage of skin problems, e.g. with chickenpox, sunburn, etc.

Modalities: Worse: warmth, heat, in the evening and from noise. Better: in the open air.

Kreosote   *Kreosotum*

This is a useful homoeopathic remedy for septic, putrid, decaying states, where there are profuse, burning discharges from any part of the body, but particularly from mucous membranes. There is a tendency to haemorrhage, and bleeding is profuse even from small wounds.

Mental and emotional indications: Irritable states to the point of violence, wretchedness, complaining that nothing is right, everyone and everything is blamed but there is little energy and not much effort is made to improve things.

Physical symptoms. Circulatory system: This is poor and there is stagnation in the venous system.

Digestion: Kreosote is the remedy for stomach troubles which cause bad temper. There is undigested food, water tastes bitter, and there is burning pain in the stomach soon after eating, with a sense of dullness and nausea. This is made worse by eating cold food and improved by eating warm foods. Use for children who suffer from summer diarrhoea, especially if they are teething.

Mouth and face: There are often problems in the mouth with an increase of saliva, which makes the lips and corners of the mouth raw. The gums bleed easily and become raw, swollen and sore. Toothache during pregnancy. Children's teeth decay when they come through. Nosebleeds. The skin looks yellow and blotchy red.

Skin: There can be puffy swellings and discolouration, ulceration and oozing blood (*see also* lachesis), and burning pains.

Women's complaints: It is a good remedy for symptoms centred around the female generative area. There is a fear of intercourse. Leucorrhoea is gushing, offensive, excoriating, causes itching and stains clothes yellow. Periods are heavy, intermittent, too early or too late, and clotted. The blood can be black, offensive and burning and can lead to soreness and swelling. There can be a sudden desire to urinate and the urine burns and smells.

Modalities: Worse: during teething, pregnancy, from rest or lying down and eating cold food. Better: warmth and hot food.

Lac Caninum   *Lac caninum*

An excellent homoeopathic remedy for women, particularly useful to help stop milk production in breastfeeding mothers.

Mental and emotional indications: This homoeopathic remedy is marked by changeability and extremes. The person will want company or seek death; they can be excitable and angry as well as sad and depressed. Children shriek and are easily startled or can be weepy. They may be nervous, restless, sensitive, absent-minded and make mistakes in writing and speaking. They can suffer from intense despondency and depression with outbursts of rage. There is a fear of solitude or death, insanity, snakes, vermin or falling down stairs. They may think that their disease is incurable.

Physical: Symptoms are erratic. They can be on alternate sides, occurring from the left side to the right and back again, returning every few hours or days. When the picture of lac caninum fits it can be given for rheumatic pains which move from one side to another.

Colds: One nostril is blocked and one is clear, and this alternates.

Throat: Give for sore throats that are sensitive to touch, where the pain extends to the ears and is made worse by empty swallowing. There can be glistening patches of whiteness on the tongue and throat. Consider this remedy for tonsillitis or diptheria, or sore throats that begin and end with the period. The tongue is often white with bright red edges. There is a desire for milk and spices. Often there is a real hunger even after eating. A sinking faintness in the stomach may occur.

Women's complaints: Symptoms include periods that are too early or too profuse, the blood gushes and is bright red and stringy and it feels hot. Breasts get swollen, painful and sensitive before and during the period. Sexual organs tend to be very sensitive and are easily excited. There is flatus from the vagina. Lac caninum helps to dry up milk when weaning if this is necessary. It can also be given after a late miscarriage or the death of a baby.

Modalities: Worse: being touched, jarring, during periods, cold wind and air. Better: open air, cold drinks.

Lachesis   *Lachesis*

This homoeopathic remedy, made from the venom of the snake, is a good remedy of the heart and circulation. Blueness is the first indication for lachesis, whatever the complaint.

Mental and emotional indications: These are significant for this remedy. Lachesis people are competent types – they like to be in control, they are self-sufficient. They nearly always feel worse in the morning when they wake up. In the morning the symptoms will be worse, and mentally they will feel confused and anxious. They are generally lively and talkative. They have abundant ideas and change quickly from one idea or topic to another; they have very good thinking processes but are often unable to synthesize them. They are intelligent gossips with vivid imaginations and can be clair-voyant. They are passionate people and often very sexual, tending to be possessive and have great attachment to things and people that they love. This can lead to jealousy and violence. They have strong instincts and are ambitious. They can be cold, ruthless, suspicious and critical of others, although they find it difficult to accept criticism themselves. They can frighten people with their sharp tongue and power to be manipulative or vindictive. They are also generous, vivacious, excitable, nervous people that can rapidly become stubborn, sulky or bad-tempered. They have a great fear of snakes.

Physical: A lachesis person is easily over-stimulated and needs to seek an outlet for her energy. This can result in hot flushes, constipation, high blood pressure or haemorrhages. Lachesis can be used for varicose veins, palpitations and piles. Use for bites or stings which become blue at the edges. Also for injuries which are slow to heal and look bluish. These people cannot stand any pressure, particularly around the waist or throat. They cannot sleep on the left side and all complaints are left sided or go from left to right, except sciatica which is usually on the right.

Headaches: This is the remedy when they are pulsating, throbbing, bursting, also for left-sided migraines.

Respiratory system: Difficult respiration feels worse sitting bent forward; the person wakes from sleep with a sensation of choking.

Stomach: The person desires food containing flour, coffee, alcohol and especially red wine, which brings on headaches. There is pain in the abdomen which feels worse with tight clothing.

Throat: Symptoms include a sensation of a lump and tonsillitis; it is sensitive to the slightest touch, feels worse after sleep and with hot drinks, and feels better swallowing solids.

Women's complaints: There are PMT headaches before the period. Lachesis is an excellent remedy for symptoms that come on during the menopause: piles, haemorrhages, hot flushes, perspiration or burning sensation on top of the head. Lachesis can be used where there is profuse bleeding, slow oozing bleeding, a retained placenta, sepsis, gangrene of the mouth and extremities or a weak heart.

Modalities: Symptoms tend to recur at yearly intervals and are much worse on waking in the morning. Worse: heat, summer, sun, hot winds, constriction, touch and pressure, during the menopause, from suppressed discharges, alcohol and before periods. Better: in the open air, with discharges, from cold drinks and hard pressure.

Lady's Mantle   *Alchemilla vulgaris*

Parts used: Aerial parts
Habitat: Britain, Europe
Main constituents: Salicylic acid, tannins
Actions: Alterative, astringent, haemostatic, styptic
Main uses: This is a women's herb used mainly to help heavy flooding and cramping. Will increase the circulation to the reproductive organs, which make it toning and nourishing. It will restore health to blood vessels in the uterus

and to all the fragile capillaries throughout the body. Helps to improve regularity, endometriosis, fibroids. It is a warming herb taken for cold and weak conditions. Combine with crampbark and raspberry for uterine prolapse and hernias, as it will help tone the ligaments and muscles. It is said to improve fertility. Combine with marshmallow to soothe engorged breasts. Use for gastric and duodenal ulcers, colitis and diarrhoea. Good for mouth ulcers and as a gargle to relieve laryngitis.

Contraindications: Do not take during pregnancy.

Dosage: Infuse 2 teaspoons in 1 cup of boiling water. Tincture: 1:5 in 25 per cent alcohol, 2ml 3 times daily.

Lavender *Lavandula officinalis,* also *Lavandula latifolia* and *Lavandula hybrida*

Parts used: Flowers

Habitat: France and the Mediterranean

Main constituents: Coumarins, flavonoids, volatile oil

Actions: Antidepressive, antispasmodic, antiseptic, sedative

Main uses: Soothing and relaxing. Take for headaches, hot migraines, neuralgia, sleeplessness, slow circulation. Use for urinary infections and digestive problems, bloating, colic, wind. Use for stress-related respiratory problems. Helps insect bites, cuts and allergies. Combine with chamomile flowers, cleavers and rose petals in a muslin bag for a soothing bath.

There are several varieties of lavender which are readily available and they share the same basic profiles and functions. Spike lavender, *Lavandula latifolia*, is more antiseptic and antifungal, and lavandin, *Lavandula hybrida*, which is more stimulating. This is best used for respiratory complaints and muscular problems.

Contraindications: None.

Dosage: 1 teaspoon to 1 cup of boiling water, 3 times daily. Tincture: 1:5 in 45 per cent alcohol, 2ml 3 times daily. Use infusion as skin wash or combine into a salve or ointment.

Lavender Oil *Lavandula angustifolia, also L. vera or L. officinalis*

What would life be without this beautiful plant? It brings joy and its soothing fragrance to us throughout the world and it is now cultivated for distillation in every continent. This is due to lavender's functional versatility. It has the range of actions that no other oil is able to cover. It is probably universally popular as a fragrance, although native to the Mediterranean areas, where it grows wild. The plant has been used for centuries to keep insects away and for its antiseptic qualities. The Romans used lavender for washing, hence the name, *lavere* meaning 'to wash'.

Family: Lamiaceae (Labiatae)

Parts used: Slightly dried flowerheads and stalks

Main constituents: Alcohols (borneol, lavandulyl, linalool, terpinen–4-ol), esters. Spike lavender contains more ketones (15 per cent camphor) and oxides. Lavandin contains ketones (10 per cent camphor).

Fragrance: Fresh and floral. Spike lavender has a more camphoraceous smell. Lavendin is less harsh than spike but more medicinal than lavender. There are many other varieties of lavender with different and particular fragrance profiles, all dependent on their variety, distillation and growing conditions.

Main uses: Lavender has general properties that are balancing and regulating. It is cooling and will have a reviving effect initially. Used for a more prolonged time, lavender will be soothing, warming and relaxing. The nervous system becomes more relaxed and balanced. Lavender has a calming effect on the cerebro-spinal activity and will help treat depression, stress, insomnia, hysteria, shock, post-traumatic stress disorder, nervous tension. By having mild analgesic properties, lavender helps headaches, hot migraines, vertigo, neuralgia, sciatica. The oil has restorative, toning, calming effects on the heart, so it can be used for high blood pressure and palpitations. Alternatively, larger quantities will have the opposite effect. Lavender oil is an immune stimulant and can be used at the time of fevers, 'flu, earache in children. With the circulatory system, lavender helps to calm the heart and lower high blood pressure. Use for angina, palpitations, racing heart and varicose veins. The respiratory system will benefit from lavender's bactericidal and antispasmodic properties. Use for laryngitis, throat infections, asthma, whooping cough and spasmodic coughs, bronchitis, sinusitis and pneumonia. Lavender can be used to increase the gastric secretions. It is beneficial for cold, slow digestion. It will help wind, cramps, colic and through increasing bile production will assist the body in digesting fats. Use where digestive problems are stress-related – diarrhoea, dyspepsia, nausea. Lavender will calm cystitis and menstrual cramps. Use as a douche for vaginal discharges and thrush. Lavender has many properties that make it excellent for skin problems. Use for abscesses, acne, allergies, boils, dermatitis, eczema, also fungal infections, athlete's foot, dandruff, ringworm. In first aid, use for burns, bruising, sunburn and wounds. Use for insect bites where there is inflammation or infection, also for animal bites, lice and scabies. For muscular aches and pains, lavender will relieve lumbago, arthritis and rheumatism.

Safety and application: Non-toxic, non-sensitizing, non-irritant, this is one of the few oils which can be applied directly to the skin. This may be good for scalds and cuts and other localized skin problems.

Ledum   *Ledum palustre*

This is a very good homoeopathic first aid remedy for puncture wounds. These are wounds that are caused by rusty nails, wire, thorns, animal bites, insect stings, mosquito bites, splinters under the nail, etc. Ledum can be given for any shooting, pinching pains when there is a preference for cold applications rather than hot. It will help prevent sepsis, and if it is given quickly enough after an injury, it will be effective against tetanus. Ledum is particularly good for treating those puncture wounds where there is very little bleeding and the skin is cold, pale and swollen, and the pains are sticking, pricking and throbbing (compare with hypericum). It is good for a black eye which is bloodshot and bruised and the eyelids are purple and puffy. It is noticeable that even though the damaged area can feel cold to the touch, the person will experience intolerable heat. Ledum can be used for rheumatoid arthritis particularly when the pain starts in the smaller joints and moves upwards.

Modalities: Worse: warmth, wine, movement. Better: cold air, cold bathing.

Lemon Balm   *Melissa officinalis*

See Balm.

Lemon Oil   *Citrus limonum*

This well-known fruit has been a part of natural healing for centuries. The oil, expressed from the rind of the fruit, comes from Sicily and southern Europe. It is preferable to obtain an organic oil to ensure that it is free of pesticides and other chemical residues.

Family: Rutaceae

Parts used: Rind

Main constituents: Alcohols, aliphatic aldehydes, coumarins, esters, lactones, monoterpenes (limonene, etc.), sesquiterpenes

Fragrance: Citrus, fresh, sharp, reminiscent of the fruit

Main uses: This is one of the best detoxifying oils. It has strongly toning and antibacterial functions. It has a refreshing effect on the nervous system. It protects the body against diseases and infections by stimulating the production of white blood cells. When there is fear of a contagious disease, try a massage containing lemon oil. Lemon works for the circulation by breaking down the sclerotic deposits in the blood. Good for high blood pressure, arteriosclerosis, sluggish circulation. It is traditionally used for treating broken blood capillaries. As a cleansing oil, lemon will clear the skin. It has a moving effect on the digestive system, helps indigestion, gastro-enteritis and wind. It is excellent for respiratory complaints, colds, 'flu, asthma, catarrh and bronchitis. Use for water retention, also for skin problems. Traditionally it was said to remove warts and verrucas, if applied frequently and neat. Good against fleas, ants and other insects.

Safety and application: Lemon oil is great to combine into a rich floral blend to lift and lighten it. It adds a toning effect, acting as a 'messenger' to the blend. This is a strong oil; do not use in dilutions greater than 1.5 per cent. Lemon is slightly phototoxic; do not apply before going out into daylight. Possible sensitization, non-toxic.

Lemongrass Oil   *Cymbopogon citratus*

A strong lemony oil that is produced from rampant tropical grass, well known as an insect deterrent.

Family: Poaceae

Parts used: Freshly dried grass

Main constituents: Alcohols, aliphatic aldehydes

Fragrance: Heavy, sweet-lemony

Main uses: Antiseptic and antibacterial, this oil must be used with caution. Its main action is on the respiratory system. It will stimulate and tone. Use for colitis, gastric infections. Use to improve tone in muscles, include in any sports blend, good for pre-sports and after exercise for aching muscles. Lemongrass is excellent for the skin, has astringent properties for oily skin and skin that needs cleansing.

Safety and application: Non-toxic, possible sensitization. Do not use on sensitive skin. Do not use in dilutions over 1.5 per cent. For an insect deterrent, add a few drops of the oil to lavender water, shake well and spray over the body. It is a good oil to add to sea salts for a footbath.

Limeflower   *Tilia europea*

Parts used: Flowers and bracts

Habitat: Native to Europe

Main constituents: Flavonoids, mucilage, phenolic compounds, volatile oil

Actions: Anticoagulant, antispasmodic, diaphoretic, sedative

Main uses: A relaxing herb that is good for nervous excitability that causes palpitations and high blood pressure. It combines well with hawthorn tops and lemon balm. Use for insomnia and for hyperactive children, especially if tired, irritable or unwell. Will be helpful for early stages of fevers and colds and 'flu. Helps to reduce high blood pressure, is particularly good as a replacement for coffee or tea where there are heart problems or tension-induced digestive symptoms. Use as a wash for skin irritations.

Contraindications: None.

Dosage: 25g to ½ litre of water, to be drunk freely. Tincture: 1:5 in 45 per cent alcohol. Take 5ml 3 times daily. Macerate flowers in white wine for a soothing *apéritif.*

Liquorice *Glycyrrhiza glabra*

Parts used: Roots

Habitat: South Asia and southern Europe

Main constituents: Coumarins, isoflavones, polysaccharides, triterpenes (glycyrrhizic acid)

Actions: Anti-inflammatory, demulcent, expectorant, laxative, liver tonic, stimulant to the adrenal glands

Main uses: A well-loved herb for centuries, used for respiratory infections, coughs, catarrh and bronchitis. Good for soothing inflamed conditions of the gut and for creating a protective coating to the gut walls, so helpful for IBS. Use as a mild laxative. Detoxifying. Can be used to counter poisoning. An adrenal tonic, as well as getting the hormones to function, it has the effect of mimicking them. It is excellent for conditions that arise from stress put on the adrenal glands.

Contraindications: Overuse may cause low potassium levels resulting in oedemic swellings. Avoid use where there is high blood pressure, cirrhosis of the liver, kidney insufficiency or pregnancy. Not to be used where there are ulcers.

Dosage: Chew sticks when needed. Infuse ½ teaspoon powder in 1 cup boiling water and take 3 times daily. Tincture: 1:5 in 25 per cent alcohol, 2ml 3 times daily.

Lycopodium *Lycopodium clavatum*

This is one of the important homoeopathic remedies typified as the intellectual leading a sedantary lifestyle and suffering from flatulence.

Mental and emotional indications: The lycopodium type has a good, quick mind and is not as superficial as a sulphur-type can be. These people like to do everything properly. Often mentally bright, they are typified by the studious intellectual who is bent over a book, ignoring the need for exercise and fresh air. They are aware of the feebleness of their bodies but they take their responsibilities very seriously. This may make them very fearful of commitment, e.g. in relationships. They are prone to being tearful. They are fearful of being alone; women can be afraid of men. They suffer from anticipatory fears – fearing oncoming occasions, such as presentations, giving a lecture, exams, etc. – although they will probably do well or even enjoy the actual event. They are fearful of their own failure as they set themselves very high standards and are haunted by thoughts of financial loss and of not being able to fulfil their responsibilities.

Lycopodium types are ambitious and determined. They work hard and can appear cold, disdainful and arrogant, but this often hides a sense of insecurity. They distrust themselves and others. Their fear around their own inadequacies can make them seem cowardly and they can appear rather bossy and critical as a way of compensation. They can also be profoundly sad.

The lycopodium type is often physically slight and rather weedy. They tend to age prematurely, with wrinkles and grey hair, and the children appear 'grown up for their age'.

Physical: One of the main physical indications for this remedy is a marked aggravation of symptoms from 4 to 8 p.m., and a loss of energy at this time. Often these types are slow to wake in the morning. They can be irritable and intolerant of any pressure, whether emotional, mental or physical. Complaints tend to be on the right side of the body and may then move onto the left. They like warm drinks and feel worse with cold drinks or food. A lycopodium characteristic is a movement of the nostrils during acute conditions. Symptoms come and go suddenly, pains are like lightning or flashes of heat, the right foot can be hot, the left one cold, burning pains feel better with more heat. There is a general dryness in the picture of this remedy: the vagina, skin, palm of the hands are dry. It is a dry, dusty remedy.

Abdomen and digestion: Symptoms include flatulence which both comes up and goes down. This is made much worse from cabbages and beans. Wind is a key symptom, with abdominal distension. These people do not like to feel constricted and will loosen their clothing especially after eating. They get indigestion if they eat later than usual and also feel sick and faint if they wait too long for a meal. They may feel very hungry but then get full up after only a few mouthfuls. They suffer from acidity, wind and bloating, and desire warm food, drinks and sweet food. Onions disagree with them. They also suffer from sluggish bowels and a distension of the bowels and colon which feel better from warm applications. Lycopodium is a good remedy for congestion of the liver when the person is feeling liverish, irritable, peevish and angry.

They may have a tendency to high blood pressure, a chronic right-sided sore throat, fibrous tumours and arthritic inflammations, which get better from movement (*see also rhus tox*). There can be amenorrhoea, and there is a tendency for impotence in men which is probably more to do with overwhelming feelings of responsibility and shyness.

Modalities: Worse: pressure, constriction of clothes, warmth, eating, between 4 and 8 p.m. Better: warm drinks, warm food, burping and movement.

Mag Phos   *Magnesium phosphorica*

This homoeopathic remedy is made from magnesium phosphate, one of the mineral salts found in the body hence called a tissue salt. It is an excellent antispasmodic remedy. It works very well in conjunction with kali phos for neuralgia, sciatica and any nerve pains that are sharp and shooting.

Physical: It is good for muscular twitching, as in the eye or face, and good for any spasm, such as hiccups, cramp or a coughing fit. Use for neuralgia where the pains are shooting along the nerves. Take for any pain that is relieved by being warm and being massaged. Use mag phos for toothache where the pain is sharp and shooting, for babies and children who are teething, and where discomfort is worse from cold air. Mag phos works for digestive pains and cramps. It can be used for colic which improves with bending double, burping and pressure. Good for muscle spasms and for cramps after prolonged exertion. It is an excellent remedy for period pains which are cramping and feel better for heat and massage, also for cramping after-pains of labour. Mag phos can be given in 200C for severe pain and cramps, and is best given in a little hot water.

Modalities: Worse: cold. Better: warmth, massage, pressure, hot drinks.

Mandarin Oil   *Citrus reticulata*

This citrus fruit is native to China and the Far East, and is so called because it was traditionally offered to the Chinese mandarins. The oil has similar properties to tangerine oil. It is one of the few oils that can be used on young children.

Family: Rutaceae
Parts used: Rind
Main constituents: Alcohols, aldehydes, esters, phenols, terpenes
Fragrance: Light, sweet, citrus, reminiscent of the fruit
Main uses: This is a toning and moving yet a calming oil, excellent for children. It has a detoxifying effect on the body and works to build up the immunity. It has calming and toning effects on the nervous system. Use for nervous tension and restlessness. Great for children that are hyperactive.

Can be used for cellulite and general slowness of the metabolism. Use for colds and 'flu. Great for skin that tends to be oily and prone to spots. Use for helping to prevent stretch marks and to tighten skin when losing weight. This oil is an easy one to blend with others, particularly spice oils (with black pepper is lovely!), clary sage, frankincense, geranium, jasmine and vetiver.

Safety and application: Non-toxic, non-irritant, non-sensitizing. Use in dilution 2–5 per cent in base oils.

Marigold   *Calendula officinalis*

Parts used: Aerial parts, harvested when flowering

Habitat: Easily grown in most soils and climates

Main constituents: Flavonoids, triterpenes, volatile oil

Actions: Antibacterial, antifungal, antiseptic, antispasmodic, astringent, haemostatic, immune stimulant, stimulates oestrogenic activity, styptic

Main uses: A very popular and cheerful herb. It is enormously useful to grow it in the garden for all skin emergencies. It can be used both internally and externally and is healing and antibacterial. Use externally for all wounds, burns, sunburn and after surgical operations, as it prevents scarring and promotes tissue growth and healing without infection. Use for babies and after childbirth for healing episiotomy or tears. Use for sore nipples and after mastectomy to help prevent the seeding of cancer cells. Care must be taken to remove stitches before the skin has healed. Excellent for measles, chicken pox, shingles. Use where there is nerve damage, especially in combination with St John's Wort (*Hypericum*). Use for stings and bites, also both internally and externally for fungal and parasitic disorders – candidiasis, thrush, ringworm. Use for digestive problems, gastric and duodenal ulcers, IBS, and where there is any internal inflammation. A cleansing herb, it will treat toxic conditions. Use for skin disorders such as acne and eczema. Use in dental preparation and mouthwash after tooth extraction. Helps reduce pains and regulate periods. Mix with witch hazel for varicose veins.

Contraindications: None.

Dosage: Infuse 1 fresh (or dried) flowerhead per cup of boiling water. Drink freely or 3 times daily. Make a tincture by covering the partly dried herb in 70 per cent vodka and leave to macerate for 3 weeks. Tincture: 1:4 in 90 per cent alcohol. Take 2–5ml 3 times daily. Combine the tincture into salves or creams, using a minimum of 10 per cent. It is also possible to include ground flowers into creams and they can form a colourful healing base to the skin preparations where oil is used. It is best to use fresh flowers and leaves whenever possible.

Marjoram (Sweet) Oil   *Origanum marjorana*

A familiar herb for cooking and native to Mediterranean areas, where it is collected from the wild. Well used in aromatherapy for its warming and relaxing properties.

Family: Lamiaceae (labiatae)

Parts used: Dried leaves and flowers

Main constituents: Alcohols, esters, monoterpenes, sesquiterpenes

Fragrance: Green, herbal, spicy

Main uses: Great for its calming and relaxing effects on the nervous system. Use for headaches, migraines, insomnia, stress and fidgety legs. Use to treat sinus pains and head colds. Marjoram tones the circulation and has a vasodilatory effect. Use for the treatment of high blood pressure, narrowing of the arteries, chilblains. For the digestive system, use this oil for colic, wind and indigestion. Marjoram is excellent to blend for muscular aches and pains, particularly those caused by overexertion. Use for strains and sprains. Great for menstrual pain and PMT, vaginal discharge.

Safety and application: Non-toxic, non-irritant, non-sensitizing. Blends well with many oils. The other herb oils, such as basil and rosemary, as well as eucalyptus, lavender and orange, all enhance its different functions. Use in dilutions of up to 3 per cent.

Marshmallow   *Althea officinalis*

Parts used: Aerial parts and roots

Habitat: Grows widely across Europe

Main constituents: Flavonoids, mucilage, tannins

Actions: Anti-inflammatory, demulcent, expectorant, laxative, soothing

Main uses: A soothing herb for all complaints of the respiratory tract. Use for sore throats, hoarseness, coughs, lung infections, encouraging the expulsion of phlegm in rattling coughs. Slightly laxative, marshmallow can be used for soothing inflammation of the digestive tract. Use for IBS, colitis. Soothing for the urinary system. Use for cystitis, nephritis, kidney stones and passing gravel. It is good for sore and swollen skin, acne and eczema. Use in a poultice to draw out splinters and matter from boils and ulcers.

Contraindications: None.

Dosage: To make syrup, combine 25g grated root with ½ litre cold water, leave overnight and strain. Boil remaining water with 300g sugar and heat till dissolved. Bottle and sterilize as with fruit in Kilner jars. Grate root and leave overnight to use to bathe the skin or drink internally. Tincture: 1:5 in 25 per cent alcohol 2–5ml 3 times daily. Combine powdered marshmallow with slippery elm to make a drawing ointment.

Meadowsweet   *Filipendula ulmaria*

Parts used: Aerial parts

Habitat: Northern Europe

Main constituents: Flavonoids, phenolic glucosides

Actions: Antacid, antirheumatic, antiseptic, astringent, diaphoretic, diuretic, stomachic

Main uses: This herb contains sodium salicylate, which is only converted into salicylic acid in inflamed tissues. It therefore has a pain-relieving effect and helps infections and inflammations. It is a specific for acid conditions, heartburn and peptic ulcers. It can protect areas that are likely to be damaged and is also pain-relieving for stomach ulcers and diarrhoea in children. Pain-reducing for arthritis, cystitis and oedema. Use for reducing fevers.

Contraindications: None.

Dosage: 1 teaspoon infused in 1 cup of boiling water 3 times daily. Tincture: 1:5 in 25 per cent alcohol, 3ml 3 times daily

Melissa Oil   *Melissa officinalis*

The oil is produced by steam distillation and approximately 500kg are required to make 100g of essential oil. It is commonly adulterated, often by lemongrass.

Family: Lamiaceae (Labiatae)

Parts used: Dried aerial parts
Main constituents: Alcohols, aldehydes (citronella), ketones, sesquiterpenes
Fragrance: Citrus-like, honey-sweet
Main uses: Although melissa oil is expensive and difficult to obtain, it is a valuable oil to have for its relaxing yet uplifting properties. As a soothing oil it works on the nervous system both on the physical and emotional levels. Use sparingly in blends for neuralgia or helping to prevent headaches. It also helps lift depression and relieve anxiety. Can be used for respiratory problems such as coughs and asthma. Reduces blood pressure and calms breathlessness. Melissa oil is excellent for bee stings. Combine in a compress or in a cream for urticaria or any kind of stinging rash. Other skin problems include allergic reactions and inflamed skin. Always use in small quantities to avoid allergic reaction. Add in a blend with rose oil for the bath for helping with relaxing for PMS and during menopause.

Safety and application: Always use this oil in very small amounts due to possible allergic reactions and sensitization. Recommended 1 per cent dilution in massage oil and maximum 3–4 drops in a bath-oil mix.

Merc Sol (Mercury)   *Mercurius solubilis*

One of the marked general indications of this homoeopathic remedy is that the individual will smell! Their discharges, whether sweat, mucus, urine, etc., will all smell strongly.

Mental and emotional indications: The temperament is hurried, restless, impulsive, suspicious and mistrustful. These people can be violent or quarrelsome. They are easily influenced – giving you what they think you want to hear. Speech is hurried, perhaps with a stammer, they have poor memories and find it difficult to apply themselves. They complain and are volatile.

Physical: All symptoms are worse at night and then improve in the morning. These include bone pains, sweating, anxiety and fears. They are worse from the heat of the bed, but better from resting. Merc sol is one of the first remedies to think of where any complaint is accompanied by profuse night sweating that does not bring relief. Sweat, breath and discharges are all foul-smelling. There is a metallic taste in the mouth. A keynote of merc sol is an indented tongue – it holds the shape of the teeth at the edges. There is trembling and weakness. Trembling is visible and is caused by any exertion. Weakness can lead to paralysis.

The main part of the body to be affected are the mucous membranes, glands and genitals. All discharges are profuse and with pus. Skin ulcerates and bleeds. There is profuse saliva out of the corner of the mouth, dribbling during sleep, and a heavily-coated tongue. Also, sore gums which bleed easily, can feel spongy and recede, and offensive breath. Teeth decay easily. There can be toothache, with tearing, shooting pains which feel better from the warmth of a bed. Also catarrh, with sneezing, mouth ulcers and yellowy-green ulcers in the nose, and painful sore throats with foul-smelling breath. It is a good remedy to consider for measles, especially where there are complications and earaches. Merc sol is good for ear problems in general, and where there are sharp pains or boils in the ears. It is also good for mumps with swollen glands, smelly breath and feverishness. Use for catarrhal conditions where the mouth tastes horrible and discharges are thick and smelly.

Abdomen: Digestion is poor, there are stomach ulcers, a swollen and sore liver, and gall-bladder trouble. Merc sol is excellent to give for dysentery, or for diarrhoea that smells foul and burns, can be bloodstained or slimy. There is also colic and faintness. There is a constant urge to pass a stool, or a sensation of not having finished (also compare nux vom).

Women's complaints: Leucorrhoea is acrid, burning, itching; it causes rawness which is worse at night or with ulceration. Morning sickness with profuse salivation. Painful breasts during periods. Symptoms also include swollen joints and rheumatism, which gets worse at night accompanied by profuse, oily sweat. They desire bread and butter and fatty foods, are averse to sweet things, and very thirsty.

Modalities: Worse: night, wet or damp weather, from sweating, lying on the right side, in draughts, heat, changes of temperature or weather. Better: moderate temperatures, rest, intercourse.

⚘ Milk Thistle *Silybum marianum*

Parts used: Seeds, flowers

Habitat: Waste ground around the Mediterranean

Main constituents: Lactones, lignans (silymarin), mucilage, sesquiterpenes

Actions: Carminative, diaphoretic, febrifuge, galactogogue, tonic for the spleen

Main uses: Used mainly for its action on the liver. Research has shown that the seeds have a protective action, help cell renewal and stimulate the metabolic processes. Use for hepatitis, jaundice. Will help the liver to recover from chemical treatments, alcohol or drug damage. Good for stress, wind, digestive problems that are related to liver problems, gall-bladder disorders. Traditionally the flowerheads were cooked and eaten as artichokes.

Contraindications: Can cause vomiting in large doses. Avoid in pregnancy, or where complaints are caused by acidity.

Dosage: Infuse for 15 minutes, 1 flowerhead to 1 litre of boiling water. Take 1 cup 3 times daily. Tincture: 1:5 in 25 per cent alcohol, 5ml 3 times daily.

Mints   *Mentha piperita, Mentha pulegium, Mentha spicata*

Parts used: Aerial parts

Habitat: Europe; commercially grown in China and the USA

Main constituents: Flavonoids, terpinoids, volatile oil

Actions: Anti-emetic, carminative, diaphoretic, digestive, emmenagogue, insect repellent

Main uses: There are many different members of the mint family and they broadly share similar properties, with peppermint (*Mentha piperita*) being the most widely used medicinally. This is readily available in teabags and can be used as a digestive tea after meals. It is effective in aiding the digestive processes, helping travel sickness, colic and loss of appetite. Use to increase sweating at onset of fever. Pennyroyal (*Mentha pulegium*) is particularly used for fevers, colds, worms and respiratory complaints, and can also be used as a digestive. It is stronger than peppermint due to the volatile oil containing menthol and pulegone, and must therefore be used with care. Garden mint or spearmint (*Mentha spicata*) is a milder mint and used more in cooking. This, however, still makes a pleasant after-dinner tea, flavours water in summer and can be used as a mild antiseptic in a dental mouthwash. All mints can be made into effective repellents for fleas, mice, mosquitoes, midges, etc.

Contraindications: Do not use mint in therapeutic doses if pregnant or breastfeeding. In particular, avoid pennyroyal completely, as it is toxic and can cause damage to the foetus or infant. Avoid with kidney disorders.

Dosage: Peppermint teabags to infuse as required. Tincture: 1:5 in 45 per cent alcohol. Take 2ml 3 times daily.

⚶ Motherwort   *Leonurus cardiaca*

Parts used: Aerial parts
   Habitat: Native to Asia, Europe
   Main constituents: Alkaloids, flavonoids, rutin, tannins
   Actions: Antispasmodic, emmenagogue, sedative
   Main uses: Traditionally used to soothe the nerves and as a heart remedy, particularly for palpitations. Use for menopausal symptoms, hot flushes, dizziness and mood swings. It stimulates the uterine muscles and can be used for PMT and painful periods.
   Contraindications: During pregnancy or heavy bleeding.
   Dosage: Infuse 1 teaspoon dried herb in 1 cup of boiling water. Take 3 times daily. Tincture: 1:5 in 25 per cent alcohol, 2ml 3 times daily.

⚶ Mullein   *Verbascum thapsus*

Parts used: Leaves and flowers
   Habitat: Europe
   Main constituents: Flavonoids, rutin, tannins, triterpenoid saponins
   Actions: Anti-inflammatory, demulcent, diuretic, expectorant, soothing
   Main uses: Soothing to the respiratory tract and lung infections and helps reduce phlegm. Will soothe and loosen a dry cough. Reduces inflammation. Particularly good for ear infections, for which a macerated oil can be combined with garlic. Mullein can also be used externally to heal wounds, ulcers and piles.
   Contraindications: None.
   Dosage: To make the macerated oil it is best to use the flowers and macerate in olive oil. Put 2–3 warm drops of oil into the ear to bring relief. Infusion: 1 teaspoonful of dried herb in boiling water. Drink 3 times daily. Tincture: 1:5 in 45 per cent alcohol, 2ml 3 times daily. Mullein can be used with aniseed and horehound to make a syrup or add garlic for earache.

⚶ Myrrh   *Commiphora myrrha*

Synonyms: Commiphora molmol
   Parts used: Gum resin
   Habitat: Native to Northeast Africa

Main constituents: Gum, resin, volatile oils

Action: Analgesic, antibacterial, antifungal, anti-inflammatory, antiviral, astringent, bitter, carminative, deodorant, diaphoretic, emmenagogue, expectorant, vulnerary

Main uses: Stimulating the production of white blood cells, it is excellent against viral and infectious diseases. Use both internally and externally for its antiseptic properties. Good for ulcers, wounds, boils, acne, ringworm, etc. Use as a douche for candidiasis. Use as a mouthwash. Combine with lavender and sage as a gargle and mix with marigold and witch hazel for boils, etc. Lowers high cholesterol levels. Relieves pain and swelling by eliminating blood stasis. Traditionally used to improve the brain and act as an antiseptic.

Contraindications: Pregnancy.

Dosage: Tincture: 1:5 in 90 per cent alcohol. Take 3 times daily.

Myrrh Oil   *Commiphora molmol*

A sticky resinous oil, steam distilled from myrrh resin collected in Somalia, the Sudan and Ethiopia.

Family: Burseraceae

Parts used: Resin collected from incised shrubs

Main constituents: Alcohols, aliphatic aldehydes, ketones, phenols, sesquiterpenes

Fragrance: A balsamic, caramel, dark golden liquid smell

Main uses: Traditionally used as a medicine and as an incense, both for its highly antiseptic properties, myrrh acts as a tonic to stimulate the immune system, is antiviral and helps to increase antibodies. It is well known for its use for respiratory complaints, asthma, bronchitis, catarrh, coughs and sore throats. Anti-inflammatory. Can be used for fungal infections such as thrush and candidiasis. Myrrh has strong disinfecting properties. It can be used on the skin to treat all infections that are fungal or parasitic, such as ringworm, scabies and gangrene. Dab neat oil onto ulcers. It is excellent to include in mouthwashes or dental pastes, due to its antiseptic properties, also to use as a preserving agent in creams, bodycare and other cosmetic preparations.

Safety and application: Blends well with frankincense, lemon and sandalwood. Use in inhalations or massage blends. Dilution maximum 2 per cent in base. Non-toxic, non-sensitizing, non-irritant.

❋ Nat Mur   *Natrum muriaticum*

Nat mur is one of the main homoeopathic remedies. It is also a tissue salt, being one of the minerals, common salt, found in the body. It can be used where discharges are watery or like uncooked eggwhite. It is a popular remedy for colds, headaches, constipation, cold sores and dry skin problems.

Mental and emotional indications: These are marked by extreme sensitivity and a marked ability to not show feelings. It is a good remedy for the ill-effects of grief and love affairs These people feel weepy but are unable to cry, then may weep without any apparent cause – often sobbing rather than crying. They do not like sympathy; they have a belief that they 'must be strong'. They do not generally like going to parties. They do expect recognition and if they do not get it, they feel resentful. They are deliberate, self-conscious people. Adults and children dislike physical contact. They can easily get hurt and remember grudges and hold grievances. They lack humour. They are not particularly easy to live with due to their unstable moods and impatience. They are not the type to just drop by, they walk fast with a purpose and if they visit you it has taken a lot to get them there. They get worse from attention and superficial chat and improve greatly with talking for a long time, when they will open up and feel a lot better afterwards. They appear serious, poised and cool but feel depressed and tremulous or become bitter under the surface.

Physical: Nat mur is a good remedy for coughs and colds where the discharges are profuse. The hacking cough is worse in the evening. The nose drips like a tap. Sweating helps. Nat mur can be used to treat hayfever if the rest of the indications are present. The nat mur individual is often suffering from exhaustion, they feel tired and drained, especially in the evening. It is a good remedy for insomnia if it is caused by grief or loss. This is a major remedy for cold sores that often arise from suppressing hurt or grief. Urination can be difficult, especially in the presence of others. Stools are dry, hard, crumbling with a sticking pain in the rectum. There can be anal herpes.

Digestion: A Nat mur type will tend to be slim, these people emaciate easily. They experience a sinking, empty feeling from hunger at around 11 a.m. or after a meal. A good remedy for indigestion where they desire salt and fish and are averse to rich, fatty foods, bread, meat or coffee.

Head: These people often wake up with a headache which will get worse in the morning and then improve throughout the rest of the day, or it will stay over the eyes on the left side of the head. The pain is bursting, like a thousand little hammers, with flashing lights, zigzagging before the eyes; headaches come on after being in the sun, and get worse from noise. Schoolchildren's headaches, migraines. The eyes are sensitive to light and get watery in the wind. The tongue is mapped with red and white patches and there is a sensation as if a hair is on the tongue (*see also* silicea). The tongue is dry maybe with blisters.

Skin: Acne; itchy, scaly eruptions along the nape of the neck and the hairline, which becomes red. There may be cracks in the centre of the lower lip, herpes, thrush, cold sores on the lips and mouth. Urticaria becomes worse after exertion. The nails crack easily and the skin around the neck is dry.

Women's complaints: Periods often come late and are accompanied by a headache. There may be vaginal dryness or thrush with white discharges and a low libido in both men and women. Nat mur can be good to give for oedema in pregnancy.

Children: May be slow to talk and walk. Fearful dreams are particularly about burglars.

Modalities: Worse: from 9–11 a.m., in the sun and heat, from sympathy, at puberty, from exertion of the eyes, talking, writing and reading. Better: open air, from sweating and from talking in depth.

Nat Phos   *Natrum phosphoricum*

A homoeopathic remedy made from natrum phosphate found in the body which forms one of the 12 biochemic tissue salts. It helps the body to break down lactic acid, an excess of which results in too much sugar, leading to acidity and sourness. Sourness is the keynote of this remedy.

Mental and emotional indications: Marked by irritability and touchiness. There is indifference, mental and nervous weakness and these types become frightened easily (especially at night). They are frightened that something will happen, are generally apprehensive and fearful. They tend to be forgetful.

Digestive symptoms: Sour risings and belches (described as having a coppery taste), flatulence, nausea and heartburn. Desire for strong-tasting foods like eggs, beer and fried fish and an aversion to bread and butter. The back of the tongue is yellow. Nat phos will tend to neutralize too much acidity and will help where there is too much uric acid or gallstones in the kidneys. Use for gout, pains in the joints, rheumatism and pains in the balls of the feet, knees and ankles.

Headaches: Mainly at the front of the head, they come on from mental exertion. There is dizziness with cutting pains in the temples, feelings of pressure and headache on top of the head. The nose can be sticky with yellow, thick, offensive mucus. A child will pick her nose.

Women's complaints: Sour creamy leucorrhoea that is acidic and watery. Morning sickness and sour vomiting. Nat phos is really helpful for heartburn during pregnancy.

Modalities: Worse: sugar, fats, thunderstorms, intercourse. Better: in the cold.

Nat Sulph   *Natrum sulphuricum*

A homoeopathic remedy that is made from a mineral found in the intercellular fluid of the body and known as a tissue salt. The remedy aids the regulation of excretion and helps rid the body of superfluous water. Its action is opposite to that of nat mur which attracts water to be used. Nat sulph attracts water to be eliminated. It has an effect on the liver and the pancreas. Keynotes for nat sulph are piercing pains and yellow, watery discharge from the skin or in the stools. Pus is thick and yellowy-green.

Mental and emotional indications: Nat sulph people are affected by the moon, especially a full moon, when they feel increasingly unbalanced because the fluid level rises up the spine and causes pressure and compression in the brain. They have vivid or frightening dreams, feel disheartened and sad, unable to talk. This can become extreme, with bouts of wildness or insanity. There is a desire to jump from heights, suicidal tendencies. They are suspicious and very sensitive, easily startled by sudden noises and generally irritable and melancholic. There may be mental or behavioural problems which can be traced back to a head injury during infancy – the head has 'never been right since'. It is good to give nat sulph immediately to anyone suffering from a head injury.

Physical symptoms. Headaches: Violent, pulsating, worse on the top of the head. There is vertigo with gastric problems, excess bile, a brownish, green-coated tongue, a bitter taste and sick headaches with bilious diarrhoea or vomiting of bile. The scalp can feel sensitive with burning at the top of the head. Acute photophobia. The face is sallow and yellowish with biliousness.

Digestion: Symptoms include a disordered stomach, vomiting of greenish/brown bile, sour risings, heartburn, flatulence, an engorged liver with cutting pains which get worse when lying on the left side and gallstones. Tight clothes around the waist are intolerable. Stools are loose and dark or green.

There are rumbling, gurgling bowels, spluttering stools, foaming yellow diarrhoea mixed with green slime. Loose stools in the morning driving the person from bed, but afterwards they feel better in themselves.

Respiratory system: Nat sulph can be used for asthmatic conditions which get worse in wet weather. It is good for damp, rattling mucus in the chest, such as bronchial catarrh, where there is a heavy weight on the chest and a loose cough with thick, ropey, greenish expectoration. The respiratory symptoms are often much worse from living in a damp environment, e.g. a basement. There is soreness of the chest made worse by coughing. Breathlessness is worse in damp weather and the bronchial catarrh is worse in the early morning. The nasal discharge is thick and yellow/green.

Skin: There is a tendency for warts. Eruptions on the eyes, scalp, face and chest. Yellowy, watery secretions. Nat sulph can be effective for ringworm and inflammation in the root of the nails. There are also stiff joints that crack with motion, and arthritis that gets worse with damp.

Modalities: Worse: damp, lying on the left side, injuries to the head, late in the evening, eating vegetables and fruit, cold foods and drink, light, music. Better: open, warm, dry air, lying on the back.

Neroli Oil   *Citrus aurantium* subsp. *amara*

A delightfully light and cooling oil and one of the mildest oils. Can be applied neat to the skin or diluted for babies and children. It is an expensive oil which is comparatively easy to produce synthetically, so buy only from a reputable supplier.

Family: Rutaceae

Parts used: Sweet orange blossom

Main constituents: Alcohols, aliphatic aldehydes, esters, monoterpenes

Fragrance: Fresh, floral, light, delightful

Main uses: A wonderful oil for the skin, for cooling children's fevers and for uplifting the spirits. It is tonifying for the reproductive system. Acts as an antifungal for skin conditions and as a bacteriocide for coughs and infections. Use to balance the hormones and regulate periods. Its marked calming effects will help relieve stress and problems resulting from tension. Use for skin complaints. Excellent to include in anti-ageing creams for the hands and face. Excellent for broken capillaries, varicose veins and haemorrhoids. It is very appropriate to use during pregnancy. It will help prevent stretch marks and have a calming, relaxing effect.

Safety and application: A safe oil to use even undiluted, although always blend in maximum 1 per cent for children. Will lend a refreshing, lifting beauty to most blends.

❋ Nettles   *Urtica urens* or *U. dioica*

Parts used: Aerial parts and root

Habitat: Waste places in temperate climates

Main constituents: Amines (acetylcholine, histamine, serotonin), ascorbic acid, flavonoids, minerals (iron, potassium, calcium, silicea), vitamins

Actions: Alterative, antihaemorrhagic, antiallergenic, antirheumatic, astringent, blood tonic, circulation stimulant, decongestant, diuretic, expectorant, haemostatic, hypoglycaemic, hypotensive, immune-stimulant, nutritive, vasodilator, reduces inflammation of the prostrate

Main uses: A really useful and easily found plant with a well-known sting, the nettle has been used for centuries as a nutritive and detoxifying tonic. It can be drunk in combination with raspberry leaf during pregnancy to ensure the vitamin and mineral levels are sufficient. Use especially in the spring for cleansing and making a fresh start in the year. Nettles are rich in iron and other minerals and vitamins and are an excellent tonic for detoxifying or for use where the body is depleted, as with anaemia. They help weak digestive systems during convalesence, can be used for high blood sugar in diabetes, and also strengthen the liver, spleen and kidneys. This is also demonstrated by nettles' diuretic action and their proven use in treating rheumatism, gout and skin problems. Use to treat allergies, as well as for nettle rash; can help eczema, bites and stings, hayfever and asthma, as well as allergic reactions to various foods. Nettles are astringent and can be used for stopping bleeding, both internal and external. Use for prolonged and heavy periods as well as for nosebleeds. Use externally for burns and wounds, nappy rash and bedsores. As an immune enhancer, nettles have been used in cases of cancer and the root has been used to treat prostatitis, also vaginitis and vaginal discharges. Use to increase the flow of milk in breastfeeding mothers.

Contraindications: Overuse of nettles may create an allergic reaction. Be careful before you embark on a cleansing programme!

Dosage: Drink nettle tea as required, or at least 3 times daily for cleansing.

Teabags are available or use 1 teaspoon per cup of boiling water. Fresh nettles are best picked in spring. Use just the young top leaves. Make soup, combining them with other vegetables or combine in risotto! Make fresh juice by liquidizing the leaves for external applications or combine the juice into a cream base. Use dried leaves or tincture to make a salve. Infuse 2–3 handfuls of fresh leaves with 3 litres of boiling water to make a final rinse for the hair. The same can be used as a fertilizer for the garden or plant pots. Tincture: 1:5 in 25 per cent alcohol. Take 2–6ml 3 times daily.

Niaouli Oil *Melaleuca viridiflora*

Part of the tea tree family, this oil is still somewhat under-appreciated. An excellent antiviral, antifungal, antibacterial oil, it is more easily tolerated than eucalyptus or tea tree.

Family: Myrtaceae

Parts used: Twigs and leaves

Main constituents: Alcohols, esters, oxides, monoterpenes

Fragrance: Fresh, green, herbal, cold, medicinal

Main uses: It can be used to treat burns and all infected skin conditions. This is an oil which increases antibodies. It is said to be helpful with HIV. As a tonic, it will help memory loss and aid concentration. Has a toning effect on the skin. Use for all septic and damaged skin conditions, particularly for burns and scalds. Use to combat infections of the respiratory system, asthma, bronchitis, catarrh, coughs and pneumonia. Use as a gargle for sore throats or where the mucous membranes are infected. Tonifying for the digestive system. Excellent to use as a douche or wash for genital infections and herpes.

Safety and application: Non-toxic, non-irritant. Use in dilution, not more than 2 per cent.

Nit Ac *Nitricum acidum (Nitric acid)*

This homoeopathic remedy is appropriate for people who are very irritable and suffer from sharp stitching and pricking pains.

Mental and emotional indications: These people are prone to be very touchy, cold and often angry. They can be very easily provoked and fly into a rage over anything, and then weep. They may become so angry that they tremble, and feel hateful and vindictive. This can be due to lack of sleep, e.g. with young children, or PMT. They can swear and curse and refuse consolation. They become tired of life, despondent and sad. One of the significant features of this remedy is extreme anxiety, especially over health. Such people may despair of improvement and are terrified of dying, of being left alone and of the future.

Physical: The most noticeable physical indication is of being cold; compare with arsenicum album, nux vomica and hepar sulph, which are the three other main remedies where this is such a significant feature. There will be a tendency to smell foul, the urine will be very offensive and the smell will linger; feet, nasal discharges and sweat will all be offensive. Other aspects of this remedy are joints which crack. All discharges are thin, offensively acrid and either brown, green or yellowish. Nit ac is very good for treating thin, watery, brown, smelly leucorrhoea.

Abdomen: There may be diarrhoea, or the passing of a stool will seem incomplete even if accompanied by straining. There may be great pain, as if the rectum is torn, which it may well be, and the pain will remain for several hours. This remedy is really effective for anal fissures. There are piles which are very painful and bleed.

Pain: The pains of this remedy are pricking and sticking and appear to come and go. There may be a sensation of a tight band around the head or bones. The person in need of nit ac is very sensitive to pain, and this may come on during sleep and be accompanied by frightening dreams.

Respiratory system: Use for the sore throat or common cold where there is acute sensitivity, ulceration and burning of the mucous membranes.

Skin: It can be very effective for all parts of the skin which meet with mucous membranes. The skin is dry, cracked and may ulcerate and bleed easily at the corners of the mouth, nose, vagina or anus. These areas can become red and swollen and are very sensitive. Ulcers look raw and warts can bleed.

Modalities: Worse: being touched, cold or cold air, after 2 a.m., jarring movements, draughts, any additional slight burden. Better: mild weather, gentle movement.

Nux Vomica   *Nux vomica*

A major homoeopathic remedy, nux vom works effectively for a very wide range of mental, emotional and physical symptoms. The picture of the person that suits this remedy has traditionally been seen as masculine, but it is not exclusively for men or women. In the last century, when homoeopathy first became used in its present form, nux vomica was seen as a remedy for those who abuse the body and mind on all levels and for ailments stemming from excessive behaviour, generally male behaviour. Women were expected to be acquiescent supporters of the aggressive male role.

Mental and emotional indications: It is one of the most appropriate remedies for the type of person who lives hard, for people who are seen to have a strong character, who are forceful, charismatic, work too hard and drive themselves beyond their own limitations. They become people who have 'the right impulse but the wrong expression', and through driving themselves become irritable, fault-finding, nagging and quarrelsome hypochondriacs. They can become violent, very reactive and self-willed. They may particularly dislike being questioned and having to be responsive to others. In extreme cases they can get suicidal, but they are also afraid of death.

Physical: They are people who chill easily, and are prone to ailments that come on from getting cold. These people feel worse from coffee, tobacco, alcohol, drugs, highly-spiced food (all of which they tend to crave), overeating, mental overexertion, lack of exercise and loss of sleep. It is a good hangover remedy.

Abdomen and digestion: Nux vomica works for nausea after eating, in the morning or from smoking, with a feeling that vomiting would ease the discomfort. There may be burping after eating, with sour and bitter risings, heartburn and a sensation of pressure in the stomach for 1 or 2 hours after eating, with a desire to loosen clothing. There may be pains that go into the back and chest, flatulent colic and bruised soreness in the abdomen. The person can feel sleepy after dinner – maybe finding it difficult to think – and also after feeling anxious or worried. Nux vomica can be very good for nausea and vomiting in pregnancy, especially where the nausea is temporarily relieved by vomiting. There is constipation with a frequent desire to pass stools but these then recede, and may alternate with diarrhoea. There may be a tendency to faint after passing a stool or vomiting. It is a good remedy for those who have used laxatives for years. Nux vomica is good for piles that itch or bleed and get better with cool bathing, also for varicose veins which are black, hard and look like cords; these have probably come from sedentary habits. It is a very good remedy for hernias.

Catarrh: Symptoms include a nasal discharge which flows during the day and is dry at night. It is worse in a warm room and gets better in cold air. Nux vomica is good for infants who have constant snuffles (especially if the mother is very active and stressed). It is also good for babies with an umbilical hernia.

Coughs: These are marked by their violent paroxysmal nature, often accompanied by a splitting headache with the need to hold the head. It is good for whooping cough or asthma where there is a sensation as if something has torn loose in the chest. There may be a desire to eat during a coughing fit. There will be hoarseness and painful roughness in the larynx and chest.

Women's complaints: This is the remedy to take when periods come on too early, are profuse or too long. They may be irregular and are prone to stopping and starting. Use nux vomica where labour pains are violent and spasmodic, and there is an urge for a bowel movement or to urinate.

People who need this remedy find sleep irresistible when they return home from work or in the early evening – they may sleep for a while or just benefit from catnaps, and then be wide awake at bedtime, unable to sleep and finally drop off just before it is time to rise in the morning. They will awake feeling tired and weak. They may have sexual dreams or nightmares about being chased. They may also cry or talk during sleep. A nux vomica type of person often has strong sexual impulses. They are very sensitive to pain.

Modalities: Worse: early morning, cold, open air, draughts, after excesses, pressure (physical), any incidents however slight. Better: hot drinks, warmth, free discharges.

⚘ Oats *Avena sativa*

Parts used: Seeds and stalks

Habitat: Native to northern Europe, grown commercially as a crop throughout the world

Main constituents: Alkaloids, minerals (calcium, iron, zinc), proteins, saponins, starch, vitamins

Actions: Antidepressive, cleansing, nervine, nutritious, tonic

Main uses: A great tonic for the nervous system, oats improve nervous weakness, depression, anxiety and stress. Good for overwork, tension, headaches, insomnia. Helpful when trying to break an addiction, e.g., smoking, alcohol, drugs, tranquillizers. As a food, oats are very nutritious, being a source of vitamins, especially the B group. Use when recovering from illness. An important remedy in the treatment of anorexia nervosa. They will help restore the appetite and lower cholesterol, help prevent hardening of arteries and heart problems and strengthen the muscles and stamina. Good for strong physical exertion. Oats can be used as a substitute for soap – they are cleansing and good for allergic skin conditions. It is easiest to put them into a muslin bag and rub it onto the skin.

Contraindications: Where there is sensitivity to gluten.

Dosage: Make a habit of eating soaked muesli or porridge every day. Infuse 1 teaspoon oats in a cup of boiling water. Take 3 times daily. Tincture: 1:5 in 45 per cent alcohol. Take 1–5ml 3 times daily.

Olibanum   *Boswellia thurifera*

See Frankincense Oil.

Orange (Bitter)   *Citrus aurantium*

Parts used: Flowers, fruit, peel, seeds

Habitat: Asia, Mediterranean areas

Main constituents: Coumarins, flavonoids, vitamin C

Actions: Antibacterial, anti-inflammatory, aromatic, carminative, digestive

Main uses: This is a calming herb for the digestive system, particularly where ailments arise from nervous causes, indigestion, wind and bloating. The peel can be used to help relieve headaches and tension. It is excellent to include a small amount of dried orange peel in herbal blends, as it adds flavour and imparts a soothing aspect to the functioning. This tree also is known for its fragrant flowers (blossom) which are made into neroli oil *(see page 319)*. The residue water from the distillation, orange flower or floral water, has been traditionally used for centuries as a cosmetic and food flavouring. Orangeblossom is used as a herb for its antidepressant qualities.

Contraindications: None.

Dosage: When mixing a blend of herbs, add a teaspoon to a 25g mixture. Use 1 teaspoon to cup of boiling water.

Orange Oil (Sweet) *Citrus sinensis*

A familiar citrus oil, easy to use in blends or in cooking as a refreshing, lifting fragrance or flavour. Try to purchase an organic quality, as this is an oil expressed from the rind and it is important to avoid any pesticide residues.

Family: Rutaceae

Parts used: Rind of fruit

Main constituents: Alcohols, aliphatic aldehydes, ketones, monoterpenes

Fragrance: A sweet, fresh fragrance, like the fruit

Main uses: This is an oil that is both calming and stimulating. Use in blends for depression, stress and tension. It will help relieve indigestion, constipation and wind. Helps as a decongestant for bronchial problems. Warming for colds and 'flu. Use for detoxifying, water retention and tendency to obesity. A good oil to combine in skin and bath preparations for its cleansing properties.

Safety and application: Non-toxic, non-irritant in dilution. Do not use in the sun, possibly photosensitizing. Use in dilution maximum 2 per cent.

Parsley *Crispum petroselinum*

This herb, as we know, is widely used in cooking. The leaves, root and seed can be used. The leaves contain vitamin C and iron; the herb is nutritious and extra amounts can be added to the diet for people who are anaemic. It stimulates the stomach juices; for this reason it is contraindicated where there are stomach ulcers. It helps digestion, it is a carminative herb and soothes colic and flatulence. One of the main medicinal uses for parsley is its diuretic action. Use where there are problems with fluid retention and for helping arthritis, osteoarthritis and for the passing of urinary stones. Parsley also stimulates menstruation, making it good for dysmenorrhoea (pain during periods) and amenorrhoea (absence of periods), but it is contraindicated during pregnancy in medicinal doses.

Dosage: Take 1 teaspoonful to a cup of boiling water 2–3 times daily.

❋ Parsley Oil   *Petroselinum sativum*

The volatile oil is distilled mainly from the seeds. It contains apiol and this is an abortifacient, so it is important not to use parsley oil during pregnancy. It can be used for similar reasons to the herb, but is mainly used for its diuretic value. It can be diluted (use a dilution of 0.5–1 per cent) and massaged in, or use a drop in the bath when you are feeling particularly bloated before a period.

❋ Parsley Piert   *Aphanes arvensis*

This herb acts on the kidneys, it is a soothing diuretic and can help dissolve stones and gravel. If it is taken over a long period of time it helps to restore normal functions to the kidneys and is good for oedema (water retention). Combine this herb with pellitory of the wall and hawthorn to support the kidneys and the heart.

Dosage: Use 1 teaspoonful of herb to a cup of boiling water and drink 3 times a day, or 2ml of tincture diluted in water 3 times daily.

❋ Passiflora   *Passiflora incarnata*

Parts used: Aerial parts

Habitat: Native to the USA, now grown throughout Europe

Main constituents: Alkaloids, flavonoids, rutin

Actions: Analgesic, antispasmodic, sedative, tranquillizer, vasodilator

Main uses: Known as a tranquillizing herb, it is good to use where the brain is over-active, preventing sleep and causing anxiety, also for restlessness and for over-active children. It will help to reduce pain. Give before going to the dentist, for PMT, neuralgia or headaches. Assists withdrawal from drugs or alcohol.

Contraindications: None.

Dosage: ½ teaspoonful infused in boiling water, 3 times daily. Tincture: 1:8 in 25 per cent alcohol, 2 ml 3 times daily.

❧ Pellitory of the Wall   *Parietaria judaica*

Parts used: Aerial parts
   Habitat: Europe
   Main constituents: Flavonoids, minerals
   Actions: Demulcent, diuretic, tonic for the kidneys
   Main uses: A herb that has been traditionally used for centuries as a sooth-
ing diuretic. Useful for dissolving stones and gravel. Good to use for inflam-
mation, cystitis, pyelitis. Externally, can be used as a soothing balm.
   Contraindications: Do not take if suffering from hayfever.
   Dosage: Infuse 1 teaspoon of fresh herb (if possible). Take 3 times daily or as
required. Take for an extended period of time for results.

❧ Pennyroyal   *Mentha pulegium*

See Mint.

❧ Peppermint   *Mentha piperita*

See Mint.

❧ Peppermint Oil   *Mentha piperita*

A traditional oil produced in the UK. The well-known 'Mitcham' peppermint
is now grown and distilled over the world. Native also to Mediterranean areas,
cultivated in the USA. A popular flavouring.
   Family: Lamiaceae (labiatae)
   Parts used: Aerial parts
   Main constituents: Alcohols, esters, ketones, monoterpenes, oxides,
sesquiterpenes
   Fragrance: Penetrating, lingering, minty, menthol, fresh
   Main uses: This is a strongly stimulating oil, which causes the blood capillaries to expand and so increases circulation and cools down the body. It is
primarily stimulating and warming, although on the skin's surface it will feel
cooling and refreshing. It will induce sweating in fevers and for the nervous

system it is refreshing. Use as a compress for headaches, tiredness, vertigo, neuralgia, tension. It is well known as an aid to digestion. Use for indigestion, constipation, wind, colic, nausea, travel sickness. Helps to digest fats (hence peppermint oil being a perfect mix with chocolate). Good as an expectorant. Use in a chest rub as a decongestant for coughs and colds and to relieve blocked sinuses. Use for bad breath or for mouth infections. For muscles, aches and pains, use to relieve muscle fatigue and aching feet. Also has deodorizing properties, which makes it excellent for foot treatments. Use as an insecticide, against ants in particular.

Safety and application: Although this oil is not known to be toxic or an irritant or sensitizing, it is known to have quite dramatic effects. Avoid in pregnancy, anxiety, neurosis and nervous excitability. Use with care and do not use in dilutions over 1.5 per cent. Do not use before going to sleep, due to its stimulating effects. Not suitable for young children or for use in steam inhalations.

Phosphorus   *Phosphorus*

An effective homoeopathic remedy for people who are commonly identifiable types. They are excitable, outgoing, lively people who burn out quickly. They are weak, chilly and prone to coughs.

Mental and emotional indications: These people are usually full of vitality, quick moving, bright and intelligent. They are alert, they sit forward in their seats, and are expressive and sensitive to surroundings, people, noise, odours, light and atmospheres. They can be tense and restless, become fidgety, impatient, anxious and very fearful. They can have a sense of dread or feel nervous without knowing why, overshadowed by fear. Tension tends to increase in the afternoon and symptoms are at their worst around twilight. They fear the dark, being alone, disease and death. They have an impending fear that something will happen. When they are unwell they become very demanding and attention-seeking.

They can be sensitive on the psychic level, tending to be clairvoyant, vulnerable or impressionable. They are often very sympathetic to the needs of others and will go out of their way to help. They are warm, friendly, affectionate and extrovert. They love being touched, stroked or massaged. They can get over-concerned for the welfare of others. They are easily influenced and reassured; they like sympathy themselves, and have vivid imaginations, often being artistic and musical. They are daydreamers.

Physical: Generalized by chilliness. There is great weakness and trembling accompanying all symptoms. The circulation is unstable and becoming easily flushed is an indication of this remedy – hot, spicy foods, temperature changes or even strong ideas will cause flushing. A phosphorus type will become easily and quickly exhausted, they can be said to be 'running on their nerves'. They have short, intense bursts of energy and then need to rest. There may be a feeling of burning along the spine, in the feet, in between the shoulder blades, on the palms and in the chest. Phosphorus is a very good remedy for haemorrhage, post-partum haemorrhage (here is good to use 200C), where small wounds bleed easily and profusely, and when the blood is bright red, and for nosebleeds. There is a tendency to anaemia, and there can also be hair loss. Use for hair loss after an acute illness.

Abdomen: Stools are slender, tough and dry, and there may be bleeding from the rectum. There is profuse, exhausting diarrhoea, like water. It pours out but is painless. It can come on after a fright or nervousness. There can be an involuntary stool, with weakness afterwards. Haemorrhoids which bleed.

Coughs: A dry, tickling, hard, racking cough which is exhausting and accompanied by a bursting headache *(see belladonna and nux vom)*. A tightness of the chest which is improved with pressure. There is trembling when coughing. Expectoration is yellow, bloody, rusty-coloured and salty. The cough gets worse from laughing, talking, eating, lying on the left side, from the open air and going from warm to cold or vice versa *(see also rumex)*. Coughs are often brought on by a cold going down to the chest, leading to bronchitis and pneumonia.

Head: Throbbing violent headache with hunger or preceded by hunger, or mental exertion. Violent, neuralgic pains darting and shooting. Symptoms get worse from light, heat, motion and lying down. They improve from cold and rest.

Skin: Wounds bleed excessively. They may heal and then break out and bleed again.

Sleeping: Generally on the right side. The person is better from taking naps and from sleeping. Sleepy during the day, restless at night. Vivid dreams.

Stomach: Symptoms include a liking for chocolate, spicy food, fish, salt and ice-cream. A thirst for cold drinks which, during illness, are vomited up once they get warm in the stomach. There is post-operative vomiting. The remedy can be indicated for nausea after anaesthesia. Also, ravenous hunger, burning in stomach, stomach ulcers, an empty, hollow feeling and waterbrash.

Throat: Frequent soreness, inability to talk as the larynx is so painful, swollen tonsils, voice loss.

Women's complaints: Periods of bright red blood may be frequent, scanty, can go on too long or there may be bleeding in between periods, amenorrhoea. Uterine polyps, fibroids. Leucorrhoea can be burning and replace menses. Strong sexual desire which increases during pregnancy and breastfeeding.

Modalities: Worse: lying on the left side or on the painful side, slight causes, cold, damp or changes in the weather, mental exertion. Better: eating, sleeping, massage, sitting, cold food, washing the face with cold water and lying on the right side.

Phytolacca (Poke Root)   *Phytolacca*

See Poke Root.

Pilewort   *Ranunculus ficaria*

Parts used: Aerial parts
  Habitat: Europe and other areas throughout the world
  Main constituents: Anemonin, saponins, tannins
  Actions: Astringent, demulcent
  Main uses: Use externally for treating piles.
  Contraindications: Not to be taken internally.
  Dosage: Use dried or fresh herb and combine into an ointment. Can also be used in a suppository.

Pine Oil   *Pinus sylvestris*

Pine is widely cultivated with many different varieties. Resin is collected and distilled into turpentine. Pine is used to fragrance disinfectants and other household items, although Scots pine oil is mainly used for bath products. Pine oil is traditionally used for easing muscle strain and for its revitalizing qualities.
  Family: Pinaceae
  Parts used: Needles and twigs
  Main constituents: Alcohols, esters, monoterpenes, sesquiterpenes
  Fragrance: Fresh, woody, resinous
  Main uses: Pine oil has a refreshing and reviving action. It is good for the

nervous system where there is exhaustion and poor concentration. Helps for stress and tension and the complaints that these create. Good for colds and 'flu in combination with other oils such as lavender and thyme. It is stimulating to the circulation and is a good decongestant and antiseptic for the respiratory system. Use for bronchitis and catarrh, coughs and sinusitis. Good for infections of the urinary tract. An excellent oil for aching, tiredness and a worn-down feeling. Use in blends with rosemary, thyme and marjoram and add to bath salts or bath-oil base for revitalizing baths. Use for sprains, strains and aching backs, rheumatism and arthritis. Use as a parasiticide against scabies and lice.

Safety and application: Non-toxic. May be an irritant. Do not use in quantities over 1.5 per cent dilution.

Plantain   *Plantago major*

Parts used: Leaves

Habitat: Throughout Europe

Main constituents: Flavonoids, iridoids, tannins, vitamins

Actions: Antibacterial, antihistamine, astringent, lymphatic, styptic, tonic

Main uses: It is healing and stops the flow of blood. Use externally to treat wounds and as a cleansing wash for damaged tissue, also for treating torn ligaments and broken bones or for areas where the nerves are damaged. Internally, use as a diuretic, for cystitis and blood in the urine, and for involuntary urination. Use for treating digestive disorders, IBS, diarrhoea, ulcers. Its cooling, drying action on the respiratory system will help coughs, catarrh and bronchitis. Use as a mouthwash for bleeding gums. Excellent for treating bites and stings, especially good for relieving the itching of mosquito bites.

Contraindications: None.

Dosage: Fresh is best! Combine liquidized leaves into an ointment or poultice for external use. Infuse 2 teaspoons of herb to 1 cup boiling water for cleansing wash or for internal use. Take 3 times daily. Tincture: 1:5 in 25 per cent alcohol, average dose 2–4ml.

❋ Poke Root   *Phytolacca americana*

This is a plant known and used by both herbalists and homoeopaths. It was at one time widely used by Native Americans to treat fevers, aches and pains. Homoeopathically, the mental and emotional indications are not particularly marked, although there may be a reluctance or indifference towards work and a general sadness.

Physical: Homoeopathically, Phytolacca affects mainly the tonsils or mammary glands, and works on inflammation of bones and glands in general. It helps: pains that come and go suddenly or those that move from spot to spot; pains that are shooting or feel like electric shocks; weakness; feeling faint on rising. Pains feel worse on the right side. The body feels chilly but the head and face can feel hot. There may be thirst, with frequent yawning and a restlessness from pain. The person may wake feeling very weak. She feels tired and worn out and wants to lie down. There can be aching all over the body, with a bruised feeling, and painful throat that is inflamed or swollen, dry, rough, bruised and smarting, as if a ball of red hot iron is lodged in the throat – it feels full and choking. There can be pain at the end of the tongue and pain in the ears when swallowing. There is a sensation of a lump when swallowing or when the head is turned to the left. Phytolacca is a good remedy to try when bryonia and rhus tox fail, for rheumatic pains and stiffness in the muscles, when the joints are swollen and hot and the pains are like electric shocks. It can help right-sided sciatica.

Mumps: Phytolacca is a useful homoeopathic remedy for mumps where there is inflammation of the submaxillary and parotid glands, especially when they are hard like stones and there is pain shooting into the ear when swallowing.

Women's complaints: Use for the breasts – when they become sore and lumpy, particularly before or during the period. It can help where the lymph glands are enlarged in the armpits and when the pain shoots all over the body. It is good for nipples that have become very cracked and sore and sensitive during breastfeeding. The breasts feel better from firm pressure. It is a good remedy for mastitis, when the breast becomes hard, painful, purplish and very sensitive.

Modalities: Symptoms get worse on exposure to damp, cold weather or a change of weather, on getting up, from motion, swallowing hot drinks, heat, menses and rain. They improve in dry weather, from rest, lying on the abdomen or on the left side.

USING THE HERB

As a herb, poke root stimulates the lymphatic system. It is a good herb for glandular fever or colds, or where there are accompanying swollen glands in the neck and armpits. It can also be given for the treatment of mastitis. Use poke root for respiratory complaints, especially chronic colds and where there is inflammation. Although poke root is a very effective herb it must be given with caution. It is not advisable to use it as a general lymphatic cleanser. It is not a gentle herb, such as cleavers, and should not be taken over a long period of time. It is not to be used during pregnancy and breastfeeding.

Dosage: Dilute 1ml of tincture in water and take 3 times a day, or decoct 25g (1oz) of root to 570ml (1 pint) of water and take a tablespoonful 3 times a day. Do not take for more than 3 weeks at a time.

Prickly Ash   *Zanthoxylum americanum*

Synonyms: Toothache tree
  Parts used: Bark, berries
  Habitat: Native to North America
  Main constituents: Alkaloids, lignans, oil, tannins
  Actions: Alterative, bitter, carminative, diaphoretic
  Main uses: A great herb for warming and moving the circulation, particularly helping blood to go to the brain. Stimulates the circulation to the joints and muscles, therefore good for rheumatism, arthritis and cramping pains. Also good for colds and 'flu and for toning the digestive system.
  Contraindications: Do not take during pregnancy or if there is inflammation of the gut.
  Dosage: Make a decoction using 1 teaspoon in 250ml water. Simmer for 5–10 minutes. Take 3 times daily. Tincture: 1:5 in 45 per cent alcohol. Take 2ml 3 times daily.

Psyllium   *Plantago psyllium*

Synonyms: Flea seed
  Parts used: Seeds or husks
  Habitat: South Europe, India, Africa
  Main constituents: Mucilage, oil, starch

Actions: Antidiarrhoeal, demulcent, laxative

Main uses: Both the seeds and husks are used for their mucilagenous nature and therefore soothing properties. They are highly absorbent and swell to create bulk that will increase the bulk of the stool and stimulate the colon to contract. Use as a gentle laxative during pregnancy or chronic constipation and IBS. The mucilage absorbs toxins as it passes through the gut. It is good for infections and can also be used for diarrhoea and dysentery. Use for soothing gastric ulcers, haemorrhoids and urinary infections. Externally, psyllium can be used in a poultice to help draw out toxins.

Caution: Always ensure that sufficient water is drunk when taking psyllium.

Contraindications: Stenosis of the oesophagus or the gastrointestinal tract

Dosage: Macerate the 25g seeds in 250ml water for 10 hours. Drink at bedtime. Take 2 capsules at night accompanied by 750ml of water.

Pulsatilla   *Pulsatilla vulgaris*

A homoeopathic remedy well known for women and children marked by a need for company and great sensitivity.

Mental and emotional indications: The general indications are marked by changeability and a softness which puts up no resistance to confrontation. These people will tend to shape themselves around what they think will please. They have very little sense of self, no opinions of their own. They are easily dominated, being timid, shy and often embarrassed. Their emotions are quickly aroused, they can go from tears to laughter very quickly. They will cry when reading and feel much better for it, they can easily feel very sorry for themselves and will tend to whine and grumble, but they improve greatly with consolation and feelings of compassion.

Pulsatilla types usually have a strong sexual desire but sometimes they have a dread of the opposite sex. They may be sensuous, but needy and overdependent. This can lead them into being possessive and becoming victims of their own jealous feelings. They can be very demanding although are not aggressive or malicious. They can become easily offended, irritable, touchy or angry through their lack of self-confidence. It is often possible to trace their symptoms back to a time when they felt abandoned and forsaken. They have a strong desire for company, and have fears of being alone, death, the dark and insanity, all of which increase in the evening. In women, hysteria, sadness and depression get worse before their period. A pulsatilla person will crave the open air and hate stuffiness and although she can be chilly, she is averse to heat. It is one of the main remedies for babies and children where cold drinks or ice-cream tend to upset the digestion.

Physical: The changeable temperament is matched by changing symptoms. Pains shift rapidly and are erratic. Pulsatilla is indicated for pains in the extremities which rapidly shift about. Joints can be painful, red and swollen. There is a thirstlessness with nearly all complaints. Headaches pulsate and are bursting. Nervousness from overwork is improved by walking in the open air.

Children: It is a good remedy and often indicated for chickenpox, measles, etc. The child will become weepy, irritable and clingy during the illness. Use for children who wet the bed when sick. Also can be indicated when the child is teething, but made better by cold water.

Digestion and Abdomen: Gastric disorders come on from rich, fatty foods such as pork, sausages, pastry and ice-cream. Nausea and heartburn are symptoms of pulsatilla, and so is vomiting food that has been eaten hours before. Digestion is slow and the stomach feels weighed down with an 'all gone' sensation. The person feels hungry but they do not know what they want. The abdomen is distended, stools are changeable in appearance, and diarrhoea can occur after a fright during the night. Diarrhoea is watery, greenish-yellow and can also arise from eating fruit, ice-cream or cold food. There can be piles which tend to improve during the menses. Cystitis can occur if the person lies on her back, and there may be involuntary urination during sleep or in pregnancy.

Ears: Earaches occur after colds, there is yellow-green discharge from the ears. Impaired hearing with catarrh of the Eustachian tubes. Earache is worse at night, and causes the child to become weepy and clingy.

Eyes: Symptoms include a thick yellow-green, profuse, bland discharge. There is a tendency to develop conjunctivitis from a cold or have recurring styes.

Mouth: It is a common feature in many pulsatilla cases to have a crack in the centre of the lower lip *(see Nat Mur page 316)*, and there is a great need to lick the lips. This is often accompanied by an offensive taste in the morning when waking. There may be toothache which gets better with cold water held in the mouth. There is a marked thirstlessness, but a dry mouth. Use for fevers that are burning but the person is also feeling chilly, often moaning. Pulsatilla can be used for chilblains.

Nose: Loss of smell with catarrh, nostrils blocked with yellowish, bland discharge. These symptoms are worse when lying down and better in the open air.

Respiratory symptoms: Pulsatilla is good for coughs when they are dry at night and then loose in the daytime. The cough is exhausting and racking. It gets worse at night and causes the person to wake up and then feels she must sit up. Coughs get worse with exertion and heat. There can be yellowish-green expectoration. It is a good remedy for coughs that come on after measles.

Women's complaints: Symptoms include amenorrhoea which comes on after getting the feet wet, or where there was debility and anaemia at puberty. Pulsatilla will generally regulate or bring on periods. It is a good remedy for late, irregular, scanty periods, clotted, dark, thick blood, and where there are changeable, bearing-down pains or cutting, griping pains during periods. It can help bleeding between periods and is good for PMT when the person is nervous, touchy, restless, weepy, depressed and has headaches and swollen, tender breasts. It is a frequently-used remedy for breast problems: mastitis, swollen or cracked nipples, swollen breasts during breastfeeding, for thin, watery milk, and when the mother gets weepy every time the baby is at the breast. It can be used if the milk continues after weaning. Use for leucorrhoea that is acrid and cream-like or milky and thin. There may also be polyps in the vagina. Pulsatilla can be given to help correct the position of the foetus in pregnancy, for false labour or where the labour contractions are ineffectual and spasmodic. This remedy includes stinging and painful varicose veins that are worse during pregnancy.

Modalities: Worse: warmth, warm air, a warm bed, wet feet, in the evening, rich foods, ice-cream, eggs, at puberty, during pregnancy, before periods. Better: cold, fresh, open air, gentle motion, erect posture, after crying, pressure, lying down with the head up.

Purple Coneflower   *Echinacea angustifolia* or *Echinacea purpurea*

See Echinacea.

✳ Raspberry   *Rubus idaeus*

Parts used: Leaves, fruit

Habitat: Europe and Asia; thrives in damp soil where it can grow wild

Main constituents: Leaves: flavonoids, polypeptides and tannins; fruit: also pectin and vitamins

Actions: Astringent, toning

Main uses: This is one of the best herbs for toning the muscles. Use during any fitness regime or when dieting, as it will help tone slack muscles. As a uterine tonic it will help tone the uterine muscles and will prepare the body for an easier labour. Take for 3 months before giving birth. During labour, drink raspberry-leaf tea to help prevent haemorrhage and then continue drinking for 2–3 weeks after the birth to help contract the muscles and resume the normal shape. Promotes milk production. Combine with motherwort for threat of miscarriage. Use for PMT or for prolonged periods. As an astringent this herb can be used as a mouthwash or a gargle for mouth ulcers, hoarseness and sore throats. Externally, raspberry-leaf infusion can be used as an eyewash for conjunctivitis. The fruit is used less medicinally, but is more nutritious and has a cooling action.

Contraindications: Not to be used in the first 3 months of pregnancy.

Dosage: Infuse 25g to 500ml boiling water. Drink freely or 1 cup per day for the last 3 months of pregnancy. Tincture: 1:5 in 45 per cent alcohol, 2ml 3 times daily.

Red Clover   *Trifolium pratense*

Parts used: Aerial parts
  Habitat: Temperate climates; grown as a green manure for its nitrogen-fixing abilities
  Main constituents: Coumarins, flavonoids, isoflavones, minerals, vitamins, volatile oil
  Actions: Alterative, antispasmodic, phyto-oestrogenic, sedative
  Main uses: One of the main herbs used in blood purifying. Good for skin problems and for cleansing the lymphatic system. It has been used for mastitis and the prevention of cancer. Used in the treatment of tumours, in particular for breast cancer, and to relieve menopausal symptoms, including those where the heart is affected. Can be used as a mouthwash for ulcers and sore throats.
  Contraindications: Not to be used during pregnancy.
  Dosage: Infuse 1 teaspoon to a cup of boiling water. Drink 3 times daily. Tincture: 1:5 in 25 per cent alcohol, average dose 2ml 3 times daily.

Red Sage   *Salvia officinalis*

See Sage.

Rhubarb (Chinese)   *Rheum palmatum*

Parts used: Bark, rhizome
  Habitat: Native to Asia, grows near wet areas
  Main constituents: Anthraquinones, flavonoids, rutin, tannins
  Actions: Anti-inflammatory, antiseptic, astringent, bitter, laxative, tonic
  Main uses: In larger doses, rhubarb root will have a laxative action; in smaller doses it will tend to be more constipating, due to the level of tannins. This herb therefore can be used in either case to regulate bowel movements. In the treatment of constipation, it is especially useful where the muscles of the colon are weak. Use also for complaints of the liver and gall bladder. It is toning for the digestive tract and an appetite stimulant.
  Contraindications: Do not use during pregnancy or when breastfeeding, during periods or where there are kidney stones.

Dosage: Take 2–3 capsules at bedtime or decoct 25g in 500ml of water and drink before bedtime.

❈ Rhus Tox   *Rhus toxicodendron*

This homoeopathic remedy affects the fibrous tissue and covers rheumatic symptoms of the ligaments or joints. It is good for aching, sore joints and muscles.

Mental and emotional indications: There can be mental restlessness, with a feeling of despondency, sadness, anxiety and depression which gets worse in the evening; also a tendency to weep without knowing why and a desire to be alone. These people can be forgetful, and there is a fear of being poisoned and of drowning. In children, there can be rigidity and anxiety, while being in the cold and damp makes them feel mentally worse.

Physical: Pains are tearing, sticking and shooting, and they get worse at night. It is difficult to find a position to rest in. The key indication to this remedy is that the symptoms are worse from rest and at the start of movement. They improve with prolonged movement. It is excellent for sprained ankles and wrists, strained ligaments and tendons around the joints or strained and pulled muscles. Symptoms get worse in cold, wet and damp conditions; they improve from the heat.

Rhus tox is a good remedy to use whenever there is pain and stiffness that compels movement. Movement brings relief until exhaustion forces rest, but rest then makes the symptoms start up again. It can be a remedy for heart trouble due to overexertion. A rhus-tox fever is very hot with a high temperature, even though the person feels cold and needs extra covers. There is restlessness and slight relief comes from shifting positions, but the person may be motionless from exhaustion. Headaches feel as if a board is strapped to the forehead. Dreams are often of work and things that need to be done.

Rhus tox is a remedy that follows arnica well (see pages 198–9 for the homoeopathic dosage).

Digestion: There is hunger without appetite, an empty sensation in the stomach but no desire for food. Drowsiness after eating. A craving for cold drinks and ices, but these will create nausea after eating.

Fibrous tissues: This is the remedy when they are inflamed from overexertion, ligaments feel strained. Symptoms include slipped discs, back pain, arthritis, lumbago in the small of the back, pains from trying to get up and stiff neck and back pains that are worse from cold and better from warmth.

Skin: Dry, hot and itchy. A triangular red tip to the tongue is a key indicator for this remedy. Rhus tox is good for eruptions of vesicles, as in chickenpox and shingles. Itching is not relieved by scratching. There can be moist eruptions which are worse on hairy parts. Swelling of the joints. Red, spotty, itchy skin rapidly progresses to vessication and swelling, and then into yellow pus and scabs with surrounding yellow skin, which looks red and angry (as in chickenpox). Eczema, particularly of the face, neck and genitals. Eruptions are dark red. Swollen glands particularly under the arms (*see also* graphites). The eyelids are inflamed red, stiff and gluey.

Modalities: Worse: rest, at the beginning of movement, overexertion, damp, cold and wet. Better: continued motion, heat and hot baths, massage, rubbing, changing position.

Rose   *Rosa* x *damascena, R. gallica, R. rugosa*

Parts used: Petals

Habitat: Cultivated throughout the world

Main constituents: Volatile oil

Actions: Antidepressant, antiseptic, astringent, tonic

Main uses: Roses can be added to a blend of herbs both for added taste and for their gently toning properties. Combine with elderflower and marshmallow to help with eczema and other skin conditions. Give with motherwort for menstrual or menopausal problems. Add to lavender to help sleep. The tincture has been shown to have antimicrobial properties. Use diluted as a vaginal wash for pruritus and discharges.

Contraindications: None.

Dosage: 1 teaspoon in a cup of boiling water. Tincture: 1:4 in 60 per cent alcohol, average dose 2–4ml 2–3 times daily.

Rose Oil   *Rosa damascena* or *Rosa centifolia*

The queen of the oils, rose has been used for centuries for medicinal purposes and as a perfume. It is available as an absolute (solvent extracted) or the very costly rose otto (essential oil). It is wonderful to use in floral fragrance blends, but try to use the oil rather than the absolute when creating blends for massage. It is an expensive oil, as something like 25g of oil will come from 40,000 flowerheads. Frequently adulterated with palmarosa.

Family: Rosaceae

Parts used: Flowerheads collected at dawn

Main constituents: Alcohols, esters, monoterpenes, phenols, sesquiterpenes

Fragrance: Richly floral. Softer, less sweet and heavy when diluted.

Main uses: This oil has a well-known effect on the emotional and mental levels. It is soothing, uplifting and balancing. It has been used as an aphrodisiac. It has a regulating effect on the hormones and is excellent to use for PMT or irregularities of women's cycles. Said to help with infertility. It can be used to help mood swings, irritability and depression during the menopause. Use to tone the uterus before and after pregnancy, also for post-natal depression and where there is a lack of confidence. Rose oil has antiseptic properties and can be used for burns and cuts. Excellent for skin complaints, is toning and good for broken capillaries. Use for respiratory problems and as a tonic to the digestion.

Safety and application: As a pure oil this is non-toxic and non-irritant. Combine in creams for the face, into bath bases and massage oils, particularly with evening primrose oil for very dry skin and skin troubled from stress and transitions.

Rosemary   *Rosmarinus officinalis*

Parts used: Top cuttings, leaves and twigs

Habitat: Native to the Mediterranean areas.

Main constituents: Diterpenes, flavonoids, rosmarinic acid, volatile oil

Actions: Antibacterial, antioxidant, antispasmodic, nervine, sedative, tonic

Main uses: Traditionally known to increase the circulation, especially to the head, hence its reputation in helping to improve the memory. Good for poor circulation and fainting, giddiness. Use to aid concentration. Good for pre-exam studying and to help with stress and nervous debility. It stimulates and nourishes the nervous system. Can be good for depression, headaches and migraines that improve with heat. Warming and stimulating for the digestion, will increase the appetite and relieve wind. Improves cramps. A tonic for the elderly. Use for insomnia where the cause is nervous exhaustion. Strengthens blood vessels, good for weak capillaries. Good for hair growth. Make a strong infusion of rosemary (infuse 100g to 2 litres of boiling water, leave to brew for at least 20 minutes) to create a strengthening bath to revive the body and lift the spirits.

Contraindications: Avoid in in therapeutic doses in pregnancy and with high blood pressure.

Dosage: ½ teaspoon to 1 cup of boiling water. Drink 3 times daily. Tincture: 1:5 in 45 per cent alcohol, average dose 2–4ml 3 times daily. Rosemary wine is a warming tonic. Drink 5ml daily.

Rosemary Oil   *Rosmarinus officinalis*

Wonderfully fragrant, evocative of the Mediterranean, rosemary has been traditionally used for centuries for medicinal purposes. Steam distilled in many countries on both the north and south sides of the Mediterranean, the oil varies considerably in quality and it is difficult to obtain a true fragrance. It is added to many commercial products.

Family: Lamiaceae (labiatae)

Main constituents: Alcohols, esters, ketones, monoterpenes, oxides, sesquiterpenes

Fragrance: Herbaceous, green, sweet, can be camphoraceous

Main uses: A strongly stimulating oil known for its warming action on the circulation and nerves. Helps relieve depression, headaches, neuralgia, mental tiredness, poor memory, stress and vertigo. Will aid concentration. Use to help with exams and driving tests! As a tonic, rosemary will have a beneficial action on the heart, helping to regulate the blood pressure. Use for arteriosclerosis, for coldness of the extremities and poor circulation. Rosemary will have an anti-septic and decongestant effect on the respiratory system. Use for coughs, asthma, whooping cough and chronic lung problems. Promotes the flow of bile and helps painful digestive problems. As a diuretic, use for cystitis and oedemic swellings. Apply in a massage oil to relieve painful periods. Combine in a suppository for vaginal discharges and fungal infections. An excellent oil to include in blends for arthritis and rheumatism. Good for stiffness, sports preparation and muscular weakness. As an anti-inflammatory it will bring relief to muscular aches and pains. Rosemary is well known to add a shine to hair. Combine with cedarwood and lavender in coconut oil as a treatment for hair loss.

Safety and application: Non-toxic, non-sensitizing. Use in dilution of 2 per cent in blends.

Ruta   *Ruta graveolens*

This is a good homoeopathic remedy to use alongside arnica.

General symptoms: It can be given for injured or bruised bones, fibrous tissue, tendons, cartilage or periosteum (tissue covering the bone), tendonitis or whiplash injuries. The injuries tend to be very painful. This remedy is indicated where there is injury and sprain, particularly when it involves the periosteum and wrists and ankles. Pains are sore, aching and bruised, there is a feeling of restlessness. It is an ideal remedy for treating strains around joints. Use for persistent stiffness after a sprain or strain. Give ruta when rhus tox fails to work. Limbs can feel heavy and weak, legs give way on getting up or going up the stairs. There are pains in the hips and bones of the legs. There is unsteadiness when walking and extreme weakness of the legs after straining the back, weariness and feelings of intense weakness and despair. Affected parts become sore even in bed. There may be a general feeling of dissatisfaction and a fear of anything new.

Eyes: Ruta is a good remedy for the eyes or eye strain which is then followed by a headache. Eyes can be red, hot and painful after reading small print or reading in a dim light. This remedy helps weak eye muscles.

It is indicated for 'housemaid's knee', 'tennis elbow' and rheumatism, especially if due to strain or overexertion. It is particularly indicated when the bony parts are affected. Use for sciatica which is worse from lying down or in the evening and gets better during the day. Give ruta for osteoarthritis which comes on from an old sprained ankle or knee.

Use for prolapse of the rectum which has occurred on stooping, after delivery or during a stool. Ruta helps to strengthen prolapsed muscles.

Modalities: Worse: lying, sitting, eye strain, cold air, wind, damp, sprains, injury from overexertion. Better: warmth, massage, lying on the back.

✳ Sabadilla   *Sabadilla officinarum*

This is a homoeopathic remedy which is often used for hayfever, 'flu or conditions affecting the mucous membranes.

Mental and emotional indications: These are not very marked; the main ones are fears, confusion and fixed ideas, which are often to do with the state of the body.

Physical: Persistent, spasmodic sneezing, with itching or tickling in the nose. The nose may be blocked or dry or with a profuse nasal discharge. The person may rub or pick the nose. The eyes may be watery or red, with discharge, which will water when sneezing, coughing, yawning or walking in the open air. A distinctive indication of this remedy is an acute sense of smell. The nasal discharge will get worse with the smell of flowers. The face is hot and red, it burns as if scalded, the lips feel hot. The soft palette of the mouth itches. A sensation of a lump in the throat makes the person swallow constantly. Sabadilla is a remedy for worms where the symptoms are a craving hunger for sweet food and a crawling, itching anus, alternating with itching in the nose and ears. Sexual desire may increase with worms.

Modalities: Worse: cold air, drinks, periodically, during a full and new moon. Better: open air, heat, warm food and drink, eating and swallowing.

✳ Sabina   *Sabina*

This is a homoeopathic remedy useful to help stop bleeding in the uterus. This can be due to either loss of tone in the blood vessels or a miscarriage.

Mental and emotional indications: These are not marked, although there is an intolerance to music, which can lead to excessive nervousness. There may be uneasiness, restlessness and increased sexual desire.

Physical: The main area that this remedy covers is the female reproductive organs. Sabina is a good remedy for leucorrhoea which is thick, yellow, smells foul and replaces periods. It can be used for periods that are early, profuse, protracted, part fluid and part clotted, or where the flow comes in waves. It may be accompanied by labour-type pains, paroxysms or colicky pains that go from the sacrum to the pubes, or pains shooting up the vagina. Blood is hot and gushing. There may be bleeding between periods accompanied by sexual excitement. There is a tendency to miscarry, especially around the third month. It is good for haemorrhaging from the uterus which follows a miscarriage or premature labour. This gets worse from the slightest movement but gets better from walking. Use where there are intense afterbirth pains and a retained placenta. There may be itching in the genitals, increased sexual desire and itchy nipples. Sabina can be given during the menopause where there is excessive bleeding.

Modalities: Worse: night-time, heat, pregnancy, menopause, music. Better: cold and open air.

✤ Sage (Red and Common)   *Salvia officinalis*

Parts used: Aerial parts

Habitat: Mediterranean areas

Main constituents: Diterpenes, tannins, volatile oil

Actions: Antiseptic, astringent, bitter, decongestant, hormonal stimulant, reduces sweating

Main uses: The two varieties of *Salvia officinalis* can be described together, as their actions are very similar. Popular as an ingredient in cooking, sage has a long tradition as an effective healer. It has traditionally been used as a remedy for sore throats. It is effective for tonsillitis, laryngitis and gum conditions that are sore and bleeding, such as gingivitis. Sage will stimulate the circulation and warm the body. It is an excellent herb to use for the weak and debilitated, who are generally cold. As a digestive tonic, sage will increase the level of hydrochloric acid in the stomach and will help break the food down. Use where the digestion is upset or weak. It will promote absorption and help prevent putrefaction in the gut. Sage is a good lung tonic, traditionally used to treat asthma, good for cold and weakness and catarrhal respiratory problems. As a hormonal stimulant, it helps regulate periods and reduces hot flushes during the menopause, as well as reducing sweating. It will help dry up milk production. It is also excellent for slow-healing wounds. Externally, sage infusion can be used as a treatment for dandruff and as a wash for oily skin with acne.

Contraindications: Do not use when pregnant or breastfeeding. Do not use where there is high blood pressure or epilepsy. Not for long-term use.

Dosage: Infuse 1 teaspoonful of leaves to 1 cup of boiling water. Take 3 times daily. Use same as mouthwash or gargle. Tincture: 1:5 in 45 per cent alcohol. Average dose 2–4ml 3 times daily.

✴ Sage Oil   *Salvia lavandulifolia*

It is best to use a sage that has a low thujone content. Generally this is the Spanish variety (*lavandulifolia*) rather than the Dalmatian (*officinalis*).

Family: Lamiacea (labiatae)

Parts used: Leaves and woody stems

Main constituents of Spanish sage: alcohols, esters, ketones, monoterpenes, oxides

Fragrance: Herbaceous, fresh, dry; Dalmatian sage is more camphoraceous

Main uses: Sage is a powerful stimulant and can be used as a tonic for the nervous system and circulation. Use in inhalation for respiratory problems, particularly of the throat. Best use is for helping to regulate periods or during the menopause where there is accompanying depression, mood swings and hot flushes. This oil is also very effective for toning muscles. Use in a warming and softening blend for stiffness and aching.

Safety and application: Sage oil is cumulative. When in doubt, use either clary sage or rosemary oils or sage in the herb form. Do not use during pregnancy or where there is a risk of epilepsy. Do not exceed 0.5 per cent in diluted blends.

✴ St John's Wort   *Hypericum perforatum*

Parts used: Aerial parts

Habitat: Europe, temperate climates

Main constituents: Flavonoids, hyperforin, hypericin

Actions: Analgesic, antidepressant, anti-inflammatory, antioxidant, antiviral, nervine, sedative

Main uses: Much research has been done on this herb and has shown that it has a significant tonic effect on the nervous system. It is used to relieve depression with well-known and reported success throughout the world. Use for anxiety, stress, Seasonal Affective Disorder, symptoms of overwork. Take where the digestive system is affected by nervous conditions, use for peptic ulcers. Externally, apply the macerated oil *(see page 190)* for neuralgia, shingles, sciatica and shock. Use the tincture for all wounds and skin damage where the nerves are affected and for shooting, stabbing, stitching pains. Good for puncture wounds, animal bites, stings and burns. Use for toothache, extractions and joint pain. As an antiviral, St John's Wort is used for treating chickenpox, herpes and HIV. It is particularly good for emotional problems arising during the menopause, decrease in vitality, depression and mood swings. Good for the memory and clarity of thinking. Combine with rosemary and sage for senile dementia.

Contraindications: Take care when on prescribed medication, as there is a possibility of interaction. Suitable for mild to moderate depression, not suitable for severe depression.

Dosage: Infuse 1 teaspoon in a cup of boiling water. Take 3 times daily or as required. Macerate oil as directed and use as base for massage as indicated. Tincture: 1:3 in 45 per cent alcohol, average dose 2–4ml. Combine either the oil or tincture into an ointment or make a cream for external treatment for burns, etc. A classic blend is with marigold for wound and burn healing.

Sandalwood Oil   *Santalum album*

Distilled from the dried heartwood of these increasingly rare trees, this plant has virtually become an endangered species.

Family: Santalaceae

Parts used: Dried heartwood and groundroots

Main constituents: Acids, alcohols, sesquiterpenes

Fragrance: Powerful, tenacious, smooth, sensuous, woody. The oil is thick and viscous, and the fragrance really only comes out with the warmth of the skin.

Main uses: Used in traditional Ayurevedic medicine as an antiseptic and tonic, sandalwood is particularly good for the urinary system. Use also for respiratory complaints, where coughs are dry and unproductive. Sandalwood is excellent for dry or ageing skin and eczema conditions which are dry, although it is also good for oily skin as it is astringent and will help to clear acne and skin irritations. Traditionally included in soaps and men's products, this is a great oil to use in perfumes, incenses and aromatherapy blends. It is known to be an aphrodisiac and to promote relaxation.

Safety and application: Non-toxic, non-irritant, non-sensitizing. Use in dilutions of up to 2 per cent.

꙳ Sarsaparilla *Aralia nudicaulis*

Parts used: Root

Habitat: Tropical and temperate regions

Main constituents: Minerals, phytosterols, resin, saponins, starch

Actions: Alterative, anti-inflammatory, diaphoretic, hormonal balancer, tonic

Main uses: Commonly known as an ingredient for root beer and mainly used to help cleanse the body and improve the condition of the skin. Use for eczema, psoriasis, also gout, rheumatism. Traditionally used as a male aphrodisiac, it can also help depression during menopause and PMT, and act as a sexual tonic.

Contraindications: None.

Dosage: Decoct 25g root to 500ml water for 20 minutes. Drink a cup 3 times daily. Tincture: 1:5 in 25 per cent alcohol. Take 2ml 3 times daily.

꙳ Saw Palmetto *Serenoa repens*

Parts used: Berries

Habitat: Native to North America

Main constituents: Flavonoids, polysaccharides, volatile oil

Actions: Anti-inflammatory, antispasmodic, diuretic, sedative, tonic

Main uses: This herb is a good tonic, especially for the reproductive system, because it helps to regulate the functioning of the organs of both sexes. It has been used to treat infertility in men by increasing the quantity and quality of sperm. Research has shown that it is effective in reducing the enlargement of the prostate gland. Use also for infection of the prostate. It has a marked effect on the urinary system and is used to improve flow of urine and as an antiseptic. Being a tonic, saw palmetto can be used to build up strength in the body tissues and help put on weight in men and women.

Contraindications: None

Dosage: Decoct ½ teaspoon of berries in 200ml of water for 15 minutes. Drink 3 times daily. Tincture: 1:5 in 45 per cent alcohol, average dose 2–4ml.

⚜ Senna   *Senna alexandrina*

Synonyms: Cassia senna
  Parts used: Leaves, pods
  Habitat: Africa
  Main constituents: Anthraquinones, flavonoids, mucilage
  Actions: Laxative, stimulant
  Main uses: A strong laxative that is best used for occasional constipation. It is particularly appropriate where there are anal fissures and so a soft stool is important. If this herb is taken regularly it will cause a weakening of the bowel muscles. Best to prepare it with ginger root or other carminative herbs to help prevent griping. The pods are gentler than the leaves.
  Contraindications: Do not give to children, those suffering from IBS or abdominal pain, or during pregnancy
  Dosage: Soak 3–6 pods for 10 hours in a cup of warm water, strain and take at bedtime.

⚜ Sepia   *Sepia*

A major homoeopathic remedy, particularly effective in the treatment of women with hormonal problems or for female reproduction. It is made from the inky substance ejected by cuttlefish as a defence mechanism and was used as a pigment in paints.
  Mental and emotional indications: The overwhelming aspect of this remedy is of being worn out – pressure a sepia person and they will become irritable. They want to be left alone; they are indifferent to life and work and are easily offended, leading to anger and irritability. They appear to be sagging on all levels, including their spirits. Sepia is marked by sadness; there will be a tendency to cry when listening to music or when the person talks about their symptoms. They are averse to company but also dread being alone (*see also* lycopodium). There is anxiety and confusion and a poor memory as well as a sullenness which makes relationships with other people difficult. They are hardworking and refuse to give in, often to the detriment of their friendships. Their sadness can alternate with indifference and resentment. Sepia is a remedy for people who force themselves to continue through a sense of responsibility, but find no joy in living or have no energy left. These mental and emotional indications may arise during the various changes in a woman's life – puberty, childbearing, menopause, etc.

Physical: Sepia is marked by dragging-down sensations and a gnawing, weak, hollow feeling. There may be a brown mark across the nose (an indication that the liver is overloaded), and venous congestion leading to protruding veins. Sepia is to do with slow circulation and stagnation – all organs sag. There can be a pot belly, varicose veins, piles, prolapse of the uterus and vagina. There are heavy bearing-down feelings in the pelvic organs and a sensation that they will drop out. This can create a desire to cross the legs. There can be sensations of a lump in the colon, in the throat or of moving lumps in the stomach. All these symptoms are improved by exertion. Despite the worn-out emphasis of this remedy, the person who fits the sepia picture loves dancing and exercising. The sepia person can think and talk about sex but feel too tired for sex. The vagina may become very dry. Sepia is an excellent remedy for menopausal problems, especially hot flushes and loss of hair, if there is the accompanying sepia picture *(see also lachesis, page 298)*. Also effective for headaches and migraines.

Women's complaints: Give for nausea or morning sickness which comes on at the sight and smell of food; for thrush and leucorrhoea which are yellowish. Sepia 30C can be given for threatened miscarriage or where there is a tendency to miscarry between months 5 and 7 of the pregnancy. Use for period problems, periods which are early, late or absent, bleeding in the middle of the cycle and then periods which are heavy and clotted. Headaches may occur at the time of periods, either before or during, and they can be accompanied by nausea. They are usually left-sided and the eyelids feel droopy and heavy. The person is sensitive to a heavy, warm atmosphere.

Sepia will treat catarrhal complaints, especially those of a chronic nature and where cheesy lumps are coughed up. It is also good for fungal complaints such as athlete's foot and ringworm. Use for constipation where stools stay in the rectum, often as small balls which can create a sensation of having a ball in the anus; these sensations are relieved by passing a stool. These constipation symptoms can come on during pregnancy. Use for varicose veins and high blood pressure. Urine can be red with sandy sediment. There can be cutting pains in the bladder before urination, which can be involuntary, especially upon coughing, laughing and sneezing. The sepia person is prone to having droopy, lifeless hair, with sensitive roots.

Modalities: Worse: thunderstorms, lying on left side, eating, menopause, cold, cold air, before periods, during pregnancy, intercourse. Better: warmth, exercise, back massage, open air, exertion.

❋ Shepherd's Purse   *Capsella bursa-pastoris*

Parts used: Aerial parts

   Habitat: Found in temperate areas

   Main constituents: Flavonoids, histamine, polypeptides, plant acids, tyramine

   Actions: Antiseptic, astringent, diuretic, emmenagogue, haemostatic

   Main uses: One of the main herbs to help stem heavy bleeding during periods, it can also be used where there is blood in the urine. As a diuretic and astringent, shepherd's purse will help disinfect the urinary system. Controls bleeding from fibroids in the womb, vomiting blood from the gut or dysentery. Use for nosebleeds.

   Contraindications: Not to be taken during pregnancy. Use cautiously where there is a history of kidney stones.

   Dosage: Infuse 1 teaspoonful in a cup of boiling water. Take twice daily. Tincture: 1:5 in 45 per cent alcohol, 2ml in water 3 times daily.

❋ Silicea   *Silicea terra*

One of the 12 homoeopathic remedies known as tissue salts, due to the minerals from which the remedy is made. This is found in the tissues of the body. It is also an important homoeopathic remedy suited to complaints that develop over a long period of time. Give this remedy to expel any splinters or foreign objects.

   Mental and emotional indications: The silicea person lacks stamina. There is a yielding submissiveness arising from a lack of energy to hold onto their own point of view. They will not oppose anybody else, even if they think them to be wrong. They tend to be refined, intelligent, easy going, mild and reserved, although they make friends and talk about themselves easily. They are not demanding of other people's time or impatient. They do not waste time on trivia. Children will take a reprimand to heart – they do not forget it and their behaviour is easily suppressed. They can grow up with fixed ideas. Silicea is a good remedy to give for anticipatory fears, e.g. exams, public speaking, etc. The silicea person can be afraid of failing. They do well in whatever they undertake, but they get worn out, especially from a large amount of mental work. They can be obstinate and passively control others, and can be irritable to cover their underlying timidity. As children, they may learn to read and write slowly and have difficulty in understanding, they lack grit and are over-sensitive to noise, touch or light and criticism. They avoid arguments.

Physical: The children are thin and puny, often with weak ankles and a lack of stamina. They have large heads and a distended belly. The head and face or feet sweat, rather than the whole body. Symptoms often develop in cold, damp weather, although they may improve in cold, dry weather. Silicea is an important remedy for clearing up abscesses and boils. Give silicea after hepar sulph to complete the healing process. It will help eliminate foreign bodies, such as splinters, warts, pimples, pustules and suppurating cavities. It should be taken for complaints that are caused by suppressed discharges, particularly suppressed sweat.

Abdomen: Constipation, caused by inactivity of rectum, the stool is partly expelled then recedes, stools remain a long time in rectum. This is worse before and during periods.

Coughs: Dry, tickly with hoarseness, worse from cold and better for warm drinks. Green expectoration during the daytime. Colds go to the chest. If the picture fits, silicea is a good remedy for asthma, bronchitis and later stages of pneumonia.

Eyes: May have blocked tear ducts, ulcers on the cornea and styes.

Ears: Ears have an offensive thick, yellow discharge. There may be middle-ear infections, and catarrh of the Eustachian tube, with deafness. There may be hard, crusty scabs in the nose, catarrh and a loss of taste and smell.

Head: Symptoms include chronic sick headaches, with nausea and vomiting. The headache starts in the morning at the back of the head and by midday it is on the forehead. Headaches rise from the nape of the neck to one eye, especially the right eye. There are weekly headaches which are worse at night from light, noise, cold air and studying. They get better with heat, from pressure and from wrapping the head. There are profuse headsweats with headaches.

Skin: Moist and scaly, and it has eruptions. Glands around the neck tend to enlarge with a cold. Glands become enlarged and hardened.

Stomach: Hiccups, nausea, vomiting, aversion to warm food; they can also have a dislike for meat and like cold things such as ice-cream and iced water. Symptoms are aggravated by milk.

Teeth: This is the remedy when teeth tend to break and crumble. There is a loss of enamel, and mouth abscesses in gums which feel better from warmth. Also enlarged tonsils and chronic sore throats with enlarged glands.

Women's complaints: Symptoms include cysts in the vagina, fistula openings and abscesses along the vulva, if they heal they leave hard nodules. Silicea is distinguished by offensive, cheesy-smelling discharges. Periods come on from excitement or when breastfeeding. There can be profuse milky leucorrhoea, hard lumps in the breast and breast abscesses.

Modalities: Worse: cold, cold air, draughts, damp, suppressed sweat, mental exertion, pressure, nervous excitement, light, noise, full moon, alcohol. Better: warmth, wrapping up the head, summer, wet, humid weather, profuse urination.

✳ Skullcap   *Scutellaria lateriflora*

Parts used: Aerial parts
  Habitat: Native of North America
  Main constituents: Flavonoids, glucosides, iridoids, tannins
  Actions: Antispasmodic, nervine, sedative
  Main uses: One of the best sedating herbs that is also a tonic to the nervous system. Good to use for many states of anxiety and tension. Use for headaches, migraine, insomnia, PMT, depression, overwork and over use of mental energy.
  Contraindications: None.
  Dosage: Infuse 1 teaspoon to 1 cup of boiling water. Take 3 times daily. Tincture: 1:5 in 45 per cent alcohol, 3ml 3 times daily.

✳ Slippery Elm   *Ulmus rubra*

Synonyms: Ulmus fulva
  Parts used: Bark
  Habitat: Native to North America, also in Europe
  Main constituents: Mucilage, starch
  Actions: Demulcent, drawing, expectorant, nutrient, soothing
  Main uses: This herb forms a lining of the gut. It will be quickly soothing for any inflammation or ulceration. Give for heartburn or hiatus hernia. Use for any problems to do with acidity. Excellent for colitis and where there is inflammation of the bowel. Good for summer diarrhoea, gastro-enteritis, travel sickness, wind and indigestion; slippery elm is also highly nutritious. Give to convalescents and for digestive weakness. Helps to increase weight. Also good for cystitis and chronic urinary irritation. Good for respiratory problems, soothing for coughs and bronchitis. Externally, can be used as a poultice, particularly with marigold or marshmallow, on boils or infected wounds.

Contraindications: None.

Dosage: For a soothing, nutritious food, mix 1 tablespoonful into a paste before adding hot water and milk. As a poultice, mix 1 teaspoon into a paste and put on muslin, before placing over infected area.

Speedwell   *Veronica officinalis*

Parts used: Aerial parts

Habitat: Native to Europe

Main constituents: Flavonoids, glycosides, iridoids

Actions: Alterative, diuretic, expectorant, tonic

Main uses: For nervous exhaustion that prevents a good night's sleep. Helps concentration and headaches. Use for skin complaints that are itchy and flaky. Can be used as a diuretic and for respiratory problems.

Contraindications: None.

Dosage: 1 teaspoon to a cup of boiling water, 3 times daily.

Spongia   *Spongia tosta*

This homoeopathic remedy is good for hard coughs and croup.

Mental and emotional indications: These are marked by fear.

Physical: This remedy can be used for sore throats, those that have dryness in the nose and throat accompanied by sneezing. Sore-throat symptoms get worse from eating sweet things or warm drinks. The throat is sensitive to touch. It can go on to develop into a dry, hoarse and barking cough. It can be a really good remedy to give children with croup *(see aconite, page 224)*. They can have a suffocating cough which will wake them, and they will be fearful, anxious and tearful. The cough will be tight, hollow, barking or crowing, and get worse after midnight.

Spongia is good to use when breathing sounds as though it is through a sponge. It can also feel like this. There can be burning in the throat which gets worse at night. The cough does not sound bad during the day but by midnight it can sound barking and crowing. It is good for dry coughs that get worse on successive nights. Mucus can develop after several days, with a feeling of fullness in the chest; expectoration is usually easy.

Modalities: Worse: sweet food, warm drinks. Better: lying with head low.

✳ Squaw Vine   *Mitchella repens*

Parts used: Leaves and seeds
  Habitat: Native to North America
  Main constituents: Alkaloids, glycosides, mucilage
  Actions: Astringent, uterine tonic
  Main uses: A herb traditionally used to prepare the body for childbirth. Take for the final three months to tone the uterus before labour. It is good to continue after the birth to help involute the womb. Can also help to calm after birth pains. It is a uterine tonic and can be used to regulate periods and reduce heavy flow. Use for bloating, PMT. Acts as a gentle diuretic, can assist oedema.
  Contraindications: Not recommended for the first three months of pregnancy.
  Dosage: 1 teaspoon to a cup of boiling water. Take twice daily. Tincture: 1:5 in 45 per cent alcohol, 2ml twice daily.

✳ Staphysagria   *Delphinium staphisagria*

This homoeopathic remedy works for those individuals who suppress their emotions and the physical symptoms arising from suppression.
  Mental and emotional indications: These people are reactive. They can become speechless through intense feelings. They will control their emotions but then go to pieces afterwards. They may suppress their anger for a while, then when it starts to come out they will tremble with it and be unable to work or sleep. Yet this is not a remedy for the aggressive type as they are often sweet, sensitive and refined. There is, however, grief in the background, often broken relationships. They are emotionally weak, making them too receptive and eager to please everyone, in particular those that they love. They are unable to assert themselves. They become overwhelmed by a sense of their own lack of confidence. This patient will not want to cause any bother, but if given time they will open up. Although this has traditionally been a remedy for women it can also be appropriate for men hurt by relationships. Also for children with deep insecurities and fear, maybe because of parents that were abusive or bullying at school. This remedy is for victims. It will help give them confidence.
  Generally they are inhibited by their fear of hurting others and have a very low self-esteem. Even if they have an outburst of anger, it will not be aimed at anyone for fear of causing pain. When they are hurt they withdraw and feel lonely and talk to themselves, though wanting company and to be included.

Highly sensitive, they are easily embarrassed. They are sensitive on all levels. Any situation that is invasive will have a major effect – such as a surgical operation or sexual intercourse for the first time. They may say that they have never fully recovered. 'Violation' is a key word for this remedy. This is a remedy to consider giving after someone has been raped, mugged or assaulted. They will feel angry and become powerless.

Physical: The staphysagria type will find it difficult to sleep because her mind is crowded with ideas. She is wakeful at night with erotic dreams, and sleepy by day. Yawning and stretching will bring tears to her eyes.

Abdomen: Sensations of weakness and bearing down in the abdomen. Wind smells of rotten eggs. Give after abdominal operations that are slow to heal or remain painful. Good to use after surgical operations.

Cough: Worse after upsets, cleaning teeth, indignation and tobacco smoke. Croupy cough in winter.

Ears: Deafness in children accompanied by enlarged tonsils.

Eyes: Symptoms include recurring styes, nodosities on eyelids, heat and dryness in the eyeballs, blepharitis and sore, red, crusty eyelids.

Head: Headaches feel as if the forehead is about to split open and this gets worse with movement and stooping. It feels as if the brain is bruised. It improves with yawning. It can feel as if there's a ball of lead in the forehead. There is vertigo which is worse from walking and turning rapidly. Also, a tingling, tickling scalp and dandruff. This remedy has also been used to treat head lice if used in a lotion.

Mouth: The teeth are sensitive to touch; they can be black, brittle and decayed. These people cannot bear having fillings and their gums bleed easily.

Skin: There are warts which tingle like insects under the skin. Take for incised wounds, especially those from operations, causing great pain.

Stomach: Symptoms include the desire for milk, bread and soups; the person likes liquid foods, wine, brandy and tobacco. Use for severe pains after abdominal operations, hiccups, nausea that is worse in the morning and feelings of extreme hunger even when the stomach is full.

Urinary symptoms: Use for cystitis that occurs after intercourse; an urgent desire to urinate, pain after urination, pains after difficult labour.

Women's complaints: In a staphysagria woman, the suppression of anger caused by a destructive relationship may lead to breast lumps, fibroids and tumours. Later, she may become indifferent and adopt an uncaring attitude on a sexual level as well, though generally a staphysagria type is very sexually motivated. Symptoms include extreme sensitivity of genitals, sexual fantasies, mind dwells on sex, inflammation of ovaries and feelings of burning and stinging. Periods are irregular, late, profuse or scanty. There can be discharges arising from anger or indignation. A remedy to give after a Caesarean or an episiotomy where the scar is slow to heal and the area remains tender.

Modalities: Worse: quarrelling, grief, indignation, humiliation, masturbation, sexual excess, tobacco and laceration. Better: after breakfast, yawning, warmth, intercourse, rest at night.

Stone Root   *Collinsonia canadensis*

This herb, as the name suggests, has several properties which help to break up stones. These will then ease their passage away from the kidneys and gall bladder. It will help relax spasms in the ureterus and gall bladder, and has an astringent and tonic effect on the veins, making it helpful in treating piles and varicose veins. Stone root is also a diuretic and will help to flush out the urinary system.

Dosage: For all these mixtures infuse 1 teaspoon per cup of boiling water and drink 3 times a day. Using the stone root separately, use 30g (1oz) to 570ml (1 pint) of boiling water and drink a cup 3 times a day; with a tincture, use 2ml diluted in water and drink 3 times a day.

Sulphur   *Sulphur*

This homoeopathic remedy is often prescribed and is said to restore life to the spirit. It helps awaken the person to her purpose, putting her on the right path.

Mental and emotional indications: Sulphur is an excellent remedy for those who are under-functioning, ineffective and generally not getting themselves together. They tend to be unkempt and scruffy and have a disregard for their personal appearance and cleanliness. They may be great philosophers and inventors, and are unconventional, independent, inquisitive, rebellious and argumentative, but they can also be selfish, egocentric and self-satisfied. They tend to be self-deceptive and are prone to mental and physical inertia. They are daydreamers with poor memories and concentration. A picture of a typical sulphur person is of someone who is working on a thesis or project: they will start off on one thing and then pursue another idea, and then another, and the thesis will remain incomplete. They can be irritable, impatient, critical, nagging, discontented and dissatisfied, obstinate, sad or depressed.

Physical: A sulphur-type has a high-coloured face, red lips, red borders to eyelids, red ears and often stoops. Such people tend to feel hot easily. They are worse from standing and prefer to sit or lie down. Faintness or weak spells may be accompanied by great sleepiness. Sulphur is a good remedy to use where complaints get better then there are relapses again and again. Generally there is a tendency to congestion, burning, throbbing and flushes of heat. Mucus discharges are acrid, bloody, offensive and itchy. The top of the head feels hot and the feet feel cold.

Abdomen: There is diarrhoea which is offensive, watery and involuntary and worse in the early morning. Often they wake early morning (6 a.m.) and need a bowel movement. Diarrhoea alternates with constipation, when the stool is hard, large and difficult to pass. The anus is red and itchy, there may be worms, internal and external piles which are sore, bleeding, burning, itching, and worse during pregnancy. Also compare hamamelis and calc fluor.

Coughs: These tickle the larynx, they are violent and worse lying on the back or at night. There is rattling of mucus and heat in the chest, and greenish expectoration. Sulphur is often very helpful for pneumonia or bronchitis which tend to linger and are difficult to throw off. It can also help asthma and hayfever.

Head: Symptoms include headaches accompanied by nausea and vomiting. There are often headaches on Sundays (or days off) and with periods. Headaches come on if they do not eat. The nose may feel burning, produce a discharge which gets worse outside and tends to be blocked when indoors. There is frequent sneezing, and they may be very sensitive to smell, although unaware of their own, and feel nauseous about their own discharges.

Skin: Symptoms include dry, scaly, rough, raw, itchy eruptions. There is plenty of itching and it is enjoyable to scratch, although the skin condition gets worse afterwards and may bleed. Skin burns after scratching and is made worse from wearing wool. It is unhealthy, slow to heal, worse from washing, wind and air. Sulphur is a very useful remedy to give for skin eruptions that have been suppressed, such as boils or crops of eruptions all over the body. One eruption is followed by another. There can be eczema which alternates with asthma. With skin complaints, it is better to give sulphur in a low potency as it may aggravate the condition in high potency.

Sleep: There is a need to keep the feet out of bed as the soles burn. Sleep is unrefreshing; these people can be sleepy during the day but wakeful at night.

They have vivid dreams, talk, jerk and twitch during sleep and wake between 3–5 a.m., unable to go back to sleep.

Stomach: The appetite is either small or very large (sulphur-type people can be greedy). They tend to drink more than they eat, and like sweets, raw foods, beer, fat, spicy and unusual foods. There can be sudden hunger at 11 a.m. accompanied by weakness, and an 'all-gone' sensation in the stomach. There may be vomiting and nausea during pregnancy.

Women's complaints: The vulva and vagina burn, itch and are sore. Sulphur is a good remedy for thrush. There is an offensive perspiration on the genitals. Use for leucorrhoea which is yellow, burning and excoriating. Periods may be irregular, late, scanty, acrid, offensive and dark, there may be blackish blood which can bring about soreness or amenorrhoea. Use for cracked nipples, which feel sore and burning.

Modalities: Worse: using suppressive substances like anti-perspirants, medicated ointments, drugs, etc.; bathing, heat, overexertion, being in bed at 11 a.m., standing. Better: open air, sweating, motion, dry and warm weather.

Symphytum   *Symphytum officinale*

The homoeopathic remedy symphytum is one of the main remedies to help mend broken bones and fractures. It will help accelerate the growth of bone cells. Use for damaged sinews, tendons, cartilages and joints; also injuries from being hit in the eye and the area around the eye.

Modalities: Symptoms are worse from being touched.

Tarantula   *Tarantula hispania*

This homoeopathic remedy is made from the poisonous spider's bite. Traditionally the way to cure the bite was to dance all night, presumably in a state of mania. The symptoms that will indicate this remedy include great changes in temperament. The person is lively, restless and must keep moving, although this may make them feel worse. They are very sensitive to music and get excited, wanting to jump up and dance.

Mental and emotional indications: This type of person is highly strung and can become hysterical; she is uninhibited, very sensitive to touch and cold, often preoccupied with sex and her nerve endings are very sensitive. She can have orgasms without any feeling of relief and there is frequent desire for genital excitement *(consider also platina),* which can be followed by irritability and then depression. These people have a poor memory and can be cunning and underhand. The mind is not strong, they are unscrupulous and unpredictable, with no control over their emotions. They may fake illness when they want something or tend towards kleptomania. When a tarantula type is in an emotional state she trembles and can become physically violent to others as well as herself. She suffers from delusions. Laughter can swing into depression.

Physical: Pain: Pains cause twitching and jerking. The spine can be very sensitive to touch and can cause pain in the chest and heart regions; there is extreme sensitivity in the tips of the fingers, with a need to rub them. There are different kinds of pain but a feeling of burning is most common, especially in the rectum, on the palms of the hands, soles of the feet and in the uterus. Neuralgia is like thousands of needles, especially in the head. These people like having the head rubbed and their hair brushed.

Digestion: There may be an intense thirst for cold water and an empty, all-gone feeling, with burning in the stomach.

Skin: One of the main uses for this remedy is for treating sepsis, even quite severe cases, in the form of malignant ulcers, boils, anthrax, gangrene or carbuncles. The remedy helps to evacuate pus rapidly. The tissue is bluish purple or red, skin is septic with burning, stinging pains. This condition can look similar to the arsenicum or lachesis pictures. If these two remedies do not work it may be worth trying tarantula.

Women's complaints: Periods can be early and profuse, accompanied by an increase of sexual desire and irritability. There may be a sensation of something being alive in the womb – this comes on particularly after a sleep and during the time of the period. It is a remedy for hysterical pregnancies. The ovaries can feel very sensitive. There is violent itching of the genitals and this sensation can travel right up the vagina. There may be burning pains in the uterus. There is an increased dryness around the time of the period, especially in the throat, mouth and tongue.

Modalities: Worse: movement, touching affected parts, at night, bright colours, cold and damp, noise, music, intercourse, periodically once a year. Better: massage, sweating, open air, bright colours, music, smoking.

☙ Tea Tree Oil   *Melaleuca alternifolia*

Part of the eucalyptus family, this oil is generally used for its antiseptic and antibacterial functions.

Family: Myrtaceae
Parts used: Twigs and leaves
Main constituents: Alcohols, monoterpenes, oxides, sesquiterpenes
Fragrance: Medicinal, pungent, dry
Main uses: A popular oil for combating fungal, viral and microbial infections. An immune stimulant. Use for colds, 'flu and infectious diseases. It is anti-inflammatory, decongestant. Use where there is an infection of the respiratory system, coughs, bronchial infections, etc. An excellent skin oil, one that can be used undiluted to treat athlete's foot, bites, burns, ringworm and wounds, and as a deodorant. Use for veruccas, warts, callouses and corns. Tea tree is good for problems of the reproductive system, use for thrush, vaginal infections, Candida. Use as a mouthwash or in dental preparations.
Safety and application: Non-toxic externally, toxic internally. Use in inhalation, 1–2 drops in hot water. 2–3% dilution in massage oils or lotions. Dab on neat for small areas.

☙ Thyme   *Thymus vulgaris*

Parts used: Softer tops and flowers
Habitat: Native to Europe
Main constituents: Bitters, flavonoids, tannins, volatile oil
Actions: Antifungal, antiparasitic, antiseptic, antiviral, carminative, expectorant, tonic
Main uses: A highly antiseptic herb, although gentle on the skin. One of its main areas of use is on the respiratory system. It will help prevent colds and 'flu, being warming and antibacterial. It can be used for treating all mucous membranes. Use for coughs and infections where there are spasms and catarrh, also for blocked sinuses, earache and chest infections. Good where there is tiredness and debility associated with the respiratory system. Use as an infusion or as a syrup mixed with liquorice and honey. Thyme acts as a general warming tonic for the digestive system. Use for indigestion or infections, wind and diarrhoea. Can be used to dispel worms. Externally, use for ringworm, scabies, lice, stings and bites and fungal infections. Use in a douche for candidiasis and

thrush. It has been suggested that thyme is a powerful antioxidant. Drink as an infusion for its anti-ageing properties.

Contraindications: None.

Dosage: Infuse 1 teaspoonful per cup of boiling water and drink as required. For the bath, make a strong infusion using 2 handfuls of fresh thyme and 2 litres of boiling water. Leave to stand for 20 minutes. Add to the bath if feeling chilled and likely to get a cold. Thyme herbal infusion can also be used as a vaporizer for congestion. Tincture: 1:5 in 45 per cent alcohol, 2ml 3 times daily. Fresh thyme, cloves, ginger and slices of lemon can be put in a bottle topped up with fortified wine or vodka. Store in a dark place for 3 weeks and shake daily before opening. This is excellent for cold or damp winter evenings.

Thyme Oil   *Thymus vulgaris linalol*

A highly antiseptic oil from the herb which has a well-known culinary use and is native to the Mediterranean areas. There are many different varieties. It is important to know which chemotype you are purchasing, as they have varying properties and degrees of strength. The linalool chenotype is realtively mild.

Family: Lamiaceae (labiatae)

Parts used: Leaves and flowering tops

Main constituents: Alcohols, esters, monoterpenes, phenols

Fragrance: Fresh, delicate, herbaceous, spicy

Main uses: This is a stimulating oil which has an antispasmodic effect on the nervous system. Helps with fatigue and nervous debility. It stimulates the immune system to increase the production of white blood cells and combat infection. It is antiviral, and can be used against digestive colitis, diarrhoea and viral enteritis. As an antiseptic it is excellent for respiratory complaints. Use for sore throats, tonsillitis and bronchial infections. Thyme is a warming oil which will help muscular stiffness and other aches and pains of a cold nature. It is antifungal and can be used in a douche for candidiasis, thrush, etc.

Safety and application: Do not use on young children or on sensitive skin. This oil can be irritating, so always do a patch test before using. Never use undiluted. Dilution 1 per cent in massage blends or in bath bases.

✳ Turmeric   *Curcuma zedoaria*

Synonyms: Zedoary
  Parts used: Rhizomes
  Habitat: Native to Asia
  Main constituents: Minerals, vitamins, volatile oil
  Actions: Anti-inflammatory, antioxidant, bile stimulant, blood purifier, detoxifer, possibly anticancer
  Main uses: One of turmeric's main uses is as an anti-inflammatory. It has a strong effect in reducing the swellings in arthritis and skin conditions. It is used to help lower cholesterol and is important in helping reduce the risk of heart attacks. It is traditionally known to help protect the liver, help the digestive processes and help against nausea. Turmeric is a broncho-dilator and is useful to take during an asthma attack (sip the infusion). It is useful to heal skin problems, psoriasis and fungal infections and may well be good to use to combat the signs of ageing. Recent research shows that curcumin, the yellow colouring in turmeric, may be a free-radical scavenger, hence its potential use in preventing cancer.
  Contraindications: Not to be used in therapeutic doses in pregnancy. Therapeutic quantity not to be taken by people with bile duct obstruction or gall stones. Use with caution during excessive menstruation.
  Dosage: Use in cooking as an ingredient of curry. Infuse 1 teaspoonful in a cup of boiling water. Take 3 times daily. Tincture: 1:5 in 45 per cent alcohol, 2ml 3 times daily.

✳ Urtica   *Urtica urens*

As a homoeopathic remedy, urtica is mainly used for burns, scalds and hives. It can be taken to help relieve the pain of burns and scalds. It is commonly indicated for urticaria or any allergic rash with itching blotches on the skin. It can be an antidote to the ill-effects of eating shellfish. It is useful for burning and stinging pains.

Uva Ursi   *Arctostaphylos uva-ursi*

Parts used: Leaves
   Habitat: Northern Europe
   Main constituents: Flavonoids, hydroquinones, iridoids, tannins
   Actions: Antiseptic, astringent, diuretic
   Main uses: An effective urinary antiseptic, good for acute urinary infections or for cystitis.
   Contraindications: Not to be used in pregnancy or during breastfeeding. Do not use for chronic kidney disorders.
   Dosage: Infuse 1 teaspoon to 1 cup of boiling water. Take 3 times daily. Tincture: 1:5 in 25 per cent alcohol. Take 2ml 3 times daily.

Valerian   *Valeriana officinalis*

Parts used: Root, rhizome
   Habitat: Damp areas in Europe
   Main constituents: Alkaloids, iridoids, volatile oil
   Actions: Anodyne, relaxant, sedative
   Main uses: Even the smell of this plant has a heavy, sedating fragrance! A useful plant to use for overwrought people who find it difficult to switch off from their day and their thoughts. Good for insomnia, overactivity, stress, anxiety. Helps tension, especially in the muscles of the neck and shoulders. Use to relieve tension pains of headaches, PMT or anxiety symptoms during menopause. Recommended to ease withdrawal from cigarettes, drugs and alcohol. It has a pain-relieving function that can assist relaxing after injury or help where pains are spasmodic, as in colic and period pains.
   Contraindications: Not advised for depression or for heavy headaches. Do not use with other relaxing drugs.
   Dosage: Decoct 1 teaspoon of root in 250ml of water. Simmer for 10 minutes and take twice daily. Tincture: 1:5 in 25 per cent alcohol, average dose 2–4ml twice daily.

Vervain   *Verbena officinalis*

Parts used: Aerial parts
  Habitat: Europe, Africa and China
  Main constituents: Alkaloids, choline, flavonoids, tannins
  Actions: Alterative, antispasmodic, bitter, nervine, sedative
  Main uses: This is a tonifying herb, with actions on both the gut and the nervous system. It stimulates digestive functions, is toning for the liver and helpful for jaundice. Use for nervous exhaustion and where the body is suffering from long-term stress and mental illness. Use for ME, anorexia and convalescence and all cases where the digestion has been affected by the nerves.
  Contraindications: Too large doses can cause vomiting. Avoid during pregnancy.
  Dosage: Infuse 1 teaspoon in 1 cup of boiling water. Take 3 times daily. Tincture: 1:5 in 25 per cent alcohol, average dose 2–4ml.

Vetiver Oil   *Vetiveria zizanioides*

This oil is produced from steam-distilled grass roots. It is native to tropical areas, Indonesia and India, and is traditionally used to deter insects.
  Family: Poaceae
  Parts used: Sun-dried roots and rhizomes
  Main constituents: Alcohols, aldehydes, ketones
  Fragrance: A thick, heavy-smelling oil, musky, earthy, smoky
  Main uses: A calming sedating oil for the nervous system, good for relieving stress and tension. Use for depression and insomnia. Acts as a tonic to the immune system and stimulates the circulation. Good for the elderly for its warming and pain-relieving effects. In skincare, vetiver is antiseptic, good for aches, pains and acne. This is a great oil to use to create exotic blends with aphrodisiac properties. Combine with jasmine or patchouli.
  Safety and application: Non-toxic, non-irritant, non-sensitizing. Use in dilutions of maximum 2 per cent.

☙ Watercress *Nasturtium officinale*

Parts used: Aerial parts
   Habitat: Temperate climates
   Main constituents: Minerals and vitamins
   Actions: Detoxifying, diuretic, expectorant, nutritious
   Main uses: This is a plant rich in vitamins A, Bs, C and E. It also contains folic acid, iodine, iron, phosphates and sulphur minerals. It is nutritious, excellent for cleansing and detoxifying and will help build the body up after a long winter. Use for poor skin and persistent coughs.
   Contraindications: None.
   Dosage: Fresh juice is best. Liquidize ½ bunch mixed with carrots or beetroot and drink daily. Include watercress in salads. Serve with olive oil and lemon juice.

☙ White Deadnettle *Lamium album*

Parts used: Aerial parts
   Habitat: Throughout Europe and Asia
   Main constituents: Amines, flavonoids, saponin, tannins
   Actions: Astringent, diuretic, haemostatic
   Main uses: A good uterine tonic chiefly used for heavy, painful periods or intermenstrual bleeding. Also for diarrhoea, bleeding piles, varicose veins and vaginal discharge.
   Contraindications: None.
   Dosage: Infuse 1 teaspoon per cup boiling water and take 3 times daily. Tincture: 1:5 in 25 per cent alcohol, average dose 2–4ml.

☙ White Horehound *Marrubium vulgar*

Parts used: Top leaves and flowers
   Habitat: Europe
   Main constituents: Alkaloids, marrubin, volatile oil
   Actions: Bitter tonic, expectorant, sedative, vulnerary
   Main uses: The main use for this herb is as an expectorant. It works on coughs with mucus that is hard to shift. Use for asthma, bronchitis, whooping

cough, also for stimulating the appetite and improving the digestive function. Can be used to help regulate the heartbeat.

Contraindications: Not to be used in pregnancy.

Dosage: Combine in a syrup with aniseed, hyssop, liquorice or thyme. Infuse 1 teaspoonful in a cup of boiling water. Take 3 times daily. Tincture: 1:5 in 25 per cent alcohol. Take 2ml in hot water 3 times daily.

☀ White Willow   *Salix alba*

Parts used: Bark

Habitat: Damp areas of Europe

Main constituents: Flavonoids, phenolic glycosides (containing salicylic acid), tannins

Actions: Analgesic, anti-inflammatory, antiseptic, astringent, reduces fever

Main uses: Salicylic acid, now synthesized into acetyl salicylic acid, is the active constituent of aspirin. White willow acts similarly, in that it is an effective painkiller. Good for headaches, fever, backache. As an anti-inflammatory, it reduces discomfort in rheumatism, painful joints and muscles. Good for neuralgia and sciatica. Unlike aspirin, white willow does not have the side-effects of blood thinning or irritation to the stomach lining.

Contraindications: Not for those who are allergic to aspirin.

Dosage: Decoct 1 teaspoon of root in 250ml water, simmer for 10 minutes and drink ½ cup 3 times daily or when required. Tincture: 1:5 in 25 per cent alcohol, 2ml 3 times daily.

☀ Wild Cherry Bark   *Prunus serotina*

This herb can sedate the cough reflex, so it is chiefly used for dry, irritable coughs, smoker's cough or nervous and whooping coughs. When using this herb, care must be taken to also treat the underlying chest infection, as it tends to suppress expectoration. Wild cherry is a bitter and a digestive stimulant, use for people with sluggish digestions.

Dosage: Use 1–2ml of tincture diluted in water, or 1–2 teaspoonfuls of herb decocted in a cup of water. Take 3 times daily. Cherry juice is known to be specifically good for gout, drink 140ml (¼ pint) per day, or you could eat 450g (1 lb) of cherries a day and decrease the amount slowly over several weeks.

❊ Wild Indigo   *Baptisia tinctoria*

This herb is said to be an immune stimulant with a special effect on the upper respiratory tract. This makes it a useful herb to take for the treatment of sore throats, catarrh, swollen glands, coughs and colds, especially if there are accompanying headaches. The main use of wild indigo is for 'flu that is concentrated in the upper respiratory area: the head being the focus of discomfort. Take with caution, as it can cause nausea. It can also be included in a mixture for ulcers and abscesses or used for gingivitis. It can be made into a decoction or used as a douche for leucorrhoea. Avoid during pregnancy.

Dosage: 1 teaspoonful of the root needs to be decocted with a cup of water that is brought to the boil and simmered, take a tblsful 3 times a day. Use ½–1ml of tincture and take 3 times daily. Start with the minimum dose and take only for a few days as this is a strong herb that can cause nausea.

❊ Wild Yam   *Dioscorea villosa*

Parts used: Roots and tubers

Habitat: Native to North America

Main constituents: Alkaloids, phytosterols, saponins (dioscin), tannins

Actions: Anti-inflammatory, antirheumatic, antispasmodic, diaphoretic, diuretic, relaxant

Main uses: Traditionally used to treat rheumatism and relieve pain and inflammation. Helps with stiffness and aching muscles, tension and cramps in muscles. More recently wild yam has been used for gynaecological problems, especially where there are painful periods and hormonal imbalances. Use for symptoms of the menopause, combine extracts into a cream and apply externally. Also use for digestive disorders. Helps IBS, diarrhoea and diverticulitis.

Contraindications: Avoid during pregnancy.

Dosage: Decoct 1 teaspoon in 250ml water, simmer for 10 minutes and drink ½ cup 3 times daily. Tincture: 1:5 in 45 per cent alcohol. Take 2ml 3 times daily.

❋ Witch Hazel   *Hamamelis virginiana*

Parts used: Leaves, bark
   Habitat: Commonly grown in Europe
   Main constituents: Flavonoids, tannins, volatile oil
   Actions: Anti-inflammatory, astringent, bitter, haemostatic
   Main uses: Used widely for its action on the skin. Due to its strong astringency, it is used for cleansing and healing broken skin; use also where the skin is inflamed or bruised, and for eczema. Mends capillaries and damaged blood vessels. It is valuable for piles and varicose veins. Good for using on cysts and tumours. Has a contracting and drying effect on the face. Good for oily skin. Internally, witch hazel is used for any intestinal bleeding and over-secretions of the mucous membranes. Use as an eyewash for conjunctivitis.
   Contraindications: None.
   Dosage: Distilled witch hazel is obtainable for use, or infuse 1 teaspoon leaves to 1 cup boiling water. Use as a wash for external use or take 3 times daily. Combine into a cream to apply externally for piles, varicose veins, etc.

❋ Woodruff   *Galicum odoratum*

This is a herb that is good for a congested liver where there is constipation and irritability. It calms the nervous system, especially when the digestion is affected and where there is insomnia. Use when it is difficult to get to sleep or when you wake up very easily and cannot get back to sleep. Woodruff is a herb that seems more aromatic when dry, and can be used either on its own or with lavender as an insect repellant.
   Dosage: Use 1 teaspoonful of herb to a cup of boiling water and take 3 times daily, or 1ml of tincture diluted in water 3 times daily.

❋ Wormwood   *Artemisia absinthium*

Parts used: Leaves and tops of the plant
   Habitat: Native to Europe
   Main constituents: Flavonoids, lignans, phenolic acids, volatile oil
   Actions: Anti-inflammatory, bitter, carminative, digestive, febrifuge, insect repellent, stimulates bile secretion

Main uses: Useful for stimulating the appetite and for those with weak digestion. Use for anorexics and those who are convalescing. It stimulates the liver and gall bladder. Use to expel worms. Cut fresh twigs and place in between cloth and wool that are being stored to prevent damage from insects, moths, etc.

Contraindications: Traditionally included as a flavouring in absinthe in France, now banned due to its effect on the nervous system, leading to mental deterioration, epilepsy. Do not use internally during pregnancy, when breast-feeding or where there is a history of heart problems.

Dosage: Infuse ½ teaspoon in 1 cup boiling water. Drink 1 cup daily. Do not take for longer than 4 weeks. Tincture: 1:10 in 45 per cent alcohol. Take 2ml in water twice daily. Macerate 1 twig of fresh plant in vodka as an occasional *apéritif* when needed or for the elderly with poor digestion. Take no more than 1 small shot per day.

Yarrow   *Achillea millefolium*

Synonyms: Milfoil

Parts used: Aerial parts

Habitat: Native to Europe and Asia

Main constituents: Alkaloids, flavonoids, phytosterols, sesquiterpenes, tannins, triterpenes, volatile oil

Actions: Anti-inflammatory, bitter, diaphoretic, diuretic, haemostatic

Main uses: Formerly known as 'heal all' and likened to chamomile, although yarrow is less relaxing and has a more powerful effect on the lungs. It is an important herb for fevers, increases sweating and can be used in a classic combination with elderflower and peppermint for colds and 'flu. It selectively stimulates and relaxes the digestive system, improving absorption, healing gastric ulcers and internal bleeding, and toning the bowel. Yarrow has a toning effect on the blood vessels and lowers blood pressure. Give for high blood pressure when caused by stress. Use for varicose veins and piles. Helps to regulate periods and reduces pain, especially if affected by the cold. Cures nosebleeds.

Contraindications: Not to be used in pregnancy.

Dosage: Infuse 1 teaspoon in a cup of boiling water. Take 3 times daily. Tincture: 1:5 in 45 per cent alcohol. Take 1ml 3 times daily.

⚕ Yarrow Oil   *Achillea millefolium*

A dark blue oil due to the chamazulene content, similar to the blue chamomile oil, produced mainly in Europe and more recently in England.

Family: Asteraceae

Main constituents: Alcohols, esters, ketones, monoterpenes, oxides, sesquiterpenes

Fragrance: Hay-like, medicinal

Main uses: This is a tonic to the nervous system. Use for treating neuralgia and stress. Induces sweating and is an immune-stimulant useful for colds and 'flu. Decongesting for the circulation. Antiseptic. Use to treat painful periods, delayed periods and heavy bleeding. Good for menopausal symptoms, inflammation of the uterus, fibroids. On the skin, it is good for eczema, rashes and wound healing, especially where there is inflammation. Good for cleansing oily skin.

Safety and application: Not to be used in pregnancy or with very young children. Use well diluted, maximum 1 per cent.

⚕ Yellow Dock   *Rumex crispus*

Parts used: Root

Habitat: Common throughout the world

Main constituents: Anthraquinone glycosides, flavonoids, oxalates, tannins

Main uses: This is a nutritious herb that affects the liver functions, increases bile flow, helps constipation and has beneficial effects on the skin. Good for chronic, poor or itchy skin conditions – psoriasis, acne, oozing or itchy skin. Use for scabies or ringworm. A good blood-cleansing herb. Use where there is anaemia due to low iron levels.

Contraindications: Not to be taken in pregnancy or when breastfeeding. Individuals with a history of kidney stones should use this herb cautiously.

Dosage: Decoct 1 teaspoon in 250ml water. Simmer for 20 minutes. Take 1 cup 3 times daily. This herb is most often combined with dandelion and burdock root. Tincture: 1:5 in 45 per cent alcohol. Take 2ml 3 times daily.

❋ Ylang-Ylang Oil   *Cananga odorata*

A tropical fragrant tree with long, hanging blossoms. The oil is well known for its aphrodisiac properties and frequently used in the production of perfumes.

Family: Annonaceae

Parts used: Freshly picked flowers

Main constituents: Alcohols, esters, phenols, sesquiterpenes

Fragrance: Strongly floral, sweet, exotic. May be too floral and heady for some people.

Main uses: A sedating oil useful for nervous conditions, depression, anxiety, stress and tension. This is an important oil for the treatment of high blood pressure. Helps with palpitations. Excellent for relaxation and increasing libido. Good to include in exotic massage blends for infertility and suppressed sexuality. Said to help PMT, mood swings, irregular periods. It is a highly sedative oil. Recent research shows that it can benefit epilepsy.

Safety and application: Can be used in an atomizer. Combines well with clary sage, grapefruit, jasmine. Use in dilutions of 2 per cent.

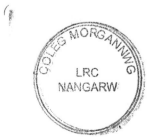

part III:

Healing Ourselves

Introduction to Healing Ourselves

To enjoy good health we need to look after the spiritual, mental and emotional aspects of our lives as well as our physical health. The flow of energy between these different aspects of our self integrates and keeps us whole; disharmony in any one of these areas will push all the others out of balance.

Daily stresses and life events tend to throw us into a state of imbalance. And if we become stuck for too long in this imbalance then we have disease. Our ability to adapt and deal creatively with life's up and downs will determine the mental and physical processes that we experience as good health. We all have an innate desire to create the conditions for balance within ourselves, and in our environment, and it is the aim of the various systems of natural healing to help us achieve this.

Our potential for good health is based on the unique mixture of our parents' genes (inherited factors), the physical and mental environment in which we were nurtured, and our individual ability to deal with all these factors. We need to strike a balance between accepting the basics of who we are, e.g. as woman/man, black/white, able-bodied/disabled, and recognizing that there are also huge areas of choice about what we can do with our lives. One of the most debilitating states of mind, and the cause of many people's depression, is to feel that there are no options to choose from. It is important to remember that there are always options, even if these are only a question of our attitude towards problems.

Knowing that we always have choices means that we also need to make decisions, and this is not always easy. As our lives have become more complex in the modern world, our choices have also multiplied. We have to make decisions continually about such things as how, when and what to eat, where to live, what to spend our money on, what paid work to pursue, whether or not or when to have children, and what kind of relationships to have. In the past, and now in less developed societies, many of these choices were restricted by environmental or social factors.

When making a decision, we can be positive by choosing the option that best supports the whole. We, in the industrialized West, have shown little concern with this kind of decision-making, and our damaged physical environment exemplifies the danger of choosing on the basis of short-term gain and exploitation. Not all societies have been so reckless. The Native American tribes, for example, placed great importance on living in harmony with their environment, and made decisions as a group aimed at maintaining its integrity and not depleting resources.

On a personal level, the principle of decision making is the same: we cannot choose personal gain or individual happiness at the expense of anything or anyone else, and at the same time sustain integrity in our life. Every time that we make a decision we can think of what best supports the whole. When we go shopping we can choose products that are environmentally sound, we can shop locally and we can encourage sustainable farming methods by buying organic products. We can work in jobs that we feel are contributing something to society as well as paying our wages.

The principles of natural medicine are based on the same idea: that we have to treat the individual as a whole and not just as a set of physical symptoms. The aims of natural medicine are to create better conditions for health to exist within the person, and to encourage them to throw off disease on every level. The disadvantage of much orthodox modern medicine is that it tends to remove a particular physical symptom without dealing with why the symptom developed in the first place. This approach not only leads to the suppression and distortion of symptoms, but also to the use of drugs which, whilst being powerful in removing one illness, cause side-effects that damage other parts of the person.

Again, the same principle applies to our emotional life: the best way of dealing with a problem is by choosing the option which best supports the whole. If we suppress our negative emotions or fail to acknowledge the aspects of ourself that we don't like, we will never come to terms with our whole self, and we will never be able to use the whole of our potential and energy. It is only by accepting our negative emotions that we can change, and use the energy that is released. This may mean taking decisions which feel like risks at the time, but which will quickly add to our experience and enrich our lives. There are many very moving and inspiring accounts of women who have suffered, for example the death of a child through a particular disease or drug abuse, who don't dwell on their anger and grief, but use the experience to help others. Their purpose in life becomes broader, they become wiser, more courageous and fulfilled and for example campaign for greater justice or set up a support group.

In this section we set out an approach to health and the enjoyment of life in the fullest sense. We examine the different aspects that make up our life experience, and show how, by seeing ourselves as part of an interconnected whole, we can both enrich our individual lives and create a better world for us all to live in.

20

Our Spiritual Selves

In this section we are going to explore what it means to be healthy in our spiritual lives and what we can do to improve things when we feel dissatisfied. As women, it is especially important to have a positive spiritual outlook because this will determine to a great extent our ability to be creative, our feelings of self-worth and the value that we put on our life experience. This, in turn, will be passed on to our children, and to all the people with whom we interact.

It is our spiritual self that links us to everything beyond the personal self; it gives us awareness of and contact with the interconnectedness of life. When we acknowledge that we are part of an interconnected whole, we realize that we cannot exploit any one person, group of people or any resource at all without damaging the balance of the whole, and in effect damaging ourselves.

Our western society, with its emphasis on exploitation of resources and material gain, has created a society in which it is very difficult to feel profoundly connected to other people and to the planet as a whole. The promotion of modern science as the answer to all our problems, both philosophical and practical, has meant that we have lost the ability to be in touch with the overview, because science always tends to focus on material gain, technological advance and the importance of research, whatever the cost to the whole. What this has led to on a physical level is a widespread depletion of resources, and pollution on a scale that now threatens our very survival. On a spiritual level it has led to very many people suffering from a sense of alienation and lack of purpose.

The environment as we know it is going to change. We are living in a world where our future is uncertain. This brings with it the challenge of alienation, despair, isolation and a sense of powerlessness. But it also presents us with the opportunity to understand what is really important for our health and well-being.

When we first wrote this book, most of us did not really appreciate the scope of environmental changes taking place in our lives. Now we can better understand how the planet works and how it can be damaged. Our actions can have global effects. Trade agreements and multinationals impact on our personal lives. We are being forced to think globally. Our perception of our world has changed. As new physics invites us to understand the dynamics of interconnectedness, it also helps us to understand that we can make an impact as individuals, or within a family. All our individual actions will affect our local community, and so on. We are starting to understand that the actions which reduce the world's ability to be well can only result in limitations for us, members of the human race.

This book contains some examples of the current issues affecting the planet. We can make choices which will contribute a positive impact on the environment. The world warmed by 0.6 per cent during the twentieth century and is likely to warm further with the continuing use of fossil fuels and other greenhouse gas processes. It is predicted that this warming process will be speeded up. We already know about the increase in greater weather extremes and rising sea levels. It is already causing suffering, and of course it will particularly affect those that are already poor or living in marginal areas.

Ozone depletion continues to cause concern to our health, making us increasingly susceptible to the UV rays of the sun. The large number of novel chemicals that have been introduced into the environment and the start of genetic manipulation will also contribute to changes in our environment.

We see how creation of waste is part of our lifestyle and we cannot find easy ways to stop. The amount of waste has increased enormously with our increased packaging. Landfills leach and the methane gas poses problems, although landfills are being phased out. After decades of filth we are finally cleaning up such things as sulphur and nitrogen. Acid rain is diminishing. Yet we continue to drive and create cars that continue to pollute. Traffic levels continue to increase. The total number of passenger kilometres per year has increased by more than six times since the 1950s. Children cannot play safely, emissions are known to damage health. It is hard not to see that our food and water are threatened.

We have been losing a great number of species in the world, although it is difficult to obtain accurate figures. We see that medicinal plants are becoming endangered, yet the real impact of monoculture agriculture, urbanization, over-population and pollution on the world's natural resources and biodiversity are yet to be really understood.

We can begin to feel hopeless with this increasing gloom in the world. Yet we believe that we, as individuals, can make a difference – in fact it is only through our individual actions that we can create a healthier world to live in. We can become guardians of nature and the natural way of doing things, living in rhythm with the whole. Become as informed as you can. The best action you can take is to choose not to buy or support products, services or companies that do not care about these bigger issues. Notice which companies pay their directors fat salaries and bonuses or are inconsistent in their export policies. The 'not in my backyard' approach is easily demonstrated by companies who sell products to the Third World which they would not like to sell in their own country, or by those governments or organizations that have policies of waste dumping in countries that are so desperate for the money that they allow it to happen. We need to be searching for fairness and those that demonstrate it in their policies. Then we can support it.

Through understanding that we are all connected, we can also realize our power to change. Our change can be small, but the effect can be big (a change in consciousness is a change in habitual process, in our attitude to health and the difference is positive, healing, miracles). We cannot avoid making the connections. And it demonstrates our lack of integrity if we avoid making positive choices for our health and for the well-being of the planet.

We believe that the following ideas are some ways in which we can make choices towards a healthier future. We can really start to make a difference if we consider and implement some of these simple ways of reducing our energy consumption:

- Be conscious of the way you travel.
- Question the benefits of long-haul holidays.
- Walk or get a bus to work or school.
- Cut down on unnecessary travel.
- Use fuel-efficient cars.
- Shop locally or get your food delivered.
- Sign up for green fuel options.
- Turn the thermostat down.
- Lag your water tank.
- Don't leave your appliances on standby, but turn them off.
- Apply draught-proofing strips to your windows.
- Insulate your home.
- Use solar cells or buy a battery recharger.
- Check your existing appliances or purchase low-energy options.

- Always use low-energy light bulbs.
- Use natural ventilation instead of air conditioning.

We use an average of 200 litres of water per person per day. This can be reduced by using low-flush toilets or putting a brick (or similar) into the cistern. If we develop an awareness of how much water we use in everyday activities, this will probably result in reducing our water usage! We waste 20 per cent of our water through dripping taps and leaks. Collect rainwater and use for the garden or washing the car.

The quantity of waste we create is growing out of control. We no longer have the space to put it, and burning it is polluting. Our problem is that our waste is not generally biodegradable. We can compost our vegetable waste, if we have a garden, and we can have a wormery, but here are a few ideas we can all act on:

- Separate out all your waste and recycle or compost where possible.
- Remind your council or MP to provide easier recycling facilities if it is difficult for you.
- Buy products that are designed to last or can be reused or recycled.
- Avoid over-packaged products.
- Reuse your carrier bags and other plastic items.
- Choose products that have minimal packing.
- Support local enterprise.
- Choose environmental options for all household items, also items for your family and clothing.

As we begin to make these choices we also learn that we are not alone. It is estimated that 25 per cent of the population are what has been termed 'cultural creatives'. If all these people work together and increase their numbers, great changes will occur. More and more people will then feel that their actions are linked to a sense of improving life and growing as people. This will create an integration between our sense of purpose and our actual life.

Being in contact with our spiritual self enables us to have an awareness beyond the mundane activities of life, and to gain insight into the larger issues of our existence: it is a source that provides us with our sense of purpose and our innate desire to be creative. The spiritual aspect of ourselves needs looking after just as much as our physical body does. We need to create time in our lives to cultivate the contact and expression of our spiritual self. It is only by continually making the commitment to allow the spiritual impulse into our lives that our daily experience is enriched with a true feeling of purpose.

The cultivation of the spiritual aspect of our lives involves the process that is known as 'becoming conscious'. This means thinking about what we do and how we live, examining all our old patterns and habits and beginning to experience life as a process of insight, inspiration and purposefulness. This may seem like a huge step to take. It need not be. We can only start from where we are, and even very small changes in our behaviour and attitudes can begin to break up the habits and personally-imposed restrictions that we all allow ourselves to fall into.

If you would like to try and set the process of breaking through some old patterns and restrictions in motion, and therefore clear a space to let some fresh insights and creative energy into your life, here are some suggestions:

- Try sleeping in a different position from your usual one.
- Give up a personal habit that has annoyed you for years.
- Eat completely differently for a while (e.g. try the cleansing diet at the back of this book).
- Make a conscious effort to do routine things a different way each day (e.g. put your socks on in a different order or get out of bed on the other side).
- Try concentrating totally on the task that you are doing at every moment of the day, and do all your tasks with enthusiasm.
- Try to start the day with a clear mind, and whenever you start thinking of something, think it right through to its conclusion.
- When you meet criticism or accusation, instead of trying to justify yourself, try to find out what gave rise to it and the point of view behind it (whether you agree with it or not).
- Try not to make an excuse of any kind for anything.
- Take every opportunity to understand someone from another culture that seems foreign and strange to you.
- Practise making a conscious effort to contact your inner source each night before going to sleep.

Try one of these exercises for a couple of weeks and then try another one. The idea is to just watch how you react to trying something different. Don't worry if it isn't easy or if you forget for a while, just observe that and have another go.

The results often appear to be truly miraculous, but as any therapist or counsellor interested in spiritual development knows, whenever a person makes a commitment to becoming more conscious, tremendous energy is released into her life, and suddenly she realizes what to do next in order to make progress. Really all that is necessary to bring ourselves more into contact with ourselves as spiritual beings is to commit ourselves to change and growth. Be committed to being true to your perceived purpose at any time, to what is best for your own growth, and to what is necessary for the development of anyone else with whom you come into contact.

It is an unfortunate reflection of our society that so many people complain of feeling purposeless, or that although they feel there may be some greater purpose for their life, they don't have a sense of what it is. Finding a purpose – your purpose – is not so much about searching around for what you think fits your expectations, but more a question of identifying where you are now and what your potential is. Lack of purpose is really alienation from society and from anything bigger than yourself; so it is also necessary to acknowledge that you, whilst being an individual, are also part of the interweaving patterns of life, and that your contribution is as important as anyone else's.

Questions like 'Who am I really?' or 'What should I be doing?' can only be answered by accepting who you are and what you are doing right now. It can feel very painful and restricting to accept that we have to start with what we are now, as opposed with what we would like to be, but from that point of acceptance we can acknowledge our strengths and our weaknesses, and then what we can change in our lives.

If you do feel totally in the dark about your purpose in life, it can be helpful to review your life up to the present time. Take time, this process can take several days. It is important not to become too attached to any one issue, or to apportion any blame to yourself or anyone else, just look at your life as if it were on a television screen in front of you. At the end of the review, consider what things have given you most satisfaction, such as caring for others, gardening, writing, teaching, being creative or physical exercise. It may be something that you have not done for a long time, if your life has gone off in other directions. But if you do realize there are some things that you find particularly satisfying, then project your review into the future and imagine ways in which you can develop this potential. Commit yourself to finding more time and chances to express these in your life, and be especially open to any chance or occasion that may arise to facilitate your chosen direction.

Another way to get in touch with a sense of purpose in your life is to spend some time doing the previous exercises to free up your habitual way of doing things. We have to make room for new experiences, and our habits, resistances and excuses for not trying something 100 per cent can block the flow of energy from our spiritual contact. The most important thing is to consciously commit yourself to cultivating a sense of purpose in your life, to be prepared to let go of how you think things should be, and to be open to change and any new opportunities when they present themselves.

You will know when you are in touch with your inner purpose because you will feel very empowered. It is the same feeling as being in the right place at the right time. When a person is acting out his purpose great things become possible, because tremendous energy flows along the channel that is created by being in line with our inner source.

It is important to remember that a particular role is only an expression of the purpose. The role itself, whether that of a plumber, doctor, mother, teacher, cleaner or poet, is unimportant unless it expresses your purpose at the time. We may need to do many different things at different times in our lives in order to stay in touch with our purpose. It is doing what seems appropriate at the time that is important.

Being in contact with your purpose is the same as being in touch with your source of energy and inspiration, or your spiritual self. This is also the source of what is called impersonal or unconditional love. Nearly all of us will recognize the experience of feeling in contact with something greater than ourselves at some time in our lives, and the aim of cultivating our spiritual life is to have constant access to this source of energy, to get it flowing through every aspect of our lives. It is this love that creates an empathy and sense of contact between people, and it brings the gift of enjoyment and well-being into our existence.

People that radiate this kind of energy come across as powerful and expansive. It is as if you can sense the love that is emanating from them. Such people are often far from 'perfect', in the sense of conforming to the ideal that society expects, and they may have some obvious shortcomings, but nevertheless other people will always be drawn to them because of their tremendous energy.

Many women and men feel at their most connected and powerful when they 'fall in love'. The outpouring of energy towards another person leads us to an experience of love filling our lives and often this creates a feeling of benignness and well-wishing on the whole world. This is a sense that could be seen as sharing some of the qualities of a profound spiritual experience. However, what we actually do is project all of our energy and emotion onto another person, who has become an 'object' of our desire. When that initial stage of infatuation passes, we return to whatever state we were in before, and do not really learn or build in any lasting qualities as a result.

The highest expression of love is of service. This concept can be hard to understand, but it means responding to your own needs, and the needs, but not necessarily the wants, of others. It implies caring about everything without expecting results, committing yourself to your purpose without becoming goal-oriented. This aspect of service is also known as unconditional love. This is not something that we can really try and achieve, but it is an ideal that we can hold in our minds and try and return to whenever we realize that we have been acting out of our own selfish wants or desires.

An experience that can both connect us with a sense of our inner energy and also create the feeling of profound contact with another person is sex. Sex can be a celebration of the link between spirit (our inner source) and matter (our body), an expression of our creative impulse and a profound exchange of energy with another person. However, our ability to 'make love' is going to be limited by any expectations or judgements, and by inhibitions on any level. Sex is an expression of ourselves, and it will reflect our limitations and unconscious habits, as well as our ability to express love and enjoyment.

When we consider commonly accepted attitudes to sex, we have another example of how we have become exploitative and self-oriented as a society. Whenever we use something for our own pleasure we denigrate it and objectify it. Women in particular have been seen as objects of sexual gratification that men have rights over. When sex becomes free of rights and obligations, and instead is valued as an exchange of intimacy and tenderness with another unique and vulnerable human being, then we can enjoy sex more fully as an expression of energy and life.

What else can we do to help us find our source of consciousness? There are many techniques that have evolved over the centuries to help us get in contact with our spiritual selves. All of these require freeing ourselves to some degree from our habitual way of responding to things and our unconscious patterns, as we have discussed. They also require us to reach beyond the rational, concrete part of our brain to the more abstract, intuitive mind, and then even beyond that. This is the aim of many self-development and meditation groups.

Meditation is a powerful tool that can enable us to calm the chattering of our brain, and create a contact with the part of our mind that uses symbols and images, and is beyond the rational and mundane. It can help us to restore our contact with ourselves, and with our real needs, so that we are motivated from inside. In this way we can have an effect on our lives and our environment, instead of being motivated only by what happens to us from the outside, and always being affected by our environment.

We have used the following meditation techniques, and if you would like to try them, then do have a go. There are lots of different kinds of meditation using a variety of techniques, although the purpose is generally the same: to open us up to an experience of ourselves that is beyond that of the petty personality. If you want to find out about different kinds of meditation we suggest you pick up one of the booklets available these days in natural health clinics, libraries and health-food shops that list local groups. Magazines such as *Kindred Spirit* and the internet also carry listings of numerous groups that practise meditation. Probably best of all is to ask people that you respect if they have ever done any kind of meditation and how they got on with it.

In common with most forms of meditation, we first suggest that you sit in a comfortable position, with your spine straight, and allow yourself to become relaxed. This can be sitting on a dining-type chair with your feet flat on the floor, or sitting on the floor cross-legged. Then breathe regularly and evenly, so that the length of the breath in is equal to the length of the breath out. Concentrating on breathing can always seem a little strange at first, but it helps to achieve a state of balance. When you get more used to it, you can try to lengthen the length of the breath in and out a little, and a deeper sense of relaxation will follow.

The next stage in this meditation routine is to bring your awareness to a focus in the centre of the forehead. In traditional terms this centre is called the 'third eye', but it is generally known as the seat of consciousness. From this centre you should be able to view things in a more detached manner. When you have become familiar with focusing your awareness on the centre of the brow, you can return there when you need to see an overview of a situation, or when you want to function on a level beyond that of the petty personality.

When you feel that you are focused in the brow-centre, use your imagination to create a circle of light travelling anti-clockwise around your head. This circle of light is a technique of the western meditation tradition, and it is the same idea as a halo, or an aura. If other people are present you can also include them in the circle of light and it will create an area of positive energy. It is also possible to imagine someone who is ill or suffering inside the circle of light, but it is important to wish nothing specific on them, just direct a sense of well-being towards them.

If you have managed to maintain these exercises, you can establish your consciousness in your spinal column by imagining that it is full of light. The lighted spine can represent your base, or your home, and you can return to this image as a way of centring yourself, or contacting your inner source.

If you want to take your meditation a step further, then you can visualize a globe of light above your head, like a sun, and bring a ray of the light down and in through the brow centre, and then down your spine. When your spine is filled with this light, you can radiate it out through every pore of your body, and fill your atmosphere with light and positive energy. When you breathe in bring down the light, and when you breathe out radiate the energy out. If at any time you feel your mind or your concentration wandering, then just bring your awareness back into the brow-centre, and start again with the basic exercises of relaxing your body and balancing your breath.

This bit of the meditation – bringing down light – is very useful for those people who need to feel inspired, and want to create a flow of positive energy in their life. For those of us who have a problem concentrating, and are prone to feeling 'spaced out', then a more useful technique can be to do the exercises including relaxing, balancing the breath, focusing in the forehead and creating a circle of light around you, but then visualize sending down roots deep into the earth, like a tree. You can then bring energy up from the earth, and up through your feet into the rest of your body. This energy can then be radiated out into your atmosphere, and it will have a more 'earthing' effect for you.

You can meditate daily, weekly or just whenever you feel like it. The meditation is not really an end in itself – its purpose is to help us to contact our source of energy and to get that positive energy flowing into every area of our life.

Another technique that can be used to open our lives up to the spiritual is ritual. There are as many variations of ritual as there are mystical philosophies and religions, but the intention is generally the same: to create a link between the spiritual and the physical. Another useful aspect of ritual is that we can use it as a set period of time in which to practise being 100 per cent conscious during every action. This can thus help us to develop an increased awareness and sense of purpose.

Some people feel very uncomfortable about ritual in general, or about ritual that is not done for them by a religious 'expert', but any action that has a symbolic as well as a literal meaning is actually a ritual. For example, decorating a fir tree at Christmas is a ritual, so is putting candles on a birthday cake or placing a wreath on a grave. In fact, other functions of ritual are that it can help us to develop an appreciation for the use of symbols, and it can also enrich our understanding of our cultural heritage.

There is a tradition of using ritual in the West that is based on the four elements. This can be done by dividing an area up into four quarters, and choosing which element to place in which quarter. Here is one suggestion:

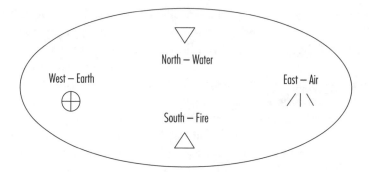

Within this space you can create a context for any activity that you consider to be sacred. For instance, it can be used for healing, meditating or creating something very special. You can divide up a room in this way, or a table top, or part of a garden, or just an imaginary space. If you want to choose symbolic objects that represent the elements to you, then you can place them in the appropriate quarter. The space that you have created can be purified by sprinkling it with water and consecrated by the burning of incense. Candles can be lit in the centre as a focus of energy and light.

To help you develop the potential of ritual, you can take any object, word or idea and consider what it means to you, both literally and symbolically. Take the example of water from the suggested layout above: water can be used as an element that represents clarity, purity, reflection and tranquillity. It is often associated with the emotions, it is generally seen as a feminine element and it is connected to the moon through the ebb and flow of the oceans.

Further illustrations can be drawn from the example above to help develop an understanding of the other elements. Air is a symbol of truth, inspiration and communication, it is associated with spring in the cycle of the year. Fire gives us courage, enthusiasm, warmth, love and is associated with midday and midsummer. Earth offers solidity, stability and endurance. From earth, we can learn about our relationship with the material world, it represents the time of the harvest. To gain a more personal understanding of these elements, and how you relate to them in your daily life, you will have to reflect on them yourself.

Everything in nature can be looked at ritually. The cycle of the seasons can be considered symbolically as well as literally. Try asking yourself what winter means to you, and then spring, summer and autumn. Consider the cycle of day and night, and what your associations are with night, sunrise, midday and evening. We can begin to see why night and winter and death have been associated with each other through the ages, likewise why spring, sunrise, the east and new life or rebirth are connected to each other. Some of the rituals that exist in our culture may then have more meaning for you. We can see, for example, why Easter eggs are given in the spring, the symbolic time of new life.

By building up our associations with the symbols that we use in ritual, we can become more conscious of our relationship with them in our everyday lives. The relationship that you have to water in a ritual, the associations that you make and the ease with which you are able to establish a contact with it, are all reflections of the role of water in your life. For example, if you find it difficult to imagine and establish a sense of contact with water during a ritual, it may be that you find it difficult to express your emotions or to feel relaxed and able to flow in your everyday life. Ritual enables us to go inside our own psyche, it helps us to understand our relationship with the world.

By means of a conclusion to this section, we would like to emphasize that we feel that cultivating contact with and expression of our spiritual selves is a very important part of developing a sense of well-being and purpose in our lives. It can also help to make us feel connected to the whole. Developing consciousness links us to both the joy and also the pain of the greater world. This sense of interconnectedness should in turn encourage a balance between the passion for our path and a tolerance for that of others.

The important thing to remember is that it is bringing the spiritual impulse into our everyday life that will create health and well-being in ourselves. There is for example, very little point in just following a spiritual trend without the experience of inner purpose enriching our day-to-day life.

When we become more confident about our contact with the spiritual part of ourselves, we find that we have more resilience to help ourselves overcome some of the traumas and painful experiences of life. If we feel connected to our own sense of being, we can draw on it as on a source in times of need. If we feel that there is more to our life than a physical body, we become less afraid of death. If we feel that we are ultimately connected to everybody and everything else, we will truly want what is best for the development of the world as a whole, even if that means re-evaluating what we think we want for ourselves.

21

Our Mental and Emotional Selves

We are going to explore what it means to enjoy ourselves in our mental and emotional life, and what we can do to improve things when we recognize that changes need to be made. The theme that we will develop is that of encouraging a healthy and well-balanced mental and emotional life by being prepared to accept and learn from the whole of an experience. This means accepting the 'good' and the 'bad', the plus and the minus, the pain and the pleasure, of all our experiences.

Firstly we will look at how 'accepting the whole' operates in our relationships with other people, because enjoying the relationships in our life is so important to our mental and emotional well-being. For example, you cannot enjoy a meaningful relationship with someone unless you acknowledge that there are things about them that you feel good about, and things about them that you find more difficult to accept, and that you will have some good times together, but also some painful and challenging times.

Every relationship with another person enriches our life, and provides a unique opportunity for us to learn and grow. We are born to certain parents, and into a certain family, at a particular point in time. These family relationships, and all the others that we go on to form, provide precisely the interaction and contact that we need in order to develop as individuals.

What is the advantage of viewing relationships as learning experiences? We need to know that we are in a relationship because we have a mutual need for that particular interaction. Once we realize this, we can both appreciate it more, and be more willing to make changes when those needs are no longer satisfied. Also, we never need to fear letting go of a relationship that we have outgrown, because we will always form others that are more appropriate to our current learning needs.

If you and your partner decide to commit yourselves to a relationship together, then you are in fact creating a third entity – a sort of pool to which you both contribute and draw out. This pool is a resource for both of you, and one that builds up over time and experiences shared together. You will develop a sense of care, respect and tolerance for the relationship itself, and it will become trusted as a source of nourishment. The partners within a relationship such as this can carry on their development as individuals, and are respected as individuals by the other partner.

However, so many relationships start out well but become stuck in a destructive process. Both parties then become judgemental, blaming and petty. If this situation is prolonged then the couple tend to support each other in their failings and weaknesses, with neither person being free to transform and grow. At the worst this leads to frustration, violence and a diseased state of mind and body.

When there are children within this failing relationship, it is important to work together to understand what is going on. Often problems arise out of poor communication skills. We have not learned to talk to each other or to be able to see what we are saying is often a result of our own conditioning. We do not always behave in a way that we want to. Whether we seek outside solutions to our problems or not, it is important to acknowledge that our children really are our future and we have a responsibility to find solutions that transform our relationships. Also, if we give up too easily on a relationship without really being prepared to look at and let go of some of our habits, we are very likely to repeat the same mistakes in our next relationship.

Developing an attitude of tolerance towards each other helps to nurture our ability to be of service to each other. We move from a selfish approach in our life to one that considers others. Our children, friends, family, our community and global issues all become more understandable and solvable.

If there is no possibilty of reconciliation consider ending a relationship and honour the rights of both individuals to change, rather than remain in an unsatisfying life. When the purpose of a relationship has ended, no matter how much effort is put in, the potential of both individuals will be unfulfilled because the relationship itself will be restrictive, rather than a source for expansion and growth.

How can we sort ourselves out and enjoy our lives to the full? How can we enjoy being ourselves, and enjoy our friendships and our relationships? This really means, how do we stay healthy? We need to appreciate our life as a process of transformation and growth. We need to allow ourselves to experience our dark side as well as our light side, to experience that aspect which we believe to be bad and wrong, that which we go to great lengths to conceal from others. We will not be able to change and grow unless we truly know ourselves, including our negative thoughts and emotions.

If we only allow ourselves to appear to be a 'nice' person or a 'good' person, and hide away the fact that we also have 'horrid' thoughts and 'bad' feelings, then we will carry what we are trying to hide around inside ourselves. We will come to feel guilty, fearful and self-critical, and lose our sense of self-worth. It is only by learning to acknowledge and accept the 'bad' as well as the 'good' in ourselves that we can come to know who we really are.

We can begin to live as a whole person fulfilling our potential only when we accept ourselves. This does not mean that we can go around projecting our bad temper, frustrations, and so on, onto other people, but we also don't have to appear nice at the expense of our health and growth. Take a risk and express some of that concealed 'bad' behaviour. You can still be sensitive to what seems appropriate and what doesn't, and to other people's reactions. You may be surprised that other people find your hidden 'vices' perfectly acceptable.

Similarly, we need to accept the right for others, and especially our partners, to be less than perfect. Others need support just as we do. Only then can we all feel less alienated and better nurtured.

We have grown up learning how to hide the bits of ourselves that are not approved of from a very early age. Babies quickly adopt strategies of behaviour as part of the process of learning how to survive in their environment. These behavioural tendencies are at first copied from one of the parents, or another available role model, and are then developed and moulded according to the feedback that the infant receives. We experience this process in action whenever we recognize that a child 'takes after' one of his or her parents.

As well as the contribution of the parents to the personality of the child, there is also the contribution from the society and the culture that the child is part of; there is the environment and the personal experiences that the child is exposed to; and there is also the innate ability and the individual characteristics of the child. It is the unique combination of these factors that will determine the habits that we develop as an individual.

What exactly do we mean by 'habits'? We mean the unconscious responses that we make to particular situations. These unconscious responses are the result of past experiences, for example if we respond in a certain way to a particular situation and we meet with a reasonable degree of success, then when a similar situation arises in the future the habitual response will be to behave in the same way again. If an infant cries when she is hungry, and as a result her mother feeds her, then she will come to associate crying with being fed. If a child initially expresses her anger and frustration visibly, but is forcibly made to be quiet and not express it by a parent, or at school, it is probable that this child will come to habitually suppress her anger.

These successful strategies become programmed-in as our methods of survival and control using the best options that we have available at the time. Our personality is built up largely from the complex pattern created by the interface between this programmed behaviour and the experiences that we are subject to. The problem is that the programming remains even when the circumstances change, and we are left stuck with a limited number of options as to how we perceive and respond to a situation. If I am an introverted young person, afraid of expressing an opinion because my parents always put my opinions down, then even when I no longer live with my parents, I am still likely to have a problem being assertive and expressing myself.

Because the experience and feedback that each individual is exposed to are completely individual, the exact pattern of behavioural habits that develops is unique to each person. These habitual responses not only affect our behaviour, but also our emotions and thoughts. If I believe it when I am told at school that I have an awful singing voice, then I will probably avoid situations where I have to sing, and I will also feel inhibited and lack confidence about my ability to sing. Thus habits can lead to inhibition, self-criticism, an absence of self-worth and the tendency to suppression.

Habitual behaviour also limits our ability to change as well as our creative potential. For example, much habitual behaviour is part of a pattern of fear: fear of change, of disapproval, of being criticized or of not being loved. These habits lead to a defensiveness that prevents us from participating fully in an experience and can also prevent us from being prepared to take the risks necessary to make a change in our lives. If I avoid asking for help when I do not understand something in a class I am attending, because I am afraid of being thought stupid, then I am unlikely to learn as much as I could, and I am also unlikely to really enjoy the class. Similarly, if I turn down a new job because I am afraid of taking a risk and making a change, then I have rejected the opportunity for growth and new experience in that area of my life.

We learn not to risk ourselves, and we learn not to be ourselves. It is this that prevents us changing our lives and from really communicating. Supporting another person in their habits, for example by allowing them to become dependent on you, is the worst thing that you can do for them. It kills their opportunity for change and growth.

When we allow our unconscious habits to repeat themselves again and again, the suppression involved is like a record getting stuck in a groove. A deeper and deeper rut is created, and it becomes more and more difficult to change the habit. Habitual behaviour comes to affect our relationships with other people, how we feel about ourselves, and all our activities. In fact it is this process of becoming stuck in habitual ways of being that creates disease. An example is someone who has got into the habit of continually worrying about work. This person will become tense and obsessive, she will alienate her family, she may become too anxious to sleep, and typically she will begin to suffer from a 'nervous' digestion, which leads to a stomach ulcer, or to develop high blood pressure.

So, how can we change habitual behaviour? Firstly, we have to realize that this will be an ongoing process; it is part of the process of becoming conscious that we described in the previous section. It is not that we suddenly stop acting out of our unconscious habits, but that we try to become more aware of when we are responding habitually, and that we continually reaffirm our commitment for change and growth.

The exercises given earlier *(see page 384)* to loosen up some of our habitual ways of doing things are appropriate here. If you feel that you really don't know where to start, there are many psychotherapists and group dynamic processes available today that aim to unravel some of the complex patterns of threads that make up our habitual behaviour *(see pages 425–41 for some suggestions)*.

A general guide to giving up a particular habit is that first we must acknowledge it, and then we must let it go. Acknowledging a habit means becoming aware that we have responded to a situation in an unconscious way. Watch yourself react. When something seems to go wrong, ask yourself why it went that way. Don't blame something or somebody else, instead check whether or not your response was appropriate to the situation. If it wasn't, consider where your reaction came from and how it could be different next time.

The motive for giving up many of our habits emerges when we realize that the pain caused by the habit is actually greater than the pain caused by giving it up. It is always difficult to give up a habit because our unconscious operates by adopting behavioural habits for survival, and so there will always be an initial resistance to change while we are retraining the unconscious to adopt a new pattern. This is why it is often the best strategy to replace an old habit with a more positive, new one. For example, if you are someone who always walks out of the room in the middle of an argument, practise instead letting go of your pride and trying to see the other person's point of view. Putting your energy into trying something new has a very different effect from suppressing an emotion: it opens the door for change, rather than closing it. You know when you have done something differently because there is a sense of freedom and excitement accompanying the action.

Another reason why it is difficult to change a habit is because the habit originated to satisfy a need and we will still have to deal with the need. If I decide to give up smoking, I will only be successful if I am confident that the benefits from giving it up outweigh the advantages or 'pay-off' of smoking. The advantages of smoking, like with many habits, are complex and subtle. There is a physical addiction to nicotine, but we know that removing the nicotine will not actually cause us any physical harm, merely some initial readjustment. What I really have to confront when I give up smoking is the removal of an emotional prop for controlling vulnerability and deflecting a sense of exposure. If I am conscious of the need behind the habit (in this case the need to hide my vulnerability), then I can at least be patient with myself if there is an emotional backlash when I try and change. In fact, trying to give up a habit is a very good way of getting to know more about yourself, and your needs and props, even if you resume the habit in the end. It seems that it is a question of intent. If you are fully prepared to understand what is needed and are able to commit yourself to the process of change, the intention is there and virtually anything is possible! Making decisions seems to be the key to becoming aware of what you are doing and what needs to be done. Check out the exercises on page 384.

So far we have dealt with how habits affect the individual. We can also see that groups and societies operate habitually. These habits need to be reviewed and changed when the damage they cause outweighs any advantages. A society where the purpose was to establish material growth and technological advance has created tremendous progress in scientific knowledge and communications. However, the habitual abuse of natural resources, so often accepted as being necessary for material growth, has resulted in widespread despoilation and pollution of the land. This has now become so damaging that we need to change our approach to materialism in order to survive. We need to build in new habits that are based on an appreciation of the balance between giving and taking. We need to become conscious of the results of our actions and be prepared to put something back in return for what we use.

How can we make these very necessary changes as a society? We can only transform a society if enough individuals recognize the need to change their personal wants and desires, and their attitude to the earth and her resources. Government legislation is necessary to enforce restrictions on the discharge of pollutants and the exploitation of natural resources. But the legislation will only come about if it is demanded by determined individuals. Business practices will only change if individual customers demand that changes are made in what they want to purchase. Every individual needs to reassess his material needs and contribution to society, in order to make change happen on a global scale.

Be wary of stereotyping people. Every time that we have an expectation about the way a certain group of people do something or feel about something or are capable of achieving something, we have limited their potential. If girls are not expected to be good at science in school, we create a reality by not encouraging them and teaching them adequately. We need to be aware of how these habitual attitudes towards people limit and damage both individuals and society as a whole. There are terrible restrictions on freedom and growth in a society that is essentially racist, sexist, classist or ageist. In fact, whenever we hear or use a word with 'ist' or 'ism' at the end we need to beware of prejudiced or judgemental attitudes.

The way that a society creates the different roles of men and women is of the most significant contributions to habitual behaviour. Gender expectations and obligations significantly form the unconscious habits of individuals, and by return, build up more entrenched attitudes and expectations for future generations to adopt. Although the rise in women's consciousness has done much to break down the habits and pressures of a male-dominated society, there is still a long way to go before both women and men are free from the limitations of stereotyped attitudes. How often do you excuse your behaviour because you are a woman?

A baby is genderized immediately from birth. The infant is reacted to differently if she is a girl or if he is a boy. Boys are expected to be aware that they are different from girls at a very early age, and that they are better at doing some things and not so good at others. They learn quickly that they are supposed to be physically adept and they are encouraged to play with constructional toys. They are also expected to be more competitive than girls and they are more likely to be encouraged to go off and explore their environment. Boys are not usually expected to read very early or to talk a lot.

As a boy grows up there is often considerable pressure on him to become successful in the world. He is generally encouraged to become achievement-oriented and ambitious. Boys are approved of if they 'go for what they can get'. They are taught to pursue what interests them and to be brave and withstand hurt. They are told not to cry and they are not generally encouraged to express more painful emotions.

As adolescents, boys are teasingly encouraged to 'prove themselves', and be good at conquering women. This attitude leads to the idea that girls are something to be possessed and taken. This unconscious process of turning girls into objects in the minds of men, creates the conditions for men to commit rape. Women have become something for men to possess. This is true with any form of pornography and sexual harassment.

How can we improve the way we bring up young men? Adolescents need clear definitions from their parents about what is right, because adolescents will, and have the right to, challenge every assumption and every dictate from authority. Honest communication and tolerance are extremely important to allow an adolescent to become an independent adult. It is important to remember that we do not own our children and that they have the right to live their own lives. It can be very difficult to be a constant source of loving support and tolerance without making it conditional.

Young men have a lot of energy, we need to provide positive and creative outlets for that energy. Violent behaviour is the outcome of frustration and a breakdown in communication. Control through fear will never create a healthy society, in the same way that suppression of an illness by drugs will never create a well person. Police and prisons are symptoms of social failure. Everybody, but especially the developing youngster, needs to know what is or is not acceptable behaviour within the family, and within society. They must learn that 'discipline' is something that comes from inside the individual. Imposed discipline can never be an adequate substitute for discipline from within.

Adolescent boys have to work out their relationships with teachers, friends, parents and society. Behind all this is the working out of their role as men. The traditional role of man is seen as the one who goes out to hunt for food to bring back for the dependent women and children. We suggest that a more empowering way of understanding this symbolic image for the man (and woman), is that of the hunter who uses his spear with choice.

In Native American society, where men and women were not in such an exploitative relationship to each other, or to the earth, as we have become, they appreciated how important it was to select the right moment to throw the spear. The hunter took only what was necessary for survival, and only that which was the most appropriate to take – the weakest of the species, so that the strongest would be left to reproduce and support its survival. He also acknowledged the life he had taken and that it was necessary for the survival of his family/group. Wielding his power as an expression of purpose and with consideration as to the result of his action, the man gains clarity, direction and the active expression of purpose. The spear is a symbol of the way man consciously exercises choice to achieve his purpose.

We can empower ourselves by having this same attitude of choosing when and how to act in our everyday use of resources. We can do this by not buying more food than we need, by supporting public transport, by using money rather than accumulating it. Native Americans never killed more animals than they were going to eat in a given period of time. This is a long way from our attitudes of accumulation and acquisition today. Try asking yourself the following questions:

- Do you enjoy work?
- Do you work just for the money?
- Do you really need the money?
- What do you need the money for?
- Do you need the money to support a particular way of life?
- Do you really enjoy your way of life?
- Does your work contribute to your sense of purpose?
- Does your job contribute to the community?
- Do you enjoy the companionship of where you work?
- Do you feel obliged to work to satisfy somebody else?
- Could you risk the disapproval if you were not the main provider/bread-winner?
- Are you still trying to fulfil your parents' or society's expectations for success?
- What does success mean to you?
- What does power mean to you?
- To what degree is material gain your purpose?

So many of us work in jobs whose contribution to our own purpose and to the well-being of society is detrimental. We feel strongly that everybody should question the integrity of the work that they do. Some of us have very little choice about our work because we do need to support our families. If you are stuck in an unsatisfying job then to some extent society is at fault because it pushes people towards material obligations and provides too few mobility opportunities. However, the more we are all aware of a need for change, the more likely is the possibility of it happening.

There is a 'grey area' of jobs that are justified by society because they are 'beneficial', that we feel are questionable in the light of our view that we should all strive for the well-being of the whole, and not for the benefit of one section or part. Much scientific research falls into this category. Animal experimentation exploits the animal kingdom for the so-called benefit of humans. Moreover, animal experiments continue despite evidence that there are frequently alternatives to using animals and also that animals are often not an exact enough substitute for the research to be of real value to humans.

It is worth remembering that 49 per cent of our genes are made up of the opposite sex. We are taught esoterically and psychologically that we are feminine and masculine on different levels. This means that we need to look at both the masculine and feminine parts of ourselves.

Girls are genderized from birth just as much as boys are. It appears that even the youngest of girls will play differently from their male counterparts. Girls tend to be less interested in constructional games and more readily involved in social and communication-oriented games. They become interested in looking pretty with the minimum of encouragement, or even at times with active discouragement. It is very difficult to identify what causes these differences in behaviour between girls and boys: it may be due to inheritance, biological make-up, parents, society, or a combination of all these factors.

A girl's development is further determined by the educational process. Girls are treated very differently from boys at school, however careful and informed the school attempts to be. They are generally considered to be easier to deal with in the classroom, they tend to apply themselves more, and they learn quickly that they get approval by being 'good'. Girls tend to mature more quickly than boys, and are usually more advanced at reading and writing than boys of the same age.

In recent years schools have generally made more effort to offer equal opportunities to both sexes. Reading material for early readers has been reviewed to remove some of the more explicitly sexist ideas. Teachers play a crucial role in society: they are the spearheads of change. Unfortunately, the power for making changes in education has been placed in the hands of politicians, whose decisions are based on votes and not vision. Our society's failure to honour the role of our children's educators is demonstrated by successive governments' persistent undermining of teachers. The teacher entrusted to be with our children must be supported and valued by parents and all the members of the community. Teachers need to be leaders within the community; their contribution towards creating our future through education is of vital importance. Children need teachers who are committed and have a sense of purpose. We need to create the conditions within our education system that allow teachers to inspire children, or at least pass on the willingness to learn.

Young people are subjected to a huge amount of advertising as they grow up. Most children also spend hours a day watching TV and playing computer games. While these provide entertainment and fill a space, they do not stimulate the creative imagination. Instead they fill the mind with a limiting set of created images and stereotypes. The media persists in perpetuating the stereotype of young women as pretty and desirable objects. A girl's sense of self-worth becomes dependent on her attractiveness and how she fits into the standards of society. The adolescent girl is desperately trying to fit in, to make herself acceptable to her peers and attractive to the opposite sex.

Adolescent girls need a lot of reassurance that they are all right, and that they are loved because they are who they are, not just because they are seen to be attractive. It is helpful to encourage girls to be self-reliant and not to be dependent on others for approval. Teach them practical things, for example, how to repair plugs, bicycles and so on, to do things around the house like putting up shelves, as well as how to make clothes, grow things and cook. They need to learn how to be independent human beings, and not vulnerable and dependent within their own environment.

Self-discipline needs to be encouraged in girls as in boys. This is not always considered to be important and as a result girls can become gullible and lack discrimination. A lack of discrimination leads to difficulties in saying no, making poor choices and the likelihood of abuse.

The choices and information available to young people these days are immense. The internet has provided a limitless resource for communication and education. However, this also requires great discrimination in its use, as much of what is available, and actually pushed in front of internet users, revolves around the lowest common denominators of behaviour, such as gambling and pornography. Although you may be able to protect your children when they are young, unless you encourage them to learn to set their own boundaries, the likelihood of them being drawn into unsavoury experiences is much higher.

Girls pick up the need to be protective from their mothers. They often enjoy caring for and nuturing animals and babies when they are still very young. This is a very fine quality, but it can develop into a tendency to overprotect and stifle other people. If mothers overprotect their sons, then the boys will grow up with a lack of independence and an inability to be creative. If mothers overprotect their daughters then girls also become overprotective and unable to let things go their own way. This is the mechanism by which girls can become emotionally manipulative and security-seeking.

Too often women seem to become over-materialistic and competitive out of a desire for control. Why do we need to control? Why do we need to stand out as special people, as 'prima donnas', queen bees or even martyrs? Because it gives us a sense of power, a feeling of being more significant than we suspect we really are. What we need to develop is a sense of our true power as women: we need to find an inner sense of worth based on our appreciation of our own strengths.

Whenever we resign ourselves to our weaknesses, or refuse to acknowledge our failings, we collude with all that is second rate in society. We accept poor-quality food, we put up with the appalling services public places provide for our children. Whenever a woman tries to prove her worth through her attractiveness she is putting down her real inner worth.

For a woman to function effectively and positively in our society, it is important not to lose touch with the positive qualities of being a woman. A positive archetype that we can draw on for inspiration is that of the Goddess. The energy of the Goddess is the earth itself; in all its abundance. The Goddess is in touch with the processes of life and death: she is the healer, the seer, the inspirer, the sister, the lover and the mother.

Too often women lack a sense of purpose. We easily confuse this with what society approves of in us, that is by being responsive and submissive. The Goddess image allows us to sense our power and our purpose, without losing touch of our femininity. If we have a sense of our inner worth, we do not need to rely on that which is external to prove our value. We need to trust the process of growth and renewal in ourselves and in the earth. The Goddess is the earth, from her and through her all life is sustained.

22

Our Physical Selves

In this section we are going to look at how we can look after our body so that we are able to resist disease and enjoy ourselves. Health has become a complex issue in recent years. Although better nutrition and hygiene did improve our health, a new and different pattern of environmental and stress-related disease has become established.

The main factors that contribute to how susceptible we are to disease today are inherited factors, individual habits, environmental stresses (including pollution), medication and diet. Our ability to be healthy depends on whether we can steer a reasonable path through these factors. We have to acknowledge that there are today a great deal more choices involved in our daily life, for example as to what we eat, how hard we work, etc., and that the choices we make influence our health.

We can all think of people who appeared not to look after themselves well, probably smoking or drinking heavily, and who thrived into a perfectly healthy old age. This kind of constitution is not so common any more. Increasingly we do need to look after ourselves in order to stay healthy. Pollution, over-medication, refined diets and stressful lifestyles have all placed a strain on our ability to eliminate toxins, adapt to our environment and remain healthy.

Maintaining our good health requires a degree of balance in our diet and the exercise and rest that we take, and we will look at all these factors in detail in this section. If we already have a specific health problem, we need to consider consulting a therapist of some kind, as well as reassessing our lifestyle and the factors in it which may have contributed to the problem.

Choosing a particular form of therapy or a therapist can be difficult just because of the wide range that are available. Probably the best way to choose is to go for one which feels to be the most appropriate for you at this moment in time. Becoming healthy is a process and this process may involve seeing more than one therapist, as well as making a variety of changes in your lifestyle. The important thing is to make a start now, and not worry if the therapy that you choose does not seem to be absolutely ideal for you, or that your therapist does not have all the answers. If you discover later that a different therapy feels better for your needs, then change, although you need to give any therapy long enough to have a fair chance of working.

Why choose holistic medicine rather than orthodox medicine? The aim of holistic medicine is to understand the process of disease and how these processes have led to a particular set of disease symptoms for an individual. Unlike orthodox medicine, the treatment will be directed at changing the disease process, not just removing the symptoms that are the end result. This is known as curing the tendency to disease, rather than suppressing the symptoms.

We described in the previous section *(see pages 392–403)* how an individual's habits can lead to disease developing in the physical body. By habit we mean any behaviour, response or attitude that prevents us from being in touch with, and expressing, our inner purpose. Curing disease requires changing the habits, which may be mental, emotional or physical. Only when the blocks to health have been removed is the body able to come back into a state of health and maintain it. Holistic medicine is one of the tools that we have available to help us become more aware of our negative processes, and to change them. At the same time, natural remedies will encourage the body to throw off, or eliminate, the symptoms of the disease.

Disease can be seen as an opportunity for growth, not by accepting the disease itself but by accepting that the process is our own, and that it is within our potential to change it. Our disease is our link with our past – we can look back at the development of the disease and see where the wrong choices were made. This can be very empowering, not if we blame anything or anyone else (or ourselves) for our disease, but if we recognize that we can make changes in our own life, and that these changes will affect our own health and well-being. Blaming anyone else, or ourselves, for our disease will create anger and resentment or guilt, which only serves to add to our ill health and further prevent our growth.

The starting-point, or the 'soil', for our health is our genetic inheritance. Not only can specific physical diseases be inherited, but so can our susceptibility to types of disease and our general constitution. Orthodox medicine was never very good at explaining or understanding how the more subtle processes of inheritance work. Traditional Chinese medicine and homoeopathy have made greater contributions to our understanding of how inherited tendencies affect our health. In recent years, however, the decoding of human DNA has led to a rapid advancement in finding the 'gene' responsible for certain inherited diseases. This information may prove very useful in pinpointing the tendency to develop a certain illness, especially if we then modify our diet or lifestyle as appropriate. It is important though that this information does not label us or limit our potential for healing.

In Chinese medicine, it is the state of the flow of body energies in the man and the woman that contribute to the health of the child. A man with a healthy and vital flow of energy will produce healthy sperm; and a woman with a healthy flow of energy will provide the right environment for a foetus to develop in the womb. In homoeopathy, the theory of 'miasms' explains how subtle characteristics are passed down in families, and the same disease tendency will crop up in different members of the same family, although the actual symptoms may differ from person to person. For example, it may be one particular miasm in the family that contributes to asthma developing in one child and eczema and hayfever developing in another child in the same family. Constitutional homoeopathic treatment aims to minimize the impact of these disease-inflicting miasms.

❋ Food and Diet

As well as our inheritance, our health will be determined by our diet, our environment and our lifestyle. Food is one of the basic necessities for life, but this basic need becomes overladen with personal and social habits and values.

Many of our eating habits stem from sharing mealtimes together. Children learn social and cultural values during mealtimes, as well as getting nourishment. This early socialization contributes to the eating habits that we develop when we are older. It is generally the mother who is mainly responsible for giving children their food. Children need to be encouraged by their mothers to be aware of food as the produce of the earth. We all need to be aware that we are fortunate to have enough to eat. Wasting food is a profound waste of resources.

Food should be appreciated, shared and enjoyed. As mothers we must be careful not to make our children feel guilty if they do not want what we think they should have. At the same time, children need to be offered nutritious food, and they need regular meals. It is a good idea to educate children about basic nutrition at home, and involve them in the preparation and cooking of food, so that they can grow up with good habits.

There is a huge amount of advertising of food products, and this is aimed at trying to prove that one brand is better than another. The food we buy is also subject to class, racial and lifestyle factors. Diet needs to be tailored to suit individual needs and tastes within broad nutritional guidelines. We do not know the full effects of living on a diet of TV dinners and refined foods on our health because they have not been around for long enough. However, there are indications that our health, and that of our children, is being seriously undermined by a modern diet of processed and refined foods. Much of our food is so highly processed that we should be asking what we are really eating. Sometimes it is hard to work out what the natural basis of a processed product really is. Always read the label and be aware of what choices you are making when you buy, for example, a highly coloured instant dessert or fruit drink!

We should also be asking questions about packaging and the effect it has on our food and on our health. Some of the processes that are now used in food preparation are damaging to the environment, but what about the effects that some of the packaging is having on our health? We do know that some types of plastic produce what are known as 'hormone disrupters' that are already affecting the hormones in our bodies. Information is being released frequently about these issues. Find out what you can. Subscribe to *Ethical Consumer* or *What Doctors Don't Tell You* or *The Ecologist*, or some of the other excellent magazines that make it their business to inform you about these matters. We believe that our power to change lies in our desire to discover the truth about what we are doing to ourselves. It is a slow process, but knowing what is going on helps us to make positive healthy choices.

In the past we have been willing to let the 'experts' decide what is good food for us and our children. Now we are becoming more aware about some of the implications of the type of food we eat, and we are starting to question those 'experts'. After 1945 great emphasis was placed on consuming sufficient milk, butter and meat. Recently there has been concern over the level of heart disease connected with a western diet that is high in animal fats. Also, children frequently suffer from allergies connected to the additives in our food.

In order to fulfil our food requirements factory farming has been developed. There have been some alarming incidents in recent years to indicate that we need to reassess our attitude to producing food. Battery-farmed chickens have led to outbreaks of salmonella. Feeding cows on an unnatural diet of meat products has led to the development of BSE (bovine spongiform encephalopathy) and CJD. The over-use of nitrates in agricultural practices has led to the pollution of our water. There are many other examples of how short-term profit-motivated ideas have led the developed world to seriously disrupt the balance of agriculture.

There is now a shift underway towards eating more of a wholefood-oriented diet, and towards producing organically-grown vegetables and free-range animal products. Children themselves are often very concerned about the welfare of the animals in factory farming and are making choices about the food they are prepared to eat. However, this recent development only applies to the western world. We still supply chemicals for intensive production of foods in underdeveloped countries. Refined foods are still very popular in less developed countries, partly as a sign of wealth, and also because food companies have looked for new markets as their domestic ones have shrunk. We need to reassess our food production practices on a global scale.

What kind of food should we eat? Basically, food retains more of its nutritional value the closer it is to its original state. Food needs to be as fresh and as unprocessed and unrefined as possible. We need, where possible, to eat the whole of the product, as with brown rice or wholemeal flour.

Food is an area where we can all have a great effect on what is produced by exercising our choice about what we buy. Women, as the main purchasers of the family's food, have encouraged supermarkets to offer more products that are additive and colouring-free by choosing brands and foods without additives and colourings. The food industry will respond to our demands if we make them known. Make a point of asking for what you want to buy, not just accepting what the retailer has decided you can have.

Refined foods are often low in vitamins, and to compensate for this some foods actually have vitamins added back in. This is a total waste of resources. The fact that intensive agricultural methods have caused a decline in the natural vitamins and minerals in our food has led some nutritionists to favour taking food supplements. There is no substitute for good, fresh food, and if we take steps to have a varied and balanced diet, with a high proportion of organically-produced foodstuffs, then food supplements may not be necessary.

If you would like to know more about what foods to eat in order to benefit from natural sources of particular vitamins or minerals, then consult the food charts on pages 420–22.

We increasingly have to make an effort to buy food that is natural and untampered with. Some food is irradiated to prolong its shelf life and to reduce bacterial contamination. We do not know the long-term effects of eating irradiated food. For several years it was said that irradiation did not alter the food in any way and you could not even tell the difference between irradiated and non-irradiated food. However, in 2002 tests were developed that can detect whether or not food has been subject to irradiation and it was announced that some foods were being sold illegally by not being marked as irradiated. Now that accurate tests are available, all irradiated foods should be labelled, and so we can choose not to buy them. If we refuse to accept food we are not confident in, then it will not be supplied.

This is equally true of genetically modified food. We just do not know the long-term health effects of eating GM food. There are suggestions that it will lead to an increase in allergic reactions as foreign proteins are inserted into foods we could otherwise tolerate. We do know, however, that growing GM crops leads to a reduction in biodiversity, the tainting of natural plant stock and the dependency of small farmers on global corporations. The most effective way to stop the production of GM food is to refuse to buy it.

If you are aware that you have not had a very good diet for some years, or that your diet is contributing to a particular disease, you should consider consulting a dietary therapist or naturopath for specific advice. The naturopathic approach to health is that we need to be able to clear out impurities or toxins in our system, rather than letting them build up and contribute to disease. If we are reasonably healthy we should be able to eliminate a small amount of additives and toxins through our bowels, bladder and skin. However, if the level of toxins in our diet is too high, or if our eliminative processes are blocked or underfunctioning, then symptoms of disease will result.

A detoxifying or cleansing diet can be a good way to clear out the system – and a good start to making improvements in your diet if you feel that to be necessary. Either consult a naturopath or dietary therapist who will guide you through a cleansing regime, or follow the cleansing diet on page 423. A traditional time to do a cleansing diet is in the spring, so that we can clear out the effects of stodgy winter foods and prepare ourselves for the new yearly cycle.

Another area related to food that has become a big issue in our society is that of body weight. We live in a society where women are expected to be nymph-like creatures, and so many of us are unhappy if this is not what our bodies are like. For some women trying to lose weight is a constant struggle and cause of anxiety; other women give up completely under the pressure, and do become obese. Neither is a very satisfactory way of being.

For some time it has been known that calorie-counting diets are rarely an effective way of losing weight and maintaining the lower weight. Calorie counting requires an attitude of self-denial and an artificial, obsessive approach to food. We need to get back in touch with what foods suit us as individual people, given our particular tastes and our lifestyle.

What is basically wrong with our attitude to weight is that being over-weight has become confused with being unfit. We often use being overweight as an excuse for not making the attempt to be fit. We can become fit by concentrating on improving the quality of the food that we eat, and by taking regular exercise. It is much more sensible and enjoyable to set your purpose at being fit than to try to live up to an image of what you would like to look like.

In addition to eating a diet based on fresh and unrefined wholefoods there are a few other general guidelines that we recommend if you are considering making improvements to your eating habits. Eat a wide variety of foodstuffs that supply a balanced range of nutrients. Eat regular meals – say, three times a day. Do not eat just before going to bed. Eat for the purpose of being healthy, and active, and to get energy, and not for other reasons. Talk to other women about your food concerns. Find a form of exercise you really want to do so that it becomes an enjoyable part of your day. Work on being positive and improving your general self-esteem, rather than just concentrating on what you look like.

Our society has attached an exaggerated importance to certain foods. These are often the ones that are likely to make us put on weight, for example choco-late, cream or sweets. These luxury foods have become readily available and commonplace, whereas once they were genuinely treats for special occasions. If we say no to these foods we can become caught up in feelings of self-denial that we may feel the need to rebel against.

The fact that so many women have eating disorders, and have even become closet eaters or anorexic, is a fundamental sign of how mixed up we are as a society about eating and weight. These kind of problems will require an in-depth assessment and investigation of the patterns behind the self-denial, and poor self-esteem, that are causing the eating disorder. A visit to a counsellor, psychotherapist or other professional therapist will be necessary to treat these more serious eating disorders.

⁂ Exercise

In order to take regular exercise we have to decide that it is an important part of our daily life. Also, we have to have developed enough self-esteem to recognize that our personal needs are important, and that one of those needs is to keep fit.

Creating the leisure time to take exercise can be a real problem for many women. If you work and have children then it is always difficult to find time for yourself. It is best to set aside a small amount of time on a regular basis – an amount that you know is realistic. There are many good exercise books and videos to help you create your own exercise routine and stick to it. It can be fun to encourage a friend to take up an exercise with you so that you can swim, jog or play tennis together.

There are many benefits to taking exercise, but generally it improves your level of energy by stimulating your vitality. Exercising also assists the elimination of toxins by increasing lymphatic drainage. It tones the circulation and improves muscle tone. Regular exercise is particularly important in women, as over a period of years exercising encourages bone growth and helps to prevent osteoporosis.

Some forms of exercise are costly, so if you are hard up you need to find ways of exercising that do not involve joining an expensive fitness club or paying for classes or equipment, and so on. Contact your local council for information about subsidized sports centres. Adult Education Institutes often offer subsidized fitness classes, or contact your local women's support group.

It is worth remembering that you can take every opportunity in your daily life to exercise and use muscles. Try running up and down stairs and walking up escalators. If you travel to work on a bus or tube, get off a stop early and walk the last bit. If you live in the city, try to set aside one day each week to go to the countryside for a walk, and if you have children, take them with you.

As we get older it tends to become even more of an effort to make sure that we get enough exercise to stay supple and fit. If we feel tired and without energy, then we may be unfit and probably lack self-esteem about our physical body. What we need is to do more exercise, but because we feel tired anyway we do less, and this vicious cycle needs to be broken. Concentrate on pleasurable exercises like walking, swimming or gardening. It is keeping moving that is important.

Getting older does require us to find different ways of enjoying life. We need to recognize that we are more than just a physical body, without neglecting our fitness. Later in life it is possible to do the things that you never had the time for during a career and looking after children. Take up those activities that you used to be interested in again, or do the things you always wanted to do. Involve yourself in the surrounding community. Try checking out your local libraries, Adult Education Institute or local council for appropriate activities. Now is the time to cultivate a special interest.

⚘ Sleep and Rest

It has been said that our bodies can only repair themselves during the hours that we are asleep. We need sleep for good physical and psychological health, although the amount of sleep needed varies considerably from person to person and at different times of our life.

Newborn babies spend the majority of their time asleep and within a few months usually become used to more regular sleeping patterns, averaging about 12 hours a day. It is very important for all children to get enough sleep to sustain their intensive growing. Most children will need about ten hours of sleep until their teens. Severely disturbed sleep in children is often caused by hyperactivity. There are many theories as to why hyperactivity occurs, and we suggest that you consult one of the hyperactive children support groups to investigate this problem further *(see page 432)*.

Sleep can become out of balance at either extreme, and may be an indication of being out of balance in other ways also. If you desire to sleep constantly, and for long periods of time, it may be that you are unwell, in which case it is normal to want to sleep more in order for the body to repair itself. If this tendency is prolonged, then you may need to find out if you are trying to avoid your daily life, and consider seeking professional advice.

If you have trouble going to sleep, then you need to assess your ability to 'let go' generally. Look at the section on Insomnia on page 88. Try to avoid stimulants such as coffee and smoking all day (not just in the evening), and make building in the time for relaxation a priority. Taking daily exercise in the fresh air can help you to sleep through the night.

Another reason that we need to sleep is to allow ourselves to dream. Dreaming is the reflective, more passive balance to the active, outgoing part of our life. Problems that have been left unresolved by our rational, conscious minds can be explored through our dreams.

We can work with our dreams to come to a better understanding of ourselves. Try writing down your dreams in a special notebook kept by the side of your bed. Recording your dreams will often increase your ability to remember them. It is worth remembering that your reaction to your dream can be as significant as the dream itself, and when you record your dream you can convey how you felt about it also. If you want to examine your dreams with someone else, then there are various forms of therapy that work with dreams; consult your natural healing centre and ask about their psychotherapists, or if they run dream workshops.

❋ Sex

Our sexual expression is an expression on one particuar level of who we are. Our sexual relationships will reflect how we relate to our bodies, and how we relate to our parents, as well as how we relate to other men and women.

Sex for procreation is natural. This is a basic urge. Sex for pleasure is a human capability, and there are a lot of opinions around, just as there always have been, about what is and is not 'right' in terms of sex. All religions have guidelines and restrictions about sex. Unfortunately, rigid guidelines and opinions will always lead to feelings of guilt in those people who do not easily conform to the prescribed attitudes. There is more sexual freedom in our society in recent years, although we still have to deal with many social expectations and opinions.

We can only experience a sense of sexual well-being if we feel good about our particular sexual needs. This does not mean devaluing sex. But we need to develop sex as an expression of love and tenderness.

Sexual intimacy gives us an opportunity to explore our inner selves and our mutual vulnerability with another person. Sex is a time when we can experience a sense of closeness with another human being. The important thing is to respect your own body, and your partner's, during sex. There are no easy solutions to the power-based struggles that often develop between sexual partners, but it is worth bearing in mind that a sexual relationship offers great opportunities for self-learning and growth.

As we get older our sexual relationships mature and our desires change. Once freed of the need or the fear of getting pregnant, we have greater opportunity to enjoy sharing our body with another. There is less pressure on achieving what you want and more of giving something to someone you love. Then sex can truly become an expression of who you are. Sex can be joyful and fun, and above all it can help create that bond of intimacy.

Our level of interest in sex does not make us more or less of a woman or man. We must guard against making assumptions about other people. When we question why some people are more interested in sex than others, we must be wary of accepting that there is a 'normal' level of sexual behaviour. Similarly, we need to be sensitive to differing sexual orientations. Any sexual orientation that is not exploitative should simply be accepted as one expression of who a person is.

Sex education in schools varies widely, but however good this education may be it can only be secondary to the openness that parents should have with their children. We need to be well enough informed to answer anatomical questions, and we should work on being close enough as a family so that the growing-up process is simply part of everyday living together. We need to impart to our children a recognition of both the pleasure of sex and the respect required, both for our own bodies and the physical and emotional needs of others.

Sex, like eating, sleeping and exercise, is part of living. Be aware of what you do and its effects, and enjoy it because you are alive.

part IV:

Appendices

Natural Remedies First Aid Kit

✳ Ointments

ARNICA
For bruising, sprains, strains and so on. Apply externally to the injured part. Do not use on broken skin.

HYPERCAL
A general purpose antiseptic and healing ointment for use on abrasions, cuts, spots and insect bites, etc.

✳ Tinctures

EUPHRASIA
A soothing and anti-inflammatory lotion made from the herb eyebright. Dilute in cool, boiled water and use as an eyewash for eye infections, sore eyes, etc. Seek medical advice if you suspect there are any particles of grit or whatever left in the eye.

HYPERCAL
An antiseptic and healing lotion. Apply neat for small cuts, bites, spots, etc. To clean wounds, dilute a few drops of the tincture in a little cool, boiled water and gently bathe the area with a piece of cotton wool dipped in the solution.

❋ Essential Oils

LAVENDER
Antiseptic and anti-inflammatory. Pour neat onto minor burns and scalds. Hold near the nose and inhale the vapours if feeling faint.

❋ Bach Flower Remedies

FIVE FLOWER ESSENCES/SOS
For shock, fear and panic. Take a few drops straight in the mouth as often as required. Alternatively, add a few drops to half a cup of water and sip as often as required. If the patient is unconscious, or cannot swallow, moisten any pulse point, e.g. temple or wrist, with a few drops of the remedy.

❋ Homoeopathic Remedies

Keep these remedies in a box and store in a dark, cool place away from strong smells. If you are taking homoeopathic remedies abroad with you, ask for them not to be X-rayed at airports, as this will reduce their efficiency.

The remedies listed below are for first aid and acute situations only. If symptoms are severe, or persist, professional advice must be sought.

For first aid and acute use, remedies in the 6th potency should be taken, one dose every two hours until there is some improvement, then dosage should be less frequent. Remedies in the 30th potency should be repeated only once or twice, preferably at eight-hour intervals. For further indications look the remedies up in the *Materia Medica* section of this book.

ACONITE 6
First stages of fever and inflammation; after-effects of exposure to a cold wind; earache; hoarse, dry cough; after-effects of shock or fright.

ARNICA 30
A very useful first aid remedy to take after any accident or injury. Helps to reduce bruising, prevent haemorrhage, and ameliorate shock; concussion; overexertion.

ARSENICUM 30
Food poisoning. After-effects of bad food or drink with diarrhoea and vomiting; great weariness; anxiety and restlessness. Acute asthmatic and allergy attacks marked by anxiety; Worse at night.

BELLADONNA 30
Fevers with a high temperature. Patient is hot, red and may be delirious. Sunstroke. Throbbing, hammering headache. Inflammation where the affected part looks red and has a violent, throbbing pain.

FERRUM PHOS 6X
For the beginning stages of a cold or sore throat; hoarseness; nosebleeds. Externally this remedy may be used by crushing a tablet and sprinkling the powder onto a wound to stop the bleeding and help prevent infection.

GELSEMIUM 30
Influenza with an aching body, heavy headache, shivering. Trembling and diarrhoea before an ordeal, or following a shock.

HYPERICUM 30
Injury to parts rich in nerves such as fingers or spine. Any injury marked by severe pain. Lacerated wounds; punctured wounds such as from a nail, needle or splinter.

LEDUM 30
Wasp, bee or other insect bites or stings. Animal, bites, such as dog bites, where there is bruising surrounding the wound. Black eyes, any injury with a lot of bruising, with swelling and puffiness. Prophylactic for tetanus.

NUX VOMICA 6
After-effects of over-indulgence in food, drink or stimulants (hangover). Irritability, nausea and headache. Any stomach disorder where there is nausea that is greatly relieved by vomiting.

RHUS TOX 6
Sprains and strains following an injury or overexertion. The painful or injured part stiffens up during rest, and is ameliorated by gentle motion. Colds or 'flu following exposure to cold, wet weather.

2

Food Charts

Chart 1: Good Sources of Vitamins

VITAMIN A
Fish-liver oils, liver, butter, egg yolk, cheese, herring, mackerel, carrots, dried apricots, kale, parsley, spinach, pumpkin, peas.

VITAMIN B1 – THIAMIN
Brewer's yeast, yeast extract, rice, wheatgerm, soya beans, sunflower seeds, broad beans, rye, lentils, chickpeas.

VITAMIN B2 – RIBOFLAVIN
Yeast extract, Brewer's yeast, liver, soya beans, wheatgerm, eggs, yoghurt, almonds, mushrooms, millet, kelp, broad beans, sesame seeds, mung beans.

VITAMIN B3 – NIACIN
Brewer's yeast, meat, liver, mackerel, brown rice, cod, peanuts, kelp, pulses, almonds, dates, millet.

VITAMIN B5 – PANTOTHENIC ACID
Brewer's yeast, liver, wheatbran, egg, lentils, cashew nuts, almonds, soya beans, brown rice, peas.

VITAMIN B6
Brewer's yeast, liver, mackerel, avocado, banana, walnuts, yoghurt, millet, rye, sunflower seeds, sesame seeds.

VITAMIN B12
Liver, fish, meat, free-range eggs, cheese, yoghurt, milk. Rarely found in cereals, fruit or vegetables, although there is a small amount in cauliflower, comfrey and alfalfa.

VITAMIN C
Blackcurrants, parsley, broccoli, green pepper, strawberries, cabbage, oranges, guava, cauliflower, watercress. You should eat vegetables raw to obtain maximum levels of vitamin C, and all foodstuffs should be fresh.

VITAMIN D
Sunshine, oily fish, egg yolk, sunflower seeds, alfalfa.

VITAMIN E
Wheatgerm oil and other cold-pressed vegetable oils, sesame seeds, tahini, almonds, wheatgerm, millet, Brazil nuts, peanuts.

VITAMIN K
Fresh leafy green vegetables, green and red peppers.

FOLIC ACID
Brewer's yeast, liver, green vegetables, eggs, lentils, milk.

Chart 2: Good Sources of Minerals

CALCIUM
Dairy products, watercress, wheatflour, cabbage, eggs, brown rice, fish, meat, sesame seeds, nuts, chickpeas, kelp, parsley, broad beans.

FLUORINE
Tea, oats, rice, watercress, most fresh vegetables, goats' milk.

IODINE
Iodized salt, white fish, yoghurt, kelp, eggs, almonds, wholemeal bread, spinach, strawberries, turnip, okra.

IRON
Liver, cocoa, treacle, parsley, lentils, dulse, kelp, sesame seeds, haricot beans, wholemeal bread, eggs, watercress, dried fruit.

MAGNESIUM
Brazil nuts, soya beans, wholemeal flour, chocolate, lentils, parsley, kelp, almonds, sesame seeds, spinach.

MANGANESE
Tea, whole cereals, beans and peas, nuts, pineapple, grapes, beetroot, watercress, kale.

PHOSPHORUS
Cheese, lentils, wholemeal bread, eggs, meat, fish, brown rice, sunflower seeds, barley, kelp, sesame seeds, almonds, rye, millet.

POTASSIUM
Brewer's yeast, dates, mushrooms, cabbage, meat, bananas, watercress, tomatoes, yoghurt, wholemeal bread, kelp, soya beans, dandelion.

ZINC
Meat, oysters, cheese, lentils, most nuts, sunflower seeds, sesame seeds, rye, olives, haricot beans, eggs.

3

Cleansing Diet

This cleansing diet is a 10-day programme which is suitable if you are basically healthy but want to clear your system out. If you have a particular health problem, you should have a consultation with a dietary therapist or naturopath before going on a special diet.

It is particularly beneficial to do a cleansing diet in the spring and/or autumn.

DAY 1
Fruit for breakfast, lunch and in the evening. Choose one fruit for each meal from the following: apples, pears or grapes. Eat as much fruit as you like at one sitting. Drink lots of mineral water throughout the day.

DAY 2, 3, 4, 5 AND 6
Fruit for breakfast. Choose one fruit each day from: apples, pears, grapes, tomatoes, kiwi fruit and grapefruit.

Raw vegetables for lunch. Make a mixture of at least five salad vegetables: mix roots (carrots, grated beetroot, and so on), sprouts and leafy vegetables.

In the evening eat cooked vegetables. Make a soup by boiling a mixture of at least five vegetables, preferably including onions. Do not add any salt or seasoning.

DAY 7, 8 AND 9
Breakfast – as Day 2.

Lunch – as Day 2, but in addition eat two slices of dry Ryvita crispbread biscuits.

Evening – as Day 2.

DAY 10

Breakfast – as Day 2.

Lunch – as Day 5.

Evening – as Day 2, but in addition eat a baked potato with a small knob of butter.

NOTES

Drink lots of mineral water every day.

If you prefer, you may add a small amount of dressing to the raw-vegetable lunch, made from virgin olive oil and a little fresh lemon juice only.

If you feel weak and very hungry between mealtimes, drink a cup of barley water made as follows: boil pot barley in lots of water until the water begins to turn pink and the barley is soft. Keep adding water if it gets low. When done, strain off the water and discard the barley. Add a little fresh lemon juice and a teaspoon of honey to each cupful. You can take this drink in a flask if you need to keep going at work.

Eat as much organically-produced fruit and vegetables as possible.

It is not unusual to get symptoms such as headaches, tiredness or skin eruptions during a cleansing diet. This is an indication that toxins are being released from the tissues and into the bloodstream before they are eliminated. If you drink enough water these symptoms should not be severe, and they usually disappear before you have finished the diet.

Important things to avoid altogether throughout the diet are: tea, coffee, smoking, salt, pepper, drugs (whether recreational or prescribed), alcohol and late nights.

Don't binge the day after you finish the diet. You will regret it. Readjust to the new range of tastes and foods available to you slowly.

Useful Contacts and Addresses

To find a practitioner of natural medicine write to the appropriate organization listed below, seek a personal recommendation from a friend or acquaintance, or look up your nearest natural health centre by looking under 'Clinics' in the local telephone directory.

In Britain, the Institute for Complementary Medicine publishes a yearbook which is a directory of practices, colleges, therapies and information. Write to:

The Institute for Complementary Medicine
21 Portland Place, LondonW1N 3AF.

ABORTION ADVICE
The Pregnancy Advisory Service
11–13 Charlotte Street
London W1
020 7637 8962

ACUPUNCTURE
The British Acupuncture Council
Suite One
19 Cavendish Square
London W1M 9AD
020 7409 1440
www.acupuncture.org.uk

AIDS
The National Aids Helpline
Freephone 0800 567 123

AROMATHERAPY
The Aromatherapy Organizations Council
PO Box 355
Croydon
CR9 2QP
020 8251 7912
www.aocuk.net

THE BATES METHOD
The Bates Association
PO Box 25
Shoreham-by-Sea
BN43 6ZE

BREASTFEEDING
La Lèche League
PO Box 29
West Bridgford
Nottingham
NG2 7NP
020 7242 1278 (24-hour helpline)
www.laleche.org.uk

CHILDBIRTH
The Active Birth Centre
25 Bickerton Road
London N19 5JT
020 7561 9006

The Association of Radical Midwives
www.radmid.demon.co.uk

The Independent Midwives' Association
1 The Great Quarry
Guildford
Surrey
GU1 3XN
01483 821104
www.independentmidwives.org.uk

The National Childbirth Trust
www.nctpregnancyandbabycare.com

CHILDREN
(see also Parenting, Teenagers)

Childline
0800 1111 (24-hour helpline for children)
www.childline.org.uk

NSPCC
42 Curtain Road
London EC2A 3NH
020 7825 2500 (child protection helpline)
www.nspcc.org.uk

CHIROPRACTIC
The British Chiropractic Association
Blagrave House
17 Blagrave Street
Reading
RG1 1QD
0118 959 5950

CITIZENS' ADVICE
The Citizens' Advice Bureau (CAB)
www.adviceguide.org.uk

COMPLEMENTARY MEDICINE
The Institute for Complementary Medicine
London SE16 7QZ
020 7237 5165
www.icmedicine.co.uk

COUNSELLING AND PSYCHOTHERAPY
The British Association for Counselling
1 Regent Place
Rugby
Warwickshire
CV21 2PJ
01788 550899

The National Council of Psychotherapists
Hazelwood
Broadmead
Sway
Lymington
Hants
S041 6DH
01590 683770

Relate (formerly The National Marriage Guidance Council)
0845 130 40 10
www.relate.org.uk

The Samaritans
08457 909090 (24-hour helpline)
www.samaritans.org.uk

The UK Council for Psychotherapy
167–169 Great Portland Street
London W1N 5FB
020 7436 3002

CRANIAL OSTEOPATHY
The Craniosacral Therapy Association
27 Old Gloucester Street
London WC1N 3XX
0700 784 735

DOMESTIC VIOLENCE
The Women's Aid Federation
Advice, refuges and support.
www.womensaid.org.uk

National Domestic Violence Helpline
PO Box 391
Bristol BS99 7WS
08457 023 468

DRUGS
Adfam National
020 7928 8900 (national helpline for friends and families of drug users)

The National Drugs Helpline
Offers free and confidential advice about any drugs issues.
0800 776600
www.ndh.org.uk

Release
020 7729 9904 (24-hour confidential helpline about drug use and legal issues)

ENVIRONMENTAL ISSUES
Friends of the Earth
56–58 Alma Street
Luton
Beds.
LU1 2YZ
020 7490 1555
www.foe.co.uk

Greenpeace
30–31 Islington Green
London N1 8XE
www.greenpeace.org.uk

The Women's Environmental Network (WEN)
PO Box 30626
London E1 1TZ
020 7481 9004
www.wen.org.uk

DRUIDISM
The Druid Order
23 Thornsett Road
London SE20 7XB
020 8659 4879

ETHICAL BANKING
Triodos Bank
0117 973 9339
www.triodos.co.uk

FLOWER REMEDIES – DR BACH
The Bach Flower Centre
Mount Vernon
Sotwell
Wallingford
Oxfordshire
OX10 0PZ
01491 39489

The Healing Herbs of Dr Bach
PO Box 65
Hereford
HR2 0UW
01873 890218
www.healing-herbs.co.uk

OTHER FLOWER REMEDIES, INCLUDING AUSTRALIAN

IFER
International Flower Essence Repertoire
The Living Tree
Milland
Liphook GU30 7JS
01428 741572
email: flower@atlas.co.uk

FOOD, ORGANIC

The Soil Association
Bristol House
40–56 Victoria Street
Bristol
BS1 6BY
0117 929 0661
www.soilassociation.org

GRANDPARENTS

The Grandparents' Federation
Room 3
Moot House
The Stow
Harlow
Essex
CM20 3AG
01279 444964

HERBALISM

The National Institute of Medical Herbalists
56 Longbrook Street
Exeter
Devon
EX4 6AH
01392 426022
www.nimh.org.uk

HOMOEOPATHY
The Society of Homoeopaths
2 Artizan Road
Northampton
NN1 4HU
01604 21400
www.homoeopathy-soh.org

HYPERACTIVITY
The Hyperactive Children's Support Group
71 Whyke Lane
Chichester
W. Sussex
PO19 7PD
www.hacsg.org.uk

MISCARRIAGE
The Miscarriage Association
c/o Clayton Hospital
Northgate
Wakefield
W. Yorks
WF1 3JS
www.miscarriageassociation.org.uk

NATUROPATHY
The General Council and Register of Naturopaths
Goswell House
2 Goswell Road
Street
Somerset
BA16 0JG
01458 840072

NUTRITIONAL THERAPY
The Institute for Optimal Nutrition
Blades Court
Deodar Road
London SW15 2NU
020 8877 9993

The Society for the Promotion of Nutritional Therapy
PO Box 85
St Albans
Herts
AL3 7ZQ
01582 792088

OSTEOPATHY
The College of Osteopaths Practitioners' Association
13 Furzehill Road
Borehamwood
Herts
WD6 2DG
020 8905 1937

The Osteopathic Information Service
Premier House
10 Greycoat Place
London SW1P 1SB

PARENTING
Gingerbread
Support for lone-parent families.
0800 018 4318

The Informed Parent
PO Box 870
Harrow
Middlesex
HA3 7UW
020 8861 1022
Publishes regular newsletters on vaccination and other issues. Send sae.

The National Council for One-Parent Families
225 Kentish Town Road
London NW5 2LX
0800 0185026
www.oneparentfamilies.org.uk

Parentline Plus
53–79 Highgate Road
London NW5 1TZ
Information and support to families.
0808 800 2222
www.parentlineplus.org.uk

REFLEXOLOGY
The Association of Reflexologists
27 Old Gloucester Street
London WC1N 3XX
0990 673320
www.reflexology.org

RAPE
The Rape Crisis Federation
Unit 7
Provident Works
Newdigate Street
Nottingham
NG7 4FD
0115 900 3560

SHAMANISM
Eagle's Wing
BM Box 7475
London WC1N 3XX
01435 810233
www.shamanism.co.uk

The Sacred Trust
PO Box 603
Bath
BA1 2ZU
01225 852615

SPIRITUAL HEALING
The Confederation of Healing Organizations
113 High Street
Berkhamsted
Herts
HP4 2DJ

The National Federation of Spiritual Healers
Old Manor Farm Studio
Church Street
Sunbury-on-Thames
Middlesex
TW16 6RG
0891 616080

TEENAGERS
The Site
Information and Advice
www.thesite.org.uk

VACCINATION
The Vaccination Awareness Network
147 Bath Street
Ilkeston
DE7 8AS
08704 440894
www.van.org.uk

Whale Vaccine Resource
www.whaleto.freeserve.co.uk

WOMEN'S ISSUES
(see also Domestic Violence, Rape)

E-quality-women
Seeks to raise awareness regarding behaviour, actions, issues, policies and
procedures that affect women.
www.e-quality-women.co.uk

YOGA
The Yoga Therapy Centre
The Royal Homoeopathic Hospital
60 Great Ormond Street
London WC1N 3HR
020 7419 7195

In Australia

Association of Massage Therapists
18a Spit Road
Mosman
NSW 2088
969 8445

Association of Remedial Masseurs
22 Stuart Street
Ryde
NSW 2112
878 2159

Australasian College of Natural Therapies
620 Harris Street
Ultimo
NSW 2007
02 212 6699

Australian Academy of Osteopathy
7th Floor
235 Macquarie Street
Sydney
NSW 2000
233 1655

Australian Federation of Homoeopaths
21 Bulah Close
Berowra Heights
NSW 2082
02 456 3602

Australian Natural Therapists Association Ltd
PO Box 522
Sutherland
NSW 2232
02 521 2063

Australian Traditional Medicine Society
120 Blaxland Road
Ryde
NSW 2112
808 2825

National Herbalists Association of Australia
14/249 Kingsgrove Road
Kingsgrove
NSW 2208
502 2938

❋ In the USA

ABORTION ADVICE
National Abortion Federation
1436 U Street, NW,
Suite 103
Washington DC 20009
202 667 5881

AIDS
National Resource Center on Women and AIDS
2000 P Street, NW,
Suite 508
Washington DC 20036
202 872 1770

BREASTFEEDING
La Lèche League International
9616 Minneapolis Avenue
PO Box 1209
Franklin Park
Il 60131-8209
708 455 7730

CHILDBIRTH
International Association for Childbirth at Home
PO Box 430
Glendale
CA 91209
213 663 4996

CHIROPRACTIC
American Chiropractic Association
1701 Clarendon Blvd
Arlington
VA 24203
703 276 8800

COUNSELLING
Association for the Development of Social Therapy
c/o Barbara Silverman
474 Third Street
Brooklyn
NY 11215
718 499 3759

DRUGS AND ALCOHOL
Alcoholics Anonymous World Services
PO Box 459
Grand Central Station
New York
NY 10163
212 686 1100

ENVIRONMENTAL ISSUES
Earth Island Institute
300 Broadway
Suite 28
San Francisco CA 94133
415 788 3666

Greenpeace USA
1436 U Street, NW,
Washington DC 20009
202 462 1177

World Women in Environment
1250 24th Street, NW,
4th floor
Washington DC 20037
202 347 1514

ETHICAL BANKING
Working Assets Money Fund (Socially Responsible Money Markets Fund)
230 California Street
San Francisco CA 94111
415 989 3200

FLOWER REMEDIES – DR BACH
Dr Edward Bach Healing Society
644 Merrick Road
Lynbrook NY 11563
516 593 2206

HERBALISM
Flower Essence Society
PO Box 1769
Nevada City CA 95959
916 265 9163

California School of Herbal Studies
PO Box 39
Forestville CA 95436
707 887 7457

HOMEOPATHY
National Center for Homeopathy
801 N Fairfax Street
Alexandria VA 22314
703 548 7790

OSTEOPATHY
American Osteopathic Association
142 E Ontario Street
Chicago Il 60611
312 280 5800

SPIRITUAL HEALING
Common Boundary Inc
7005 Florida Street
Chevy Chase
MD 20815
301 652 9495

WOMEN'S ISSUES
National Organization for Women
1000 16th Street, NW
Suite 700
Washington DC 20036
202 331 0066

National Association of Women's Centers
c/o Sylvia Kramer, Women's Action Alliance
370 Lexington Avenue
Suite 603
New York NY 10017
212 532 8330

Suggested Reading

GENERAL

Bentov, I., *Stalking the Wild Pendulum* (Destiny, 1988)
Campbell, J., *An Open Life* (Harper & Row, 1989)
Capra, F., *The Turning Point* (Wildwood House, 1989)
Capra, F., *The Hidden Connections* (HarperCollins, 2002)
Davies, N., *The School Report* (Vintage, 2000)
Elkington, J., *The Chrysalis Economy* (Capstone, 2001)
Fraser, R. and Hill, S., *The Roots of Health* (Green Books, 2001)
Gawain, S., *Creative Visualization* (Whatever, 1986)
Handy, C., *The Hungry Spirit* (Hutchinson, 1997)
Hawken, P., *The Ecology of Commerce* (HarperCollins, 1993)
Heindel, M., *The Vital Body* (Fowler, 1950)
Howe, E., *The Mind of the Druid* (Skoob, 1989)
McLuhan, T. (ed.), *Touch the Earth: A Self-Portrait of Indian Existence* (Abacus, 1973)
Myss, C., *Anatomy of the Spirit* (Bantam, 1997)
Pearson, C., *The Hero Within* (Harper & Row, 1986)
Russell, P., *The Awakening Earth* (Arkana, 1982)
Starhawk, *Dreaming the Dark* (Mandala, 1990)
Waring, M., *Counting for Nothing* (Allen & Unwin, 1988)
Wilber, K., *One Taste* (Shambala, 1999)
Zukav, G., *The Dancing Wu Li Masters* (Fontana, 1979)

HEALTH – GENERAL

Ball, J., *Understanding Disease*, (C. W. Daniel, 1991)
Chopra, D., *Creating Health* (Thorsons, 1996)
Curtis, S., *Surviving with Natural Remedies* (Winter Press, 2003)
Curtis, S., Fraser, R., and Kohler, I., *Neal's Yard Natural Remedies* (Penguin, 1988)
Dethlefsen, T., and Dahlke, R., *The Healing Power of Illness* (Element Books, 1990)
Drake, K. and J., *Natural Birth Control* (Thorsons, 1984)
Hill, S., *Oriental Paths to Health* (Constable & Robinson, 2000)

Myss, C., and Shealy, N., *The Creation of Health* (Bantam, 1991)
Needes, R., *You Don't Have to Feel Unwell* (Gateway, 1994)
Page, C., *Frontiers of Health* (C. W. Daniel, 2000)
Siegel, B., *Love, Medicine and Miracles* (New Dimensions, 1997)

WOMEN'S HEALTH
Glenville, M., *The Natural Health Handbook for Women* (Piatkus Books, 2001)
Kenton, L., *Passage to Power* (Vermilion, 1998)
McIntyre, A., *The Complete Woman's Herbal* (Gaia, 1988)
Northrup, C., *Women's Bodies, Women's Wisdom* (Piatkus Books, 1995)
Phillips, A., and Rakusen, J., *The New Our Bodies Ourselves* (Penguin, 1989)

AROMATHERAPY
Curtis, S., *Essential Oils* (Haldane Mason, 1996)
Davis, P., *Aromatherapy: An A–Z* (C. W. Daniel, 1989)
Tisserand, R., *The Art of Aromatherapy* (C. W. Daniel, 1980)
Westwood, C., *Aromatherapy, A Guide to Home Use* (Amberwood, 1991)
Worwood, V., *The Fragrant Pharmacy* (Macmillan, 1990)

COSMETICS AND BEAUTY
Kando, J., *Natural Facelift* (Thorsons, 1998)
Neal's Yard Remedies, *Recipes for Natural Beauty* (Haldane Mason, 2002)
Winter, R., *A Consumer's Dictionary of Cosmetic Ingredients* (Crown, 1999)

FLOWER REMEDIES
Bach, E., *Heal Thyself* (C. W. Daniel, 1931)
Bach, E., *Twelve Healers* (C. W. Daniel, 1933)
Barnard, J., *A Guide to the Bach Flower Remedies* (C. W. Daniel, 1979)
White, I., *Australian Bush Flower Essences* (Findhorn, 1997)

HERBS
Barker, J., *The Medicinal Flora* (Winter Press, 2001)
Bartram, T., *Encyclopedia of Herbal Medicine* (Robinson, 1998)
Chevallier, A., *The Encyclopedia of Medicinal Plants* (Dorling Kindersley, 2001)
Hoffman, D., *New Holistic Herbal* (Element Books, 1994)
Tierra, M., *The Way of Herbs* (United Press, 1980)

HOMOEOPATHY
Castro, M., *The Complete Homoeopathy Handbook* (Macmillan, 1990)
Curtis, S., *Homoeopathic Alternatives to Immunisation* (Winter Press, 2002)
Fraser, P., *The Aids Miasm* (Winter Press, 2002)
Phatak, S., *Materia Medica of Homoeopathic Medicines* (Jain, 1977)
Wells, R., *Homoeopathy* (Aurum, 2000)

PREGNANCY AND CHILDBIRTH
Balaskas, J., *New Active Birth* (HarperCollins, 1991)
Balaskas, J., *New Natural Pregnancy* (Gaia, 1998)
Gaskin, I., *Spiritual Midwifery* (The Book Publishing Co., 1977)
Kitzinger, S., *Pregnancy and Childbirth* (Penguin, 1986)

Index

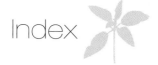

Nasturium officinale see watercress
nat mur, 48, 87, 106, 132, 156, 162, 169, 178, 316–17
Nat muriaticum see nat mur
nat phos, 53, 77, 317–18
Nat phosphoricum see nat phos
nat sulph, 9, 162, 318–19
Natrum sulphuricum see nat sulph
nausea, 236, 256, 271, 280, 291, 302, 310, 323, 330, 336, 351, 364
Neal's Yard Remedies, 204–6
Nepeta catara see catnip
neroli oil, 9, 43, 86, 87, 88, 90, 94, 101, 105, 109, 120, 139, 151, 319
nervine herbs, 185, 186
nervous system, 81–94, 186, 229, 236, 237, 255, 259, 270, 271, 278, 283, 295, 301, 303, 307, 309, 311, 324, 332, 343, 347, 354, 366, 370, 372
nettle rash *see* urticaria
nettles, 7, 15, 39, 42, 59, 62, 73, 80, 142, 164, 169, 171, 172, 311, 320–1
neuralgia, 91, 183, 256, 258, 237, 270, 301, 307, 368, 372
niaouli oil, 60, 62, 64, 67, 132, 169, 321
nit ac, 50, 321–2
Nitricum acidum see nit ac
nosebleeds, 264, 265, 275, 320
nux vomica, 30, 48, 49, 50, 51, 84, 88, 91, 104, 105, 106, 129, 145, 153, 164, 177, 322–3, 419

oats, 59, 85, 87, 93, 109, 120, 139, 151, 324–5
obesity, 284, 326

Ocimum basilicum see basil oil
ointments: aesculus ointment, 50; arnica ointment, 10; calendula ointment, 44, 54; comfrey ointment, 10, 20, 29, 118, 163; hamamelis ointment, 50; paeonia ointment, 50; rhus tox ointment, 10; tamus ointment, 44
olibanum oil *see* frankincense oil
olive oil, 10, 120, 193
operations, 234, 330, 358
orange (bitter), 85, 90, 93, 325
orange oil (sweet), 52, 69, 326
Origanum marjorana see marjoram oil
osteoporosis, 79–80, 248
ovarian cysts, 123, 145–7, 232
ovulation, 125, 133, 232, 361

paeonia, 50
pain, 260, 302, 309, 310, 368
palpitations, 43, 235, 236, 258, 278, 285, 299, 301, 314, 373
panic atacks, 236, 278
paralysis, 253
Parietaria judaica see pellitory of the wall
Parkinson's disease, 283
parsley, 42, 326
parsley oil, 327
parsley piert, 177, 327
passiflora, 85, 90, 92, 93, 135, 151, 327
Passiflora incarnata see passiflora
PCOS, 148–50
Pelargonum graveolens see geranium oil
pellitory of the wall, 177, 328
peptic ulcer, 53–4